The Heart's Code

Other Books by Paul Pearsall, Ph.D.

Superimmunity: Master Your Emotions and Improve Your Health

Super Marital Sex: Loving for Life

Super Joy: Learning to Celebrate Everyday Life

The Power of the Family: Strength, Comfort, and Healing

Making Miracles

The Ten Laws of Lasting Love

A Healing Intimacy: The Power of Loving Connections

The Pleasure Prescription: To Love, To Work, To Play—Life in the Balance

Write Your Own Pleasure Prescription: 60 Ways to Create Balance

and Joy in Your Life

PAUL PEARSALL, Ph.D.

The Heart's Code

Tapping the Wisdom and Power of Our Heart Energy

The New Findings About Cellular Memories and Their Role in the Mind / Body / Spirit Connection

BROADWAY BOOKS   NEW YORK

Library of Congress Cataloging-in-Publication Data
Pearsall, Paul.
    The heart's code : tapping the wisdom and power of our heart energy / by Paul Pearsall. — 1st ed.
        p. cm.
    "The new findings about cellular memories and their role in the mind/body/spirit connection."
    Includes bibliographical references and index.
    ISBN 0-7679-0077-4 (hardcover)
    1. Mind and body therapies. 2. Heart—Psychological aspects. 3. Mind and body. 4. Spiritual life. 5. Energy. I. Title.
RC489.M53P43   1998
616.1′2′0019—dc21   97-45968
                                                            CIP

FIRST EDITION

Designed by Pei Koay

98 99 00 01 02 10 9 8 7 6 5 4 3 2 1

For my son Scott,
whose loving heart energizes all of us

Important Note for the Reader

The material in this book is intended to provide an overview of the new research related to the role of the heart in well-being. The research is extensively referenced for readers wishing to pursue further inquiries and study. Every effort has been made to provide the most accurate, dependable, and current information. However, the reader should be aware that professionals may have differing opinions about the implications of this research, many of the theories presented here are not yet substantiated, and change is always taking place in the field of medical science. Any suggestions for techniques, treatments, or lifestyle change referred to or implied in this book should be undertaken only with the guidance of a licensed physician, therapist, or health-care practitioner. The author, editors, and publisher cannot be held responsible for the consequences of trying the ideas and suggestions in this book in a program of self-care or under the care of a licensed professional. The ideas, suggestions, and techniques in this book should not be used in place of sound medical therapies and recommendations.

Important Request of the Reader

Please consider organ donation as the ultimate gift. Register yourself as an organ donor, let your family know your wishes in this regard, and encourage others to be organ donors.

Contents

The Century of the Heart

"The Heart knows, the Thought denies, is there no other way?"

— STEPHEN SONDHEIM

Sometimes a book is written that forever changes not only the way we *think* about life, but the way we *feel* about life as well. This is *The Heart's Code*. Not only does it open our minds, it opens our hearts. *The Heart's Code* is about the gift of life as it is expressed through the intelligence of the heart—an intelligence the brain is just beginning to become aware of.

Our ancestors knew that the heart had energy—a powerful energy—and that it conveyed deep wisdom. However, as the human species developed its brain, it began to lose sight of its heart. At this point in history as we venture into space, create global communications, and invent all sorts of technological tools and toys, we are poised to destroy ourselves, our children, and everything around us. Have we simply lost our minds, or have we lost something deeper? Have we lost our hearts?

The intelligence of the brain is not to be faulted. On the contrary, as you will see as you read this book, the scientific tools created by the modern brain provide a new technology for conceiving and perceiving the energy and intelligence of the heart. While Paul Pearsall, Ph.D., the inspired author of this book, has taken the vision even beyond the current technology, he reaches this vision not only from his understanding of the ancient wisdom of his Hawaiian ancestors (the Kahuna—medicine women and men), but from his training in psychoneuroimmunology and his knowledge of modern physics, psychophysiology, and cardiology. These are big words for big ideas—but like all big ideas, they are wonderfully simple at their core.

When we began our research in 1993 on what we called "energy cardiology," we drew upon the simplest ideas in physics and cardiology and integrated these ideas with modern systems theory.[1, 2] When these ideas were married—intellectually and emotionally—the result was a veritable explosion of testable predictions that could forever change how we view not only the human heart but hearts in general—the coded pulsations emanating throughout the cosmos that give frequency and form to the universe. Heinz Pagels, Ph.D., the late great physicist, understood the deep significance of such universal codes in his book *The Cosmic Code: Quantum Physics as the Language of Nature.*[3]

Scientists and physicians tend to be conservative, fearful of saying things in print that might be challenged by their peers as seemingly "unscientific." When we began publishing our ideas and research in energy cardiology,[1, 2] we were most certainly fearful of our colleagues' emotional reactions to the inexorable logic inherent in modern systems theory. Integrity in science requires that we honor and follow *the logic of theory,* wherever it takes us, even if we do not like the implications of the predictions. Moreover, integrity in science requires that we honor and follow *the data derived from observation and experiment,* wherever it takes us, even if we do not like the implications of the findings. *The Heart's Code* honors and follows the clinical observations and empirical science suggesting, for example, that the heart stores energy and information that comprise the essence of who we are, and that sensitive persons who have received cardiac transplants may reveal the often invisible heart's code of the donor's organs living inside them.

When Gary was a professor of psychology and psychiatry at Yale University in the early 1980s, he unexpectedly discovered the logic of the "systemic memory mechanism" (an explanation for how atoms, cells, and organs such as the heart naturally store coded information) and experienced three fears. The first fear was that to determine whether the logic was truly correct, he would have to write a paper outlining the logic and share it with his colleagues. Once his colleagues knew the implications of the logic—for example, that hearts could learn and carry one's personal code—

they might question his credibility (to put it mildly). The second fear was that if the logic turned out to be wrong, this would be no small blunder (another understatement). But the third fear was the worst of all: the logic might actually be correct. If this was true, then Gary would have to dramatically change his cherished beliefs about how nature worked. How he handled these three fears was prototypic of the "sane" scientist—he didn't share the logic with virtually anyone, and kept it quiet for 12 years!

However, when he shared the theory with Linda in 1993, she said "this logic must be communicated. The logic of storing information can be extended to storing energy, which provides a key to understanding deep implications of the work we are doing in energy cardiology." We decided it was time to be brave, and we began to share the logic with those in the scientific and clinical community who were open to changing their minds.[4, 5] One of the scientists and clinicians we shared the logic with was Paul Pearsall, Ph.D.

To our delight, we discovered that our theorizing and basic science found strong support not only through Pearsall's extensive clinical observations with transplant patients, but also through his deep insights based on his cultural history, which provides a profound foundation for the new paradigm—what Pearsall calls "cardio-energetics" and "L-energy." Pearsall is especially creative and caring, and these qualities are expressed both professionally and personally.

Pearsall's focus on L-energy pushes us beyond current medical science's basic and clinical understanding of ECGs (electrocardiograms) and MCGs (magnetocardiograms). Medical science has been afraid to take the logic of the known physics of ECGs and MCGs to their inevitable conclusion. ECGs and MCGs are measured *outside* the body. This means that the heart's biophysical energy and information travel throughout the body and reaches the outside of the skin. Heart sounds, another source of energy and information, also travel through the fluids and make their way to the outside of the skin. Now, what happens to all this measurable energy and information once it reaches the skin? Does it simply stop? Disappear? Is it to be ignored? Forgotten?

Simple physics tells us that energy and information leave the body and go out into space. It reaches our loved ones and our pets and plants, it extends to the sky, and yes, logically, the electromagnetic fields expand into the "vacuum" of space at the speed of light, 186,000 miles per second.[1, 2]

Though the signal strength will obviously be very tiny, each second after our heart beats our individual heart's code has expanded and traveled 186,000 miles into space. Like star codes whose energy and information travel through space forever (and we are made of the matter, energy, and information derived from ancient stars) so too, logically, does our heart's code—the largest source of biophysical energy in the body—travel through space forever.

On first hearing this may sound fantastic if not outlandish. However, the same was once said for the idea that the earth was round, and that the earth revolves around the sun. Today we know there is more to life than our uneducated common sense teaches us. Science has taught us that the earth is not actually flat, it only appears that way until we look more closely. Science has taught us that the sun does not actually revolve around the earth, it only appears that way until we look more closely. And science is now teaching us that the heart is not without intelligence and wisdom, it only appears that way until we look more closely.

The Heart's Code points the way to a new revolution in our thinking. Metaphorically, the heart is the sun, the pulsing, energetic center of our biophysical "solar" system, and the brain is the earth, one of the most important planets in our biophysical system. One implication of the energy cardiology/cardio-energetic revolution is the radical (meaning "root") idea that energetically, the brain revolves around the heart, not the other way around.

The skeptic will be quick to say "*heart energy, heart codes, heart intelligence, heart wisdom,* these ideas are all metaphors"—and she or he will be correct. However, the same is true for ideas that conceive of creation as *big bang,* light as *massless particles,* gravity as a *force,* or thinking as *information processing.* Metaphors are stories we create, tools of the mind that help us envision and understand nature and, hopefully, live our lives with enhanced health, happiness, and success. As Marcel Proust said approximately a century ago, "The real voyage of discovery consists not in seeking new lands but in seeing with new eyes."

The question is, what kinds of metaphors or stories will foster our growth and evolution, lead us to take care of our children, our extended families, our global family, and the planet as a whole? What kinds of stories will lead us to rediscover the mystery and majesty of the pulsations of life—the intelligence behind the force, the information behind the energy, the soul behind the spirit? Can science be used to extend our current stories and create new stories that integrate knowledge and advance our species and the planet, with intelligence and compassion?

Pearsall takes such integrative metaphors and weaves a vision that is not only possible, but desirable. *The Heart's Code* is a celebration of the heart, a celebration of love, a celebration of life, and yes, a celebration of the mind that can come to know its heart.

If the 20th century has been, so to speak, the Century of the Brain, then the 21st century should be the Century of the Heart. When we say the Century of the Heart, we mean the intelligent heart, the wise heart, the heart rediscovered and reenvisioned by its most advanced planet, the brain. Energy and information, spirit and soul, this is *The Heart's Code.* May you be as challenged and blessed by this book as we have.

Gary E. R. Schwartz, Ph.D., and Linda G. S. Russek, Ph.D.

Dr. Gary E. R. Schwartz is Professor of Psychology, Neurology, Psychiatry, and Medicine, Director of the Human Energy Systems Laboratory, and Co-Facilitator of Energy Medicine, Program in Integrative Medicine, at the University of Arizona.

Dr. Linda G. S. Russek has been a Research Psychologist at the Harvard University Student Health Service and Director of the Harvard Mastery of Stress Follow-Up Study since 1978. She is also Co-Director of the Human Energy Systems Laboratory and Co-Facilitator of Energy Medicine, Program in Integrative Medicine, at the University of Arizona.

REFERENCES

1. Russek, L. G. and G. E. Schwartz. "Energy Cardiology: A Dynamical Energy Systems Approach for Integrating Conventional and Alternative Medicine." *Advances.* 12, 4 (1996a): pp. 4-24.

2. Russek, L. G. and G. E. Schwartz. "Interpersonal Heart-Brain Registration and the Perception of Parental Love: A 42 Year Follow-up of the Harvard Mastery of Stress Study." *Subtle Energies.* 5, 3 (1994): pp. 195-208.

3. Pagels, H. R. *The Cosmic Code: Quantum Physics as the Language of Nature.* New York: Simon & Schuster, 1982.

4. Schwartz, G. E. and L. G. Russek. "Do All Dynamic Systems Have Memory? Implications of the Systemic Memory Hypothesis for Science and Society." In Pribram, K. H. and King, J. S. (ed.). *Brain and Values: Behavioral Neurodynamics V.* Hillsdale, New Jersey: Lawrence Erlbaum Associates, 1997a.

5. Schwartz, G. E. and L. G. Russek. "Dynamical Energy Systems and Modern Physics: Fostering the Science and Spirit of Complementary and Alternative Medicine." *Alternative Therapies in Health and Medicine.* 3, 3 (1997b): pp. 46-56.

Acknowledgments

The possibilities suggested in this book, that the heart thinks and feels, that our cells remember, and that there is a subtle yet very powerful and pervasive form of energy that connects every thing and every person, are suggested by the creative and careful research of many scientists. I owe every idea in the following pages to these pioneers and express my gratitude for their work and help in researching this book. Many of them are my friends and I have met or spoken personally to most of them and studied for hours the publications of the others. Any errors in interpreting their work, extending the implications of their findings, or premature application of what they are beginning to discover are solely my responsibility.

Many of the central hypotheses presented in this book regarding the heart and systemic memory stem from the pioneering work of Gary Schwartz and Linda Russek. They are the founders of energy cardiology and leaders in integrating the best of modern science with the wisdom of the ancient systems of healing. The lovingly courageous Claire Sylvia and skilled and sensitive writer Bob Novak provided encouragement and support when I was not sure I should risk writing such a speculative and provocative book. Larry Dossey is a leader, guide, and teacher to thousands of us who explore the mind/body/spirit connection, and his unique take on issues in alternative medicine are sprinkled liberally throughout this book. Others to whom I owe a huge debt are Candace Pert, Bernie Siegel, Rollin McCraty, the staff at the HeartMath® Institute, and everyone at the Princeton Engineering Anomalies Research program, particularly Brenda Dunne, Robert Jahn, and Arthur Lettiere. Thanks also for the inspiring work of Stuart Hameroff, Thomas Moore, James White, James Hillman, Shirley Motz, Deepak Chopra, Stuart Nuland, Doc Lew Childre, and Rupert Sheldrake.

Thanks to everyone at Broadway Books who have been so supportive in this adventurous undertaking. I am extremely fortunate to have an editor, Lauren Marino, who is so literate in the heart's code. Thanks also to Kati Steele for her persistently patient help and for the thorough copy editing of Nancy Peske. This book would never have been possible without the faith of my agent, Jane Dystel, who knew in her heart that it was worth the risk of sharing the radical ideas in this book.

As with all of my books, I owe not only this book but my life to my wife, Celest, my sons, Roger and Scott, my mother, Carol, and the memory of my father, Frank, that still resonates in my heart. I express my deepest appreciation to all of the organ transplant recipients, donor families, and professionals who spent so much time with me sharing their feelings and experiences, but of course they are all used to opening their hearts. Lastly, each of us in differing ways owe an un-repayable debt to the deceased donors and their families who gave the gift of life. Whether or not I am right about the heart, cellular memories, and the subtle energy that drives these processes, may we always hold in our heart the memories of their gift of love and consider sharing our life energy with others who need it to survive.

The Spirit's Energy and
the Soul's Heart

"The heart has its reasons, which reason does not know."

— *BLAISE PASCAL*

LOVE-BLIND BRAINS AND HEALING HEARTS

Ten years ago in late fall, I remember thinking how the crinkled dry leaves seemed to reflect my own vague sense of internal decay. I felt weak, had an almost constant headache, and sweated so heavily at night that the bed was soaked in the morning. I often told my wife that there was some form of toxic energy in me that I could not describe, but when I told my doctors about this sense of impending doom that I seemed to be experiencing in my heart, they responded that their tests showed nothing they considered abnormal and that I was just under stress from my clinical work. My brain accepted their diagnosis, but my heart remained very worried.

As weeks went on, I became constantly nauseated, food repulsed me, and my every move was accompanied by severe pain that radiated from my pelvis and often knocked me to my knees. I often began to cry for no apparent reason and was plagued by a vague sense of dread that I kept telling my family "seemed to be my heart crying." I told my doctors that, despite their dismissal of my symptoms as being "only in my head," it was my heart that kept telling me I was dying. Their inability and sometimes unwillingness to think with their own hearts and not just their brains almost killed me.

While my brain felt and interpreted my agony, it was my heart that knew its meaning. Late at night when it was less busy with its usual ruminations, my brain could pay attention to my heart's desperate message that I was dying of cancer. In its typical rational rush, my brain had misinterpreted as signals from strained muscles of a sore back what my heart seemed somehow to know were disrupted and toxic energetic vibrations from sick cells running amuck throughout my pelvis. Because, like my doctors, I too was suspicious of the subtle messages that kept coming from my heart, I suffered and waited in vain until both my back and my psyche would become less strained.

The debate between my own heart and brain continued on for months. My brain wanted to listen to my doctor's brains, but my heart seemed to keep urging me to continue making appeals to my doctor that something was terribly wrong. After one particularly tearful discussion with my primary physician about a very sick feeling deep in my heart, he impatiently said, "I give up. I'll do a CAT scan just to put your mind at rest. For God's sake, man, you're a scientist. Use your brain, don't think with your pump."

During the CAT scan, the doctors and nurses behind the screen had their first glimpse of a soccer ball-sized tumor in my hip and cancer cells that my heart had warned had been taking over my body for months. I was diagnosed with Stage IV lymphoma, a deadly form of cancer of the lymph system. At this point it had spread into my bones and I had very little chance of surviving. Had I put more trust in my heart's code and had my doctors been more willing to listen to its lessons, I might have avoided more than two years of terrible suffering.

I learned through my cancer that when the heart speaks, it does so much as a shy child tries to get her busy mother's attention by repeatedly tugging on her skirt. Like a baby's frustrated cry as it tries to express its needs without words, my heart sobbed in a primal language that can be understood only when we allow our heart to enter into the constant dialogue between our brain and its body and when we become sensitive to a much subtler energy than the brain is used to processing. Until it has to "attack" us to get our attention, our heart has a very delicate way in which it tries to get our attention, and to hear it we must focus on our chest and not our head.

During my subsequent treatment, my heart spoke to me more like a loving grandparent than a stern teacher. It told me that my wife's and sons' hearts were sending energy that could help me heal. I could feel that energy whenever they were near me and often when they were not. My heart told me that, if I would let it, it could send energy into persons and things and extract energy from them. It told me which doctors and nurses had "good hearts" that could resonate with my own and warned me about those hearts that were not yet open or were sending a dissonant and disruptive energy that could interfere with my healing. As my brain struggled to reason its way out of my predicament, tried to fix blame, became angry at the inconvenience of my illness and the limits it imposed on its mission of self-advancement, wondered why my disease happened to its body and not another brain's body, and worked to protect its autonomy in the face of the helplessness imposed by my disease, my heart offered a gentler, more humble, patient, connected way back to well-being. It seemed to infuse me with a pervasive connective drive that counterbalanced my brain's evolutionary imperative for individuation and its built-in self-protective xenophobic orientation toward what it sees as "other."

Perhaps because of the quietness, helplessness, and months of dependent surrender imposed on my brain by the circumstances of my confirmed disease and the radical treatments it required, my heart seemed able to speak more easily and freely with me once the diagnosis was finally made. It told me that I did not have to be a passive target for the X-ray machine my doctors used to bombard and kill the overgrowing cells swarming within me. I remember thinking how ironic it was that the same doctors who so doubted an energy they could not see that seemed to come from my heart now were using an invisible energy of their own in a last ditch effort to save my life. I remember that my heart told me I could somehow actually connect with and influence the machine. It told me it could help me speak with the machine in the same subtle information-containing energy that my heart used to speak to me of my cancer. It told me that, despite what my brain said, I did not "have" cancer. It said my cells had lost their memory for how to multiply in a more connective, healthy way and, as a result, were engaging in a thoughtless "cancering." It said my cells were not getting the right information to teach them how to stay in harmony with my other body cells because they had somehow become disconnected from their coordinator of healthy energy—the heart. My cancer seemed to be the result of cells that had become heartless.

For every subsequent whole-body radiation treatment, I quieted my worried brain and allowed my heart to establish a healing energy connection with the radiation device. One radiation technician told me, "This is very, very strange, but you seem to get a much more measurable effect with much less dosage and time than most patients. What are you doing to our machine?"

When I sobbed in response to my brain's sense of total isolation, my heart spoke again, telling me it could connect with my wife's and sons' hearts no matter where they were and even though I was isolated from them by the lead walls that blocked the lethal radiation energy from escaping to affect other people's cells. When I focused on my heart and transcended my brain's fears about its body, I could feel the energy of those I loved enveloping, soothing, and healing me. I could feel the energy of my wife and sons no matter where they were and later could tell them where they had been and exactly what they had been doing while I was receiving my treatments even when their plans had suddenly changed and were unknown to my brain. My heart helped me to not only send energy to the machine but extract energy from those I loved. I was eventually cured (repaired) of cancer by the intelligence of biomedicine, the measurable energy it had learned to use, and the transplantation of healthy cells into my body that could remember how to divide in healthy harmony, but I was healed (made whole again) by my heart serving as the mediator of the new life, or "L," energy that had come with my transplanted cells.

As a cancer and bone marrow transplant survivor who has become emotionally close to hundreds of transplant patients and their donors' families, who has held a beating heart in his hand and felt its amazing spiritual essence, and who has not only read about but observed and taken part in experiments on invisible subtle energy, I have little doubt that the heart is the major energy center of my body and a conveyor of a code that represents my soul. I don't need much more convincing than my heart's victory over my cancer has already provided, so my bias in favor of the heart is clearly evident. As a scientist and clinician, however, my brain demands more evidence, and that evidence is now emerging.

FIRST SCIENTIFIC CONTACT WITH THE SOUL?

Science has recently discovered three startling new possibilities regarding how we think, feel, love, heal, and find meaning in our life. This research suggests that the heart thinks, cells remember, and that both of these processes are related to an as yet mysterious, extremely powerful, but very subtle energy with properties unlike any other known force. If the preliminary insights regarding these prospects continue to be verified, science may be taking the first tentative steps to understanding more about what shamans, kahuna, priests, spiritual leaders, and healers from ancient traditional medicines have been teaching about for centuries—the energy of the human spirit and the coded information that is the human soul.

The research and true life stories presented in this book will introduce preliminary documentation that is offering clues about the heart's code, the phrase I will use throughout this book to represent a proposed subtle life or "L" energy "cardio-cryptogram." This heart's code is recorded and remembered in every cell in the body as an informational template of the soul, constantly resonating within and from us, sent forth from our heart. Some questions about this code that will be explored include:

• Is it possible that the heart has its own form of intelligence that, because of our evolved dependence on our brain for interpretation of our experiences, we are seldom aware of?

• Although very discreetly and in a much different way than the brain, can the heart literally perceive and react on its own to the outside world, and communicate an info-energetic code of that reaction through a network of tens of thousands of miles of vessels and 75 trillion cells, which serve not only as the circulatory system but as an energy and information emitting network?

• Have we been too "brain focused" in our search for the mind, failing to see that the heart might be an informational and energetic cornerstone of a three-component or triune "Mind," made up of a heart that energetically integrates the brilliantly adaptive brain with its miraculously self-healing body?

• Is it possible that much of what our triune Mind experiences is stored within us as retrievable info-energetic cellular memories?

• Is what we refer to as the soul at least in part a set of info-energetic cellular memories, a kind of cellular soul program that is being constantly modified during the soul's brief stay in the physical body?

• Are the remarkable stories by some heart transplant recipients regarding changes in their food preferences, dreams, fantasies, and personality manifestations related on some level to the cellular memories of their donor?

• If some very sensitive heart transplant recipients can recover the cellular memories of their donor, can any of us—if we learn how to be sensitive to the heart's code—also voluntarily recover our own and our ancestors' cellular memories?

• Is it possible to tune into the codes of other people's hearts?

• Is there a form of energy—a vital life force—that humankind has sought for centuries and that science may have missed?

• Is there a subtle energy that influences our life and is free of most of the rules that limit other forms of energy?

• Is it possible that a subtle form of energy I call life or "L" energy, and which others refer to as a "healing" or "X" force, carries information and that, just as Albert Einstein showed us that energy and matter are interchangeable, information and energy are also synonymous?

• If information does ride along within energy, and because the heart is the most energetically powerful organ in the body, does every beat of our heart send a coded, faint signal from our soul to other souls?

• Can the heart send and receive some form of info-energetic message to and from nonhuman systems, including plants, rocks, trees, water, and even machines?

• If the heart thinks, cells remember, and there is a form of "L" energy that is free of the limitations of space and time, what are the implications of this heart's code for how we are connected with one another, the impact of behaviors that violate that connection, and the ways in which we become sick and heal?

The cutting-edge science that is exploring the above prospects is just entering its infancy.[1] Many old paradigms need to be challenged and we need not only to seek new answers but to learn to ask entirely new questions similar to those above. Because of the first tentative scientific steps and the creative courage of those willing to talk about their own often confusing and even frightening experiences with cellular memories and "L" energy, we can begin to learn more about whether and how the heart has and conveys its own code, and what this means for us. We may even gain the confidence and boldness to ask if it is possible that science is beginning to make its first tentative contacts with the soul.

TOWARD ONE WORLD MEDICINE

By exploring the possibility of a heart's code, we may be able to begin to build a bridge between the biomechanical wonders of modern medicine,

the spirituality of ancient traditional healing systems, the various alternative or complimentary medicines, and the wisdom of religious scholars and
spiritual leaders. It is not likely that we will be able to understand all the
forms of medicine in the world until we are willing to broaden our understanding of the world.[2] By doing so, we may not have to select from among
all the models of healing. Instead, perhaps we can combine them into one
world medicine made up of all the wisdom about the brain, body, energy,
information, the spirit, and the soul. With sufficient patience, tolerance,
creativity, a more inclusive view of the human system as it interacts with all
systems, and perhaps most of all, with a more open heart and less defensively reactive brain, we may be able to combine the rigor of science with
the subtle wisdom of the heart to answer the most important questions in
the universe: what and why is life?

THE HEART THAT FOUND ITS BODY'S KILLER

I recently spoke to an international group of psychologists, psychiatrists,
and social workers meeting in Houston, Texas. I spoke to them about my
ideas about the central role of the heart in our psychological and spiritual
life, and following my presentation, a psychiatrist came to the microphone
during the question and answer session to ask me about one of her patients
whose experience seemed to substantiate my ideas about cellular memories
and a thinking heart. The case disturbed her so much that she struggled to
speak through her tears.

Sobbing to the point that the audience and I had difficulty understanding her, she said, "I have a patient, an eight-year-old little girl who
received the heart of a murdered ten-year-old girl. Her mother brought her
to me when she started screaming at night about her dreams of the man
who had murdered her donor. She said her daughter knew who it was.
After several sessions, I just could not deny the reality of what this child
was telling me. Her mother and I finally decided to call the police and,
using the descriptions from the little girl, they found the murderer. He was
easily convicted with evidence my patient provided. The time, the weapon,
the place, the clothes he wore, what the little girl he killed had said to him
. . . everything the little heart transplant recipient reported was completely accurate."

As the therapist returned to her seat, the audience of scientifically
trained and clinically experienced professionals sat in silence. I could hear
sobbing and saw tears in the eyes of the doctors in the front row. Instead

of commenting on the story, I asked the audience if I could lead them in a prayer. I asked the technician to softly play the Hawaiian music I often use in my presentation and spoke what Hawaiians call a "pule 'ohana," a prayer in honor of our spiritual connection as family. Unlike many of the presentations, this one produced no expressions of doubt or skepticism. The very real possibility of a heart that remembers seemed to touch all of us in our own hearts.

I am a psychoneuroimmunologist, a licensed psychologist who studies the relationship between the brain, immune system, and our experiences of the outside world. I have more than thirty years of Western scientific training in how our interpretation of life events influences our health. I founded and was director of a large psychiatric clinic that treated hundreds of seriously ill patients, many of whom had received heart and other organ transplants. I was director of behavioral medicine in a cardiac rehabilitation program for heart attack victims designed to help heal their heart through significant lifestyle changes and the development of a more balanced psychological view of living, a program we called "Change of Heart." In this and my other professional roles, I have lectured around the world to various organ transplant organizations where I collected dozens of accounts of amazing stories that seemed to indicate that some type of cellular memory exists and that the heart played a major role in the recovery of those memories. I have also recorded the reports of seventy-three heart transplant patients and their families, sixty-seven other organ transplant recipients, and eighteen donor family interviews for use in preparing to write this book. I have collected many anecdotes and clinical experiences from doctors, nurses, and researchers and from professional health-care workers who attended my various presentations. I never share one of my stories about the heart's code without getting a most personal, often very spiritual reaction from my listeners. Something about these accounts seems to touch their hearts, and they often gasp and grab their chest when they hear them.

LOOK, DON'T BITE

Since I have "gone public" about my questions regarding a heart's code, I have often met with strong denial and felt the anger of those who choose—despite the increasing scientific evidence that these issues are well worth considering—not to accept the implications that may follow from these speculations. I have been told that I would do damage to the transplant movement by bringing attention to the idea that the heart is much more than a pump or that someone else's "soul stuff" could accompany a transplanted organ. I have been warned that I would lead others to donate organs for the selfish reason of attaining a kind of cellular memory immortality. I have been mocked, laughed at, and criticized for suggesting that cells can remember, even when it seemed entirely possible by every scientific standard that this prospect is well worth exploring. My ideas have been dismissed as "strange" when I speak about information stored in the energy being communicated through and from our body by our heart, even when bioscience's own measurements are already beginning to detect the effects of that energy and bioscientists' experiments have often been infiltrated and confounded by the peeking-through of that energy into their "controlled" and "double-blind" studies. Perhaps most often, I have been told that the heart transplant recipient stories, like that of the little girl above, that seemed to confirm my speculations were actually "only in the head" of those who offered them, a lingering symptom of their illness or side effect of the trauma of their transplant and the medications used in transplantation.

My scientific brain does not allow me to be certain that the above objections are not valid. It knows that, after lengthy, careful, creative study, we may discover after all that the heart is nothing more than a magnificent pump. It doubts that we will be able to show with scientific certainty that all body cells can really remember in the sense most people think about memory, or that cells are anything more than complex neurochemical containers processing biophysical energy. It seems reasonably certain that we have already identified all of the forms of energy there are in the universe and that what seems to be a more subtle, mystical, healing energy that so many alternative medicine practioners refer to is only a romantic invention. It requires that I use the phrase "subtle 'L' energy" in a provisional, metaphorical way throughout this book rather than accept its existence with confidence, as I have accepted the known forms of energy I have written about in my prior books.[3] My brain tells me that our soul is beyond its comprehension and that there are no traces or representations of it in the physical body. It says that the mind is just a manifestation of itself and that those who seem so sincere in their reports about the impact of their transplanted heart on their soul are hallucinating, having false memories, or misinterpreting a biochemical phenomenon related to their disease and treatment. I would not have written this book, however, if I my heart didn't keep gently but consistently insisting that it has its own wondrous mysteries to offer, a code that ancient healers knew and scientists may be on the verge of cracking.

My suggestions regarding a heart's code have not always met with resistance. Acceptance has been as frequent and intense as rejection, suggesting that this area of inquiry raises very deep personal concerns. I have been welcomed by the kahuna—the healers of Hawaii—whose teachers speak of two-thousand-year-old lessons of "L" energy, cellular memory, and a thinking heart. I have met with Chinese physicians who are comfortable speaking about the body as a garden full of energy.[4] I have spoken with Native Americans, the Inuit (Eskimos), and the Aborigine in Australia, all of whom seemed to wonder at the tardy appearance of Western science's interest in what to them is simple common sense. As one Apache shaman told me, "Those in the Western world often forget that they too are indigenous peoples with roots to their original land and ties to their ancient ancestors' wisdom. The modern rational brain can also learn to think with its indigenous spiritual heart."

Professional audiences have often been highly receptive to the possibility of a heart's code. I have been contacted by dozens of patients, doctors, nurses, and scientists who feel it is important not to turn away from these spiritual matters of the heart. As I was completing this manuscript, I spoke with Dr. Candace Pert, the brilliant scientist and former researcher at the National Institute of Mental Health and the author of *Molecules of Emotion.* Dr. Pert first presented the work on neuropeptides, tiny chains of amino acids that are keys to our emotional experiences that were first identified in the brain and, her work now proves, are also "bits of brain" floating all over the body. She too expressed the worthiness of testing the hypotheses that cells could have a form of memory and that the heart may be a crucial info-energetic communicator.

In addition to talking to many scientists and researchers, I have also spoken with psychotherapists and nurses working with heart transplant recipients. Many of them express their support for studying the heart's code as a means of helping them to begin to understand more about some of the unexplainable deaths and healing miracles they encounter in their clinical work and the nature of the subtle energy they said they too have suspected is involved in the making of miracles. I have spoken with Claire Sylvia, a heart-lung transplant recipient who has described her experiences of changes in her life related to her donor's energy in a wonderful book written with Bill Novak titled *A Change of Heart.*[5] Despite the strong personal criticism she sometimes receives, she persists in her belief that she received much more than a mass of biomechanical cells when she received her new heart. Her surprisingly accurate dreams about her donor, changes in food tastes and her style of dancing, and many other changes offer clues about the possibilities of cellular memories. Heart transplant recipients and donors have sent me hundreds of letters of support, often bemoaning the fact that they have become very reluctant to speak about their feelings for fear of ridicule or a medical diagnosis of a "psychiatric state." My hope is that we can work toward a better balance between realistic skepticism and adventurous curiosity in learning more about the possibility of a thinking, feeling heart as expressed by author Warren McCulloch's statement, "Do not bite my finger; look where I am pointing."[6]

THE BURDEN OF PRUDENCE

The hypotheses regarding the heart's code are without doubt among the boldest proposals any scientist could make. I offer them to facilitate more discussion and study and as new possibilities to be explored as medicine experiences its growing pains associated with the challenges in dealing with the issues of spirituality and mortality, which are of such deep concern to patients, and the lessons of so-called alternative or complementary medicines. These are proposals that many of my scientific colleagues often say they "have a very hard time accepting." Surgeon Dr. Bernie Siegel is the well-known author of *Love, Medicine and Miracles* and other books that deal with ideas about mind/body/soul interactions that many of his colleagues still refuse to accept, get angry with, and often consider strange and even crazy. He writes, "What disturbs me is the use of the word 'accept.' If we close our minds and don't accept, science and healing cannot move forward. Instead of 'hard to accept,' let us say, 'hard to understand.' "[7]

Using our current scientific way of thinking, it is very difficult to understand how the heart could have a code, a cell could have a memory, and an immeasurable form of energy could contain information about the soul. I suggest that we should study these ideas precisely because they are "nonsense." They do not make sense in terms of science's current ways of trying to explain the mysteries of life. Perhaps these new possibilities regarding the heart's code will offer some new ways to come to our senses about the meaning of life and the processes of healing.

In the mid-1800s, the idea that tiny germs invisible to the eye could make us sick was seen as "utter nonsense" by the medical leaders of that time. Based on seemingly strange but recurring reports from patients and some doctors and nurses about the suffering that seemed to be caused by dirty hands delivering babies, and thousands of needless deaths caused by the use of scalpels still defiantly sharpened on the bottom of the surgeon's boot to show disdain for the silly "germ theory," doctors began to reluctantly accept the possibility of the existence of imperceptible but deadly microorganisms. This doubting acceptance allowed the development of more understanding about invisible things causing visible consequences, and doctors began to wash their hands and sterilize their instruments before any medical procedure. Today, because of the historical prudence of their predecessors, the burden of proof has been met and doctors understand much more—but not all—about bacteria. This same cautious but accepting prudence is required if we are to learn more about the existence of a heart's code and the cellular memories it conveys.

FOUR HYPOTHESES REGARDING ENERGY, INFORMATION, AND THE MIND/BODY CONNECTION

Our understanding of the heart as a sentient organ is about where our understanding of the miraculous complexities of the brain was more than one hundred years ago. In comparison to the continuing rapid progress in study of the brain, learning about the heart as more than just a pump is developing much more slowly. The central hypotheses regarding information-containing energy communicated by the heart were initially proposed by Drs. Gary E. Schwartz and Linda G. Russek. They are as clearly stated and testable as any other set of scientific suppositions, but the ideas of a "thinking" heart and information-carrying energy seem excessively difficult for many scientists to accept as starting points for study.[8]

Dr. Gary Schwartz is a professor of Psychology, Neurology, and Psychiatry and director of the Human Energy Systems Laboratory at the University of Arizona. His associate, Dr. Linda Russek, is a research psychologist at the Harvard University Student Health Service and codirector of the Human Energy Systems Laboratory. They are a creative, energetic, sensitive research team who have always been interested in a "systems" or interactive view of how life works. They have dedicated their professional lives to the attempt to create one medicine out of the many diverse approaches to healing and have never been afraid to challenge and extend the accepted principles of psychology and medicine.[9] They have combined the fields of biology, the new physics that studies subtle energy and the invisible atomic world, and modern cardiology to help explain the info-energetic nature of the heart beyond what skeptics call the abiding impulse to mythologize the heart. They based their field of energy cardiology on what they call "dynamic systems memory theory," the idea that all systems are constantly exchanging mutually influential energy, which contains information that alters the systems taking part in the exchange. They offer four hypotheses to explain how cells might be able to make memories out of the info-energy constantly circulated through the body system by the heart. I have paraphrased and expanded their hypotheses here.

1. Energy and information are the same thing. Everything that exists has energy, energy is full of information, and stored info-energy is what makes up cellular memories. Based on theories and research from the field of biology and other sciences, all living systems are by their nature manifestations of energy that contains the information (memory) of what they are and how they function. To scientists, the word "system" refers to a set of interactions between inseparable units. From the interactions between the tiniest parts within a single cell to the exchange of information between family members at dinner to the energy bouncing back and forth between the stars and planets, everything exists in a continuous info-energetic relationship. Since all systems are information-containing energy "stuff," all systems constantly exchange memories.[10]

2. What we call mind, consciousness, or our intentions are really manifestations of information-containing energy. Based on the lessons learned from modern physics, information and mind seem to be one and the same. What I am calling "L" energy is the basic code of life and what our "system" remembers as "who" we are.[11] Energy is the ability to do work and a force that conveys our personal life code (our systemic memory) along with the information it contains. Information is what gives a system its form and structure, and energy is the force or function that moves a system, connects all aspects of a system, and helps systems communicate and connect. Since all systems are connected and share forms of the same energy, all systems share common memories.

3. The heart is the primary generator of info-energy. The heart is constantly sending out patterns of info-energy that regulate organs and cells throughout the body. Every cell in the body is literally bathed in the info-energy conducted from and by the heart. Since the heart is a primary generator and transmitter of info-energy, it is central to our system's recollection of its life—its cellular memory.

4. Because we are manifestations of the info-energy coming to, flowing within, and constantly being sent out from our total cellular system, who and how we are is a physical representation of a recovered set of cellular memories. Based on cellular biology, we know that certain molecules have very good memories because they are particularly good at storing complex coded information. For example, DNA is a nucleic acid found in all cell nuclei that contains genetic information that determines to a yet to be determined extent not only how we look but what diseases we might develop, whether or not we are grouchy or cheerful in temperament, and even how long we live. All cells have energy, so all cells contain and share information. All cells store info-energetic memories, and our heart, by nature of its immense power, millions of cells throbbing in unison, and central location in our body, is the central organ that constantly pulsates info-energy from, between, and to all other organs and cells. Because of the heart's code and the cellular memories with which it deals, every cell in our body becomes a holographic or complete representation of our energetic heart. It may take extraordinary individuals such as the little girl above and the other heart transplant recipients you will read about, or at least individuals willing to learn to employ the abilities all of us have, to be able to make our implicit cellular memories explicit. If any one of us can do it, than any of us also has the potential to be a cellular memory recoverer.

I will be using the phrase "cardio-energetics" to refer not only to Schwartz and Russek's hypotheses but to include all of the fields of study that are contributing ideas and data to the exploration of the sentient heart. When I refer to cardio-energetics, I am referring to my theories about the heart's code and not necessarily just those of Schwartz and Russek. Any errors in reasoning or other mistakes I may make regarding cardio-energetics are exclusively my responsibility.

Some of the fields contributing to cardio-energetics, such as psychoneuroimmunology, neurocardiology, and the modern physics that studies the workings of the subtle energy I call "L" energy, are themselves only a few decades old. They too are still encountering resistance from some scientists that goes beyond healthy and necessary skepticism, and some of their findings have been distorted and overextended by those with too little scientific wariness. This combination of controversial fields contributing to new and even more controversial fields, such as energy cardiology and cardio-energetics, makes the study of the heart's code very difficult.

Work in energy cardiology and cardio-energetics is complicated by the fact that many of the processes involved in the heart's code are extremely subtle and as yet immeasurable by most (but not all) of our current scientific instruments. Progress can also be slowed when overeager but well-meaning believers in the power of "L" energy and its influence make claims for which there is as yet little or no scientific documentation. Little headway is made by unfounded assertions, but even less is learned when those who should be the most cautiously curious, including scientists and others interested in learning more about the mysteries of life, are impatiently unaccepting and even put off by the elusiveness and paradoxical nature of the heart's code. It is that very elusiveness, the subtleness of the info-energy of the heart, that should most interest and attract rationally doubting but creatively accepting learners.

IT'S A BRAIN'S WORLD

Even discussing the possibility that the brain may not be the sole proprietor of our human essence can cause the arrogant brain to recoil at the possibility that contemplation, reflection, remembering, and emotionality could originate anyplace else than within itself. The brain has had things pretty much its own way for the last few centuries. Unfortunately, the brain has created an intense, complex, fast-paced, often soulless world that contributes to failing hearts, weak immune systems, and malignant cells.

The brain has devised extensions of itself, electromagnetic energy devices such as cellular phones, computers, and other increasingly rapid but less personal communication systems perfectly suited for its own enhancement and that speak in the language of its own not-so-subtle energy. The heart has been mostly left out of the alliance between the brain and its body, its pumping power admired even as its circulatory function is often overextended and abused by an ever-demanding brain. The heart's own delicate way of thinking and feeling about the world and the info-energetic cellular memories with which it may be uniquely conversant are often ignored by cardiologists trained to think about the heart but not about how the heart might think.

Progress in the study of the heart's code cannot be made if we yield completely to the brain's evolutionary imperative as displayed by our incessant cerebral-centrism. If we allow our brain to think it "is us" rather than a key part "of us," we cannot learn the true nature of what it means to be human. Survival of the fittest has come to mean survival of the smartest and the most "brainy." As a result, the brain has been left free to "do its Darwinian thing." It has created an increasingly individualistic and separatist approach to living in which many of us end up feeling overpressured and alone in our struggle for self-advancement and survival. In our striving to become more and more capable of controlling our world, we seem to have become much less connected within and with it.

The brain thinks that only its own clever competitiveness, high-level energy, and natural self-protectiveness is able to cope with the pressures of life. The idea that the heart may also be able to think is met by incredulous anger and dismissive mockery from a brain that believes that its heart, even if it does think, must be thinking much too slowly, sentimentally, and subtly to be of immediate use in its daily wars for self-preservation and enhancement.

A brain-run world may not be the world our heart desires. While we can enjoy the conveniences of the wonders of our brain's modern inventions and technology, these same accomplishments can threaten our very existence. There are two questions that the thinking heart might ask about the new millennium. It may wonder if we can survive the world our brain has created for us and the pace at which it is running us and, even if the brain is clever enough to keep us alive in its new millennium world, will we want to live in that world if we only end up feeling more disconnected, hostile, self-protective, afraid, and alone in the universe—brilliant minds lacking loving souls. An objective of this book is to offer the possibility of putting more heart into our life by learning to quiet the restless, passionate brain so it may listen for the code of a gentler, more loving heart capable of reminding it that it is supposed to not only fulfill a biological evolutionary imperative but also be an instrument for refinement and expression of the soul.

TWO INTELLIGENCES

It may also be possible that, in addition to the above difficulties in beginning to understand the heart's code, we are distracted by our struggle to make a choice that does not have to be made. Two centuries ago when science and its methods for looking for meaning emerged, an artificial choice was thrust upon us when scientific inquiry and religious faith began to come into conflict. Although Einstein warned us that science without religion is blind and religion without science is lame, we have often assumed that we had to chose between science's "hard logic" and religion's "blind faith."

Historian Sidney Mead writes, "Americans since 1800 have, in effect, been given the hard choice between being intelligent according to the prevailing stands in their intellectual centers or being religious according to the standards prevalent in the denominations."[12] More recently, this choice as to the way to find meaning in life has been played out in the often heated conflict between biomedicine and alternative medicines, between "objective" science and ancient healing systems, between rational atheism and the irrational preachings of blind faith from a religious denomination that sees itself as the only "right way" to salvation. Beginning to understand how the heart may be where the soul speaks may provide a middle ground and the establishment of a creatively tolerant meeting place for those who come from within the powerful system of the scientific method and the wisdom of the heart embraced by so many indigenous people.

We don't have to and should not give up our quest to learn more about the remarkable brain and our respect for its magnificent powers of reason in order to begin to learn more about the untapped spiritual info-energetic wisdom of the heart. An irrational world brings us only misery, but a millennium in which the gifted brain is moderated and instructed by a gentle heart could bring us a shared paradise on earth. If we are willing to try to combine the best the brain has created, and will create, with the wisdom of the heart's code that may be our soul calling out the cellular memories that give meaning to these creations, we can become much smarter than we have ever been. We can have two major intelligences and learn to adore the rational skepticism of science and still look for the energy of the soul conveyed by the heart. This is an objective of this book.

SOURCES OF SUPPORT

The ideas about the role of the heart that I present here come primarily from four sources. The first is the collection of my own personal and professional experiences that seem to illustrate and document several points about the heart's code. While I have been as careful as possible to be objective in my presentation of clinical materials obtained in my professional clinical work, what I consider to be my own lingering cellular memories of my ordeal with cancer render my personal accounts of my experiences highly subjective. When I seem excessively optimistic about the existence of the heart's code and overly defensive in my attempt to describe and document it, it is because I believe it is what I became so familiar with when I almost died. It is my hope, however, that my own story and the stories from other patients will connect with some of your own experiences so that the issues raised in this book will seem more worthy of your prolonged attention through some of the unusual and sometimes disconcerting material ahead.

A second source of support for the ideas presented here derives from the lessons from indigenous peoples who are often more comfortable and tuned in to the less blatant lessons of life and who are often very "L" energy sensitive. Based on their own form of equally important science, these lessons provide unique ways of forming new questions that may help us understand more about the heart's code.

A third source of support for the heart's code comes from stories from heart transplant recipients who provide unique insights into the workings of the heart. A small percentage of these patients seem, like the indigenous people, to be extremely "cardio-sensitive" to their "L" energy and cellular memories. Like the little girl who helped catch her heart donor's murderer, they are able to produce very accurate accounts of changes in their personalities that correspond with the personality and memories of a donor about whom they would seem to have no way to know anything. As with my own story, I do not offer these accounts as proof of the existence of a heart's code or cellular memories but as clinical evidence that much more is going on in transplantation that all of us may learn from whether or not we have a new heart placed in our chests.

The fourth source of support comes from the theories and research of scientists contributing to energy cardiology and cardio-energetics, the many new fields of scientific inquiry that deal in different ways and to varying degrees with concepts related to the idea that energy and information are one in the same. You will read about research at major centers by highly respected scientists who are offering strong hints regarding the possibility of "L" energy and the heart's code and about what physicians and nurses have to say about a thinking heart.

By combining aspects of all of the above sources of support for the possibility of the existence of a heart's code, you can make your own judgment as to whether further study of its existence is merited, and you can chose whether or not to be alert for what your heart has to say about the way you live, work, and love.

AN INVITATION TO JOIN THE HYGEIAN HEART CLUB

Using only the words from my brain, I am not able to completely tell you how, but your heart will understand what I have said above about how my heart and other hearts saved my life. Through my illness, chemotherapy, bone marrow transplant, and near suffocation from the tightening of my lungs caused by an opportunistic deadly virus, my heart kept saying, "You'll be OK. It's all right. You'll live to write a book about all of this. You must write a book about this. You must tell others. You will heal so you can help heal others." The more I focused on my chest and my heart, the calmer and more confident I became. One afternoon when they came to wheel me out of what they called "the chamber," where I was drenched in lethal radiation, a nurse said, "You're breaking my heart. You're smiling and yet you're crying such big tears. What's wrong?"

I looked into her eyes and took her hand. I began to try to explain, but I was too weak to talk. She looked down at me, smiled, gently tapped her chest, tears came to her eyes, and she said, "It's OK. I understand. I feel it right here. You don't have to say a word."

I spent months in the hospital, isolated from the outside world with dozens of other transplant patients, including heart transplant recipients. I have walked with the other "pole pushers" leaning on the stands carrying bags of lifesaving medications that dripped into our veins. I have marched in the parade of pale, weak, almost inanimate dying patients waiting to be re-animated and re-energized by an infusion of energy of another person's vital life force. As a bone marrow transplant recipient myself, I have spent hours sitting in a wheelchair in quiet, darkened halls whispering with other transplant recipients. We often talked late into the night about the energy of the heart and how that energy might contain information converted to memories and stored in the cells of our body. We cried and laughed together about the remarkable implications of "L" energy and its cellular memory manifestations, but we learned to do so out of earshot of our doctors for fear we would be diagnosed as suffering from medication-induced delusions or be visited by some "heartless" psychiatrist who would prescribe medicine to numb our brain from the signals from our heart.

We often spoke of doctors who seemed to have a "good heart" and others who seemed "heartless" or who had a "cold heart." The more we talked, the more nurses joined us. The nurse I mentioned who pointed to her chest and said she knew how I felt after my radiation treatments became a charter member of what we came to call our Hygeian Heart Club, named after the Greek goddess of a vital loving and healing force, the counterpoint to her father, Asclepius, the more heartless Greek god of repair and fixing the body back to mechanical function. Because many of us were hospitalized for nearly a year without seeing the light of day or feeling a gentle breeze on our face, our club grew in size. Stories were shared by patients, doctors, and nurses about transplant recipients getting the memories of their donor, "feeling" physical health threats in the heart before any doctor could detect them, and "knowing" in the heart when death was imminent or a miracle was about to take place even when all biomedical tests indicated otherwise. Some of the stories you will read about in this book came from the meetings of the Hygeian Heart Club, and while they are only anecdotes, they provide a very personal side to why it is important to try to understand the heart's code. It is my hope and the hope of all the charter members that, after careful consideration by your brain and subtle connection with your heart with the material to follow, you yourself may consider becoming a member of the Hygeian Heart Club.

Part One

Heart, Soul, and Science

"Human love is not a substitute for spiritual love.
It is an extension of it."

— EMMANUEL

CHAPTER ONE

Breaking the Lethal Covenant

"At the earliest moment at which we catch our first glimpse of Man on earth, we find him not only on the move but already moving at an accelerating pace. This crescendo of acceleration is continued today. In our generation it is perhaps the most difficult and dangerous of all the current problems of the human race."

—ARNOLD TOYNBEE

WHERE ARE YOU?

The first thing I ask my patients to do in order to begin considering the presence and impact of the heart's info-energy is to locate the self. I want to illustrate to them that while they almost always spend most of their time focused on or focused by their brain, there may be another more neglected side to their life and another source of information by which to guide their decisions about what, how, and how much to do. As you read these words, take one hand from this book and point to yourself. Where is your hand pointing? Most people find their hand touching the area of their heart. With some cultural exceptions, such as some Japanese who may point to the general area of their nose, almost every person I have asked to point to himself or herself points to the general area of their heart. No matter how important it thinks it is, the brain that is coordinating the pointing movements seems to know where a major component of the "self" it shares with the body resides.

When we are surprised with very good or bad news, we usually place one or both hands over our chest. We seldom say we love someone with all of our head, send brain-shaped candy on Valentine's Day, or tell our lover that we want to give our brain to them. We may sometimes intentionally try to be sensitive to the heart's code, such as when a major work or life decision is pending and we seek guidance from our heart to tell us what to do even though our brain has already rationally made its decision. Although the brain is often locked in a hectic two-way conversation with its body, "L" energy, the constant oscillating code coming from the center of our being, may also offer lessons that give spiritual perspective to what the brain so urgently makes us do. It may also bring up cellular memories of what it would be like to lead a more patient, connected, blissful existence.

Once I have my patients' attention about at least the possibility that there is a different way to think and place from which they may think, we then discuss the nature of the brain's point of view regarding the world. In effect, I teach them the brain's code to compare and contrast with the heart's code. Whether or not my patients accept the idea that their heart "thinks," that we have cellular memories that can guide us to a healthier life, or that there is a subtle "L" energy that connects us all, is less relevant than that they learn that their health depends not only on looking at numbers representing their cholesterol count but on developing another perspective for looking at their life.

CONSTANT COGNITIVE CHATTER

In its potentially lethal covenant with its body, the brain never shuts up. It is designed to constantly be on some level of alert. Even as you dream, it tries to get your attention. It is in a state of perpetual readiness to react, defend, or attack when it or its body senses threats—real or not—to its self-enhancement. The brain itself never truly falls completely asleep. It has different levels of vigilance, but it never gives up its hold on the body. In a sleeping disorder called sleep-maintenance insomnia, or sleep apnea, the person falls asleep and stops breathing. After about ten to sixty seconds, the ever-alert lower brain jars the person awake to breathe for a while until sleep returns.[1] The brain/body covenant is one designed primarily for staying alive, seeking stimulation, doing, and getting. In effect, the brain "drags" your body with it to do its bidding, hauling you and your heart along on its rough ride, whether or not you are sure "in your heart" that you want to go where it is taking you.

CEREBRAL SELF-PRESERVATION

The brain is mortality phobic. Its greatest fear is its own end or any consciousness state that seems to approximate the selflessness that the brain may experience as the end of its existence. It resists states such as deep meditation, says you "are killing me" when your uncontrollable laughter makes you lose all self-consciousness, and tolerates only brief sexual orgasm, described by some romantic authors who have lost themselves in sexual ecstasy as "the mini-death."

The brain is afraid of cognitive darkness. It constantly seeks input and feeds on new, different, intense stimulation. For the brain, old news is no news at all. Like a child waking in a night terror, it often jolts you back to its form of reality from a peaceful brief reverie. It resists beauty that "arrests" its attention from self-survival. Its primary value is "self-health" not splendor, going and not being, and grit rather than grace.

TYPE A BRAIN, TYPE B HEART

The brain is not easily distracted from its lethal alliance with its body. It compulsively sticks to its task of trying to win the "human race." Author Thomas Moore writes of the Latin word "vocatio"—meaning to briefly pause from the pressures of daily living to wonder at being alive.[2] Because the brain is primarily programmed to seek success and not the connection the heart craves, it barely tolerates such vacations.

By nature of its primary vigilance role in the brain/body alliance, the brain is the ultimate "type A," as in type A behavior pattern, which is associated with heart disease. The brain is always in a hurry, preparing its body to go somewhere and uncomfortable with "just being" anywhere. It may resent being slowed down by what it sees as annoying interference and demands from other brain/body systems. The heart, however, seems to think in a more "type B," gentle, relaxed, connective way and is in search of connecting its subtle "L" energy with other hearts as a means of establishing lasting relationships and intimacy. The brain seems to want to "have a blast" while the heart needs to "have a bond."

THE TERRITORIAL BRAIN

The brain is self-protective and territorial. Its code is "I, me, mine." A natural pessimist, it evolved to expect and anticipate the worst as a form of self-defense left over from our primitive ancestors' necessary constant vigilance for outside threats.[3] Psychologist Mihaly Csikszentmihalyi asserts that the brain has an evolutionary bias toward pessimism and that unhappy, pessimistic, vigilant negativism helped our ancestors maintain an environmentally adaptive "ready to defend" posture in order to survive in a hostile environment. He writes that the pessimistic brain, by dwelling on unpleasant possibilities, is "better prepared for the unexpected."[4]

The energy that attracts and comes from the brain seems to be a darker, ready-to-fight, more negative energy than that of the heart. Dr. Larry Dossey, writing about the role of unhappiness in health, points out that, "It is as if all our potential thoughts are a roulette wheel of possibilities, with only a single red, positive slot amid thousands of black, negative ones."[5]

Because we tend to be so cerebral-centric and driven by the brain's constant search for the negative, we gawk at an auto crash, race to witness a disaster in progress, and are drawn to television shows that show "real life" crises. Even though it may "break our heart," our brain seems to seek the sad and terrible. While the brain may consider sameness boring and predictability dull, the heart is constantly on the lookout for the wonderfully simple pleasures of life.

Some of the most creative works of the cynical cortex tend toward the more grotesque. Philosopher Alan Watts observed that our brain's natural inclination toward the more hideous side of life is reflected in paintings such as Hieronymus Bosch's *Gates of Hell,* with all its sinister details, and the great literary works that typically deal more with human frailties and tragedies than gentle, nonproblematic loving.[6] By learning to contrast the brain's and heart's distinct codes, we may be able to more easily recognize which of our cultural creations are serving the objectives of the more selfish brain and which promote the more altruistic agenda of the heart.

ALL THOUGHTS ARE SECOND THOUGHTS

This is a book for those who are willing to respect the magnificence of the brain while considering that it is a remarkable partner with, but not the master over, the body and heart. The brain is primarily designed as a reactive health maintenance system, not as a contemplative, feeling system. The thinking centers of the brain have been evolutionarily crumpled up and crammed in above the more dominant and primitive brain systems that tend to take up most of our cerebral time. Our more rational higher brain is often taken hostage by the hypersensitive lower brain, resulting in a lowering of any emotional intelligence the brain inherits from our heart.[7]

The brain is more protectively reptilian, paleomammalian, and immaturely emotional than it is reflective, considerate, and patient. The brain thinks and seems to know it thinks, but thinking is not its primary evolutionary imperative. Rational thinking comes second to the brain's reactive survival instincts, and enhancing the self takes precedence over regard for the welfare of others. The primary mission of the brain is to keep us alive and to make our individual life as physically pleasurable as possible. Connection, loving, and caring are the brain's second thoughts usually seeping through the din of its urgent energy as expressions of the heart's code.

The brain tends to see the world and other people as food for its thought and means to its personal and individual ends. You will read later about the dangerous consequences of the neglected heart syndrome and the health effects of the abuse, deprivation, and exploitation of the heart by a compulsively driven cortex, but you can see its results all around you now. We all experience the impacts of an increasingly heartless world of alienation, disconnection, depression, failed and often abusive relationships, violence, discrimination, sexual harassment, environmental pollution, and an accelerating life pace that leaves us too busy trying to stay alive to have the time to reflect on the joy of being alive.

BYPASSING OR CONNECTING THE HEART

Once the brain has abused the heart with its deadly, cynical code of self-preservation above all else, and driven the heart beyond its physiological limits, it can burn out its own life-support system. The heart is the most powerful muscle in the human body, but even it can be strained and torn by the pressures applied by a stressed and stressful brain. Our brains have even managed to devise ways to bypass the hardened and dystrophied heart or arrange to have another previously owned replacement heart installed. I have the deepest respect and appreciation for the modern medicine that the brain has created and for its rigor and power. It helped save my life and put my parts back together again, but as with Pinocchio, in the final analysis it seemed to be the energy of my heart that gave my spirit and soul back and made me human again. Putting the heart back into our life can not only help save and prolong our life but make our life and all of the life around us more hardy—and "hearty"—for everyone and everything.

ARE YOU GOOD-HEARTED?

What is your cardio-temperament? Would those who know you the best say you have a good heart? Would they say you are a nice, caring person who is a real pleasure to be around? Would your family say your mere presence seems to bring peace and harmony to their home? Would your colleagues at work say you are a total joy to work with, always willing to help out, honest, and free of pettiness? Are you the kind of person you yourself would want to live, work, love, and play with every day? The answer to these questions may reveal the nature of "L" energy your heart is sending to your own cells, showering on those around you, and available for use in mitigating the lethal brain/body covenant.

One of my heart transplant patients discussed "L" heart energy when he said, "I don't know whose heart I got, but it sure is a relaxed one. I've never felt calmer and people seem to be more relaxed around me and drawn to me more. Maybe its because I'm in a much better mood now that I'm not dying and maybe it's because I got the heart from a good-hearted person. It's probably both." Like this man, many of my heart transplant patients spoke at length about a change in the nature of their general life energy that they attributed to their new heart.

GOOD OR BAD VIBRATIONS

Most of us have heard descriptions of people who seem to give off "good" or "bad vibes." Consider two people described to me by two of my patients. The first is a ninety-two-year-old grandmother and the other is a forty-seven-year-old male accountant.

"She really brightens up a room as soon as she walks in," said her grandson. "My grandma is ninety-two years old, but whenever I'm around her, I feel younger, happier, and more energetic. There's just something about her. She has such a good heart you can feel it in your own heart. Nothing gets going when the family gets together until grandma comes. When she gets there, the family lightens up right away."

The second description from the wife of the accountant reveals a much different type of energy. "He is just a downer. He's always angry and thinks he has to control everything, and when he can't, he just brings all of us down. We know when he's down even before he walks in the door. Even the dog can feel him coming and hides. We say that he's PMS: pretty mean spirited."

While most doctors ask, "How do you feel?" cardio-energetic medicine asks, "How do you make others feel?" The best monitors of the nature of your heart energy are the people who live and work with you. From the point of view of cardio-energetics, psychological, spiritual, and physical well-being is less a matter of personal fulfillment than being in energetic balance with all of the hearts and energy around you.

MEDICINE'S OLDEST IDEA

For twenty-three centuries, one of the oldest forms of medicine has focused on the heart as the center of the spiritual energy that expresses our soul.[8] While modern biomedicine grew from the Newtonian mechanical model of the body, Chinese medicine derived from a view of the body as an energy-driven ecosystem in which health depends on a proper balance of energy forces flowing throughout that system. Talking about and trying to measure life energy is not something modern Western medicine is comfortable with, but Chinese medicine, like almost every other older form of medicine, has always emphasized an energetic approach to understanding disease and healing.

A Taoist text reads, "The universe produced Qui" (spiritual energy, pronounced "chee").[9] This is a view of energy and mass as forms of the same cosmic stuff. While biomedicine sees the heart as a powerful pump constructed of passive, inert cells sending nurturing "stuff" to other passive, static, receptacle cells, the old and longest tested energetic medicines of the world have no trouble seeing the heart as both stuff and energy and particles and waves at the same time.

Sinologist Nathan Sivin points out the Qui (the Chinese version of subtle or "L" energy) is both ethereal [wave] and substantive [particle] at the same time. (brackets mine) He says that we moderns tend to divide the world into either substance (mass) or function (energy) and, therefore, have a great deal of difficulty accepting the fact that the body is mass, energy, and information all at the same time. Sivin observes that "Qui," or subtle energy, is what makes life happen and, at the same time, what is happening to make life.[10] As illustrated in the principles of the "L" energy of the heart, which will be presented in chapter 2, this quantum matter/energy/information interchangeability is the fundamental nature of the subtle energy the heart sends through and from us.

MONITORING THE ENERGY OF THE HEART

Until we can find other ways to measure "L" energy—we must use a brain-oriented means to try to access our heart's code and to interpret the behavioral signs in our body that reflect the nature of the energy of and from our heart. As physician W. Brugh Joy writes, "The magnificence of the heart perspective of awareness is the direct connection to the Divine aspects."[11] From the time the stethoscope was invented in 1817 through the advent of

X ray in 1895 to the ultrasonic and electromagnetic instruments of today's modern cardiology, we have been trying to determine if we have a "good heart." Cardio-energetics suggests that we simply ask it. By reflecting on the nature of the energy the heart seems to be sending through us and resonating out to other hearts, we can tap the force that bonds us as the created with our Creator.

TAKING THE H*E*A*R*T*

In my clinical work, I have used the following Heart Energy Amplitude Recognition Test (H*E*A*R*T*) with over one thousand patients in the United States, England, Germany, Spain, Norway, Switzerland, Italy, the former Soviet Union, and a "control" group of indigenous people from my native Hawaii who have their own version of "Qui" called "mana," and their version of the quantum wave/particle duality in the heart, which they call a lump of energized water or "pu'uwai." I used the test more as a teaching tool than a research instrument in an attempt to show my patients how they could be more aware of the quality of the energy they are sending out to their world and to help them recognize by which code they are primarily living their life—the brain's or the heart's. It is a crude, brain-designed instrument, but it is one way to begin to attend to more than just the heart's neuromuscular power. A copy of H*E*A*R*T* is provided below.

The Heart Energy Amplitude Recognition Test

Dr. Paul Pearsall—President & CEO—Ho'ala Hou (To Reawaken), Inc.

SCORING

0=Never   1=Almost Never   2=More Than Sometimes   3=A Lot   4=Almost Always

_____ 1. Are you in a hurry? (Have you looked ahead on this test?)

_____ 2. Are you so busy that others are afraid to "bother you"?

_____ 3. Would others say that you walk, drive, or move quickly?

_____ 4. Do you like to "save time" by doing many things at once and/or thinking one thing while doing something else?

_____ 5. Does it seem that you always get in the slow line?

_____ 6. Do "unqualified express lane participants" frustrate you?

_____ 7. Do you eat quickly?

_____ 8. Do you push elevator buttons that are already lit?

_____ 9. Do you talk fast, as shown by gasping, spraying droplets of saliva, or getting tongue tied?

_____ 10. Do you try to hurry other's speaking, using "uh huh, uh huh, ya, ya, ya," or tuneless humming?

_____ 11. Are you a "disgust flasher"? (click tongue, tilt head, raise left side of mouth, sigh, hand on hip, roll eyes)

_____ 12. Do you lose your temper while driving?

_____ 13. Are you cynical and distrusting of others' motives?

_____ 14. Do you have "sleep stress"? (sleep onset insomnia, snoring, grinding of teeth, tossing and turning)

_____ 15. Do you replay angry events, rehearse sarcastic comebacks, tell "work war stories," spread rumors, and/or threaten to quit your job or relationship?

_____ 16. Do you have family or marital conflicts and/or neglect your family?

_____ 17. Do you feel a "let down" after attaining a goal or high success?

_____ 18. Do you feel that you did not or do not get enough unconditional love from one or both parents?

_____ 19. Do you have a harsh, critical, sarcastic voice quality or laughter and/or use profanity?

_____ 20. Do you clench your fist, shrug your shoulders, or make chopping motions with your hand while speaking?

_____ 21. Do you avoid public crying and/or is your laughter loud, explosive, quasi-humorous, and social more than sincere?

_____ 22. Do you react emotionally, defensively, and negatively to criticism?

_____ 23. Do you feel sleepy and/or fall asleep when sitting quietly for a period of time or become "business meeting mesmerized" at "bored" meetings?

_____ 24. Do you answer questions before they're completely asked, confront arguments before they're fully presented, and feel sure you are right?

_____ 25. Would it be tense and stressful living and/or working with you?

_____ TOTAL POINTS

(Add a five point penalty for trying to get a low score)

INTERPRETING YOUR HEART ENERGY AMPLITUDE TEST SCORE

0–5=BALANCED ENERGY (Your heart energy is in healthy balance)

6–10=OVERLY AGITATED ENERGY (You're bothering your body and other people's bodies and heart)

11–20=VERY AGITATED ENERGY (You are becoming a "real pain" to your body and other people's bodies and hearts)

21 AND ABOVE=TOXIC ENERGY (You have become a real pain to your body and other people's bodies and hearts)

UNDERSTANDING YOUR H*E*A*R*T* SCORE

The 1,000 heart patient sample who took the Heart Energy Amplitude Recognition Test averaged a total score of 66. By contrast, a 200-person sample of Polynesians to whom I gave this test during a lecture tour through the islands of the Pacific averaged 8. When I announce my test results at meetings, someone always complains that the scoring system is unrealistic. One person said, "No one could possibly score below 21 on your test. They wouldn't be normal if they did and Polynesians don't drive or have elevators—they aren't living in the modern world with all of its stress." My response is always, "That is exactly my point." What we have come to accept as "normal" life energy in our daily life is evidence of the brain's constant abuse of its body and heart. Normalcy is now the major risk to our health.

While my sampling techniques and selective administration of the Heart Energy Amplitude Recognition Test as a clinical teaching tool rule out interpreting these numbers in any way other than a general indication and picture of the heart's energy, the degree of difference in these two average scores from a Western and Polynesian group is interesting in terms of the energy ecology of island, as opposed to continental, life. Living in Hawaii, I have found that the oceanic way of life and its close connection with the energy of nature, reliance an ancient healing energy models, high degree of emphasis on family, and view of the heart and not the brain as the center of a very relaxed state of consciousness may account for the lower Polynesian score.[12]

Each item on the H*E*A*R*T* is based on the latest research from cardiac psychology.[13] It is now clear from research in the fields of psychoneuroimmunology (the study of how the brain and immune system interact with the world), social psychology (the study of how interpersonal relationships influence and are influenced by the world), health psychology (the study of how our way of thinking and behaving affects our health and the health of others), and epidemiology (the study of the origins and patterns of disease) that having less hostility and cynicism and more connection in the form of relaxed, mutually supportive social systems is an important buffer against the development of heart disease. Space does not allow a full discussion of the research basis for each item on the test, but no item was included unless its relevance was supported by at least five current research findings from the above fields. All of these fields are showing that chronic emotional reactivity to minor and unexpected stressors, free-floating hostility, and impatience seem to be the primary indicators of disrupted or unbalanced toxic cardiac energy.[14]

FIVE BRAIN FALLACIES

In my interviews with patients who took the H*E*A*R*T*, I detected five "brain fallacies" that elevated their score and reflected the selfish, controlling, reactive nature of a brain left free of the heart's moderation. The higher the score on the H*E*A*R*T*, the more the brain/body lethal covenant is intact and the less the heart's energy is available to cool a hotheaded brain busy beating up on its own body.

Brain Fallacy One: The Outside World Is Working Against Us. The high H*E*A*R*T* scorers (above 21 points) held what psychologist Albert Bandura refers to as "a belief in pure environmental determinism."[15] The brain sees the world as a problem to be dealt with, and the high scorers were misled by their brain into believing that all human behavior is a function of environmental stimuli and that we are victims of a very cruel, often unfair world. The brain is always ready to do battle with that world and protect whatever turf it can for as long as it can.

The brain has a ready answer for what Albert Einstein considered to be the most important question of all: "Is the universe a friendly or unfriendly place?" The brain is certain the universe is unfriendly and must be wrestled with in order to survive. Because of this deterministic orientation, the brain keeps telling us that we must be constantly ready to do our best against the cosmic odds stacked against us. In the ultimate mental paradox, the brain often abuses and exploits its own heart to the point that it kills itself by trying so hard to save it own life. In a form of cerebral-coronary suicide pact in which the heart is an innocent bystander, the brain becomes its own executioner.

Psychologist B. F. Skinner summarized this environmental determinism concept and absence of energetic connection and participation in the world when he wrote, "A person does not act upon the world, the world acts upon him."[16] The implication drawn by the brain is that one can control one's own life only by a complete, constant, and ever-vigilant attempt to regulate the outside world as much as possible. The result is a constantly agitated heart overburdened by a demanding brain that is starved for nutrients that enable its defensive workaholism.

The way of the heart is much less environmentally deterministic than the brain and is based on a view of the universe as essentially a friendly place. The heart speaks in the language summarized by author Elizabeth Rivers: "When something doesn't go my way, I let go of my idea of how it should be, trusting that my mind [brain] doesn't know the larger picture."

Brain Fallacy Two: Victimization. The brain has a tendency toward chronic blaming. Since it considers itself to be "us" and to be the most brilliant of all of our organs, it quickly cries "foul" when things don't seem to go its way. When the expected promotion at work, credit for an achievement, reward for a loving act, convenient parking place, or compliance by others with its expectations and need for control do not seem immediately and rapidly forthcoming, it perceives injustice. "Unfair, why you, why not me, and how could you" are its immediate responses.[17]

The heart considers itself a part of a three-part Mind, made up of brain, body, and heart, and it is ready to join with the rational power of the brain and the extraordinary senses of the body to make its soothing contribution to our daily living. While the brain uses its rational brilliance to seek reasons, the heart's wisdom teaches that the three-part Mind it is a part of can never get "its" way, only go with The Way.

Brain Fallacy Three: Hard Work Always Pays Off. Even though the brain sees the universe as a powerful and unfriendly place with which it must struggle to maintain some semblance of control in order to avoid being its victim, it is convinced it can get its piece of the pie by outworking other brains. It thinks that, with enough effort, clever maneuvering to take advantage of others, and sacrifice of those aspects of life the heart so longs for, it can keep itself alive. Many self-help books are written in the brain's code. They contain instructions for being all you can be, avoiding the errors of dysfunctionality, doing all you can do, and winning—no matter that every victory requires another person's loss.

A "self-help" book written in the heart's code would be more of an "us help" book and would provide four essential health warnings: Don't abuse your heart by allowing your brain to physically harm it by exposing it to constant stress and straining toward self-fulfillment. Don't exploit your heart by allowing your brain to misappropriate its miraculous energy for selfish purposes. Don't deprive your heart by allowing your brain's innate selfishness to distance you from the hearts of others. Finally, don't neglect your heart by allowing your brain to be so busily and reactively consumed with trying to stay alive that it forgets to allow time for your heart to proactively reflect on what purposes you chose for your living.

Many so-called self-help books offer individual strategies for escaping denial, freeing and expressing the self, and progressing into a perpetual state of recovery. Heart-coded "us help" books would be more likely to teach that you should always try to be at least a little less than you can be, try to collaborate more than compete, and pay more attention to your loving cellular memories stored within you in the form of a mature inner elder than you do to finding and indulging the often socially immature and narcissistic brain, that whining "inner child." Heart-coded books would be more likely to emphasize that, no matter how positive your attitude and how hard your brain makes you work, there are some things you can never achieve. Moreover, most achievements require you to have intimate and mutually dependent connections with others. Heart-coded books are more likely to ask readers to consider entirely new ways of understanding their own responsibilities, limitations, and emotional impacts on others than to offer a new technique for more self-actualization. Books written from the perspective of the heart's code would be more likely to be in the tradition of Franz Kafka's description of a book as "an axe for the frozen sea within us," while brain-coded books may be more likely to teach us how to spiritually ice skate.[18]

The heart knows that success cannot be pursued but must ensue as a result of a more gentle, balanced, caring, connected, and loving orientation to the world. The heart knows that there are many environmental factors that are intransigent and beyond anyone's control. It knows that some life obstacles are put there because they cannot be overcome and because they can teach us to stop trying and start being.

Brain Fallacy Four: I Can Change People. The brain tends to consider itself a very powerful and clever controller of other brains and very "self-effective."[19] It thinks it can be smart enough to get other people to change, to move in the directions it desires. When they do not, or their cardio-temperament comes through even though they have altered some behaviors, the brain becomes angry, impatient, and even urges the body to aggressive acts. The heart is wise enough to know that its brain cannot change other brains, but it also knows that, if it will listen, its brain can learn to think about other people in a more tolerant, gentle, accepting manner. The heart knows "you can't really change people, but you can change how you think about people."

The heart tends to think more in a manner social psychologists call "reciprocal determinism."[20] Psychologist Albert Bandura writes that people possess self-directive capabilities that enable them to exercise some control over their thoughts, feelings, and actions by the consciousness they produce for themselves. That consciousness can either be a brain-driven thinking about life or a brain/heart/body Mind's chorus of gentle connection with life. It is difficult to change a brain, but when we tune in to our heart, we change our Mind by introducing more balanced "L" energy into the brain/body covenant.

Brain Fallacy Five: Frustration Means Aggression. For the impatient brain, frustration of its objectives quickly leads to anger. Psychologists call this the "frustration-aggression" hypothesis. Research now shows, however, that it is not so much that thoughts of frustration lead directly to aggressive acts but that frustration provokes feelings of anger and hostility and challenges to self (read "brain") control. These unpleasant feelings in turn lead to aggression aimed at whomever and whatever is nearby. Thus, the brain's frustration turns to an anger that ignites belligerence.[21] The brain may have become frustrated at work and become angry later at home, causing disruption in the family system. This is due to the brain's displaced frustration.

HAVE A HEART

Imagine that two jumbo 747 jet airplanes full of passengers crashed every day with no survivors. That's the number of people who die of heart disease daily in the United States. We hear much about the major risk factors for developing heart disease, including high cholesterol, obesity, smoking, and high blood pressure, yet about half of those who suffer their first heart attack have none of these common risk factors, more than eight out of ten people with three of these risk factors never suffer a heart attack, and most people who do have heart attacks do not have most of the risk factors.[22] There seems to be something else at work when it comes to heart disease, perhaps the fact that the brain constantly seems to be abusing it.

By using the results of the H*E*A*R*T*, you can begin to recognize the nature of the energy of your heart and help your brain learn to sense its distress and pain. Research shows that the number of years of education a person has is a more important factor in determining risk of heart disease than all the other risk factors combined.[23] While educated people are more likely to read and understand written health warnings, they also tend to be more aware of what is going on around them and how social forces act to affect their life. The type of education I am calling for in this chapter is learning to read the subtle energetic warnings from your heart that it feels hurt when it is left out of the brain/body dialogue or is stressed beyond its limits by its demanding brain. By learning to tap into your heart's code, you may be able to prolong not only your own life but the lives of those you love. Perhaps the most important health warning of all is to "have a heart."

CHAPTER TWO

Unraveling the Mystery
of the Fifth Force

"We have reached a point in our evolution that requires us to learn to speak 'energy' fluently. Our search to understand the essence of health as well as our newfound passion to form a more mature relationship with the spiritual dimensions of our lives has led us to this crossroads."

— CAROLINE MYSS, PH.D.

GOING WITH THE FORCE

"Go with the force, Luke! Let the force be with you," urged the wise Obi-Wan Kenobi as Luke Skywalker prepared for battle in the movie *Star Wars*. Throughout history, we have been in search of this same magical invisible force that seems to offer unlimited strength and healing and that transcends all other known forms of energy. Many researchers dismiss the possibility of such a force and any need for its existence to explain how life works. They see those who assert its existence as engaging in the fantasy and illusion that renders them foolishly unscientific. More open-hearted scientists, however, are willing to entertain the possibility that an as yet unknown and immeasurable force may exist, perhaps in the form of an as yet to be documented info-energy that requires no travel time and therefore is capable of exerting its influence instantaneously across space and time with no detectable tangible traces.[1] Like most of us, however, even the most skeptical scientists seem to seek the strength of "the force" sometime in their lives in order to survive the wars of daily living.

ON BEING SKEPTICAL OF ONE'S SKEPTICISM

Less than a century ago, most scientists still believed in a life force that made living things different from nonliving things. Their belief in this force was independent of their religious convictions and they were confident that this mysterious, yet subtle, form of energy would eventually yield its secrets and be understood by natural laws. This force was named "the vital force"—a version of what I am calling the "L" or life energy that may carry the heart's code.

Those who persist in the search for a nonmaterial vital life force are called "vitalists." Vitalism is out of favor with most of today's scientists who are proud to be called "mechanists" who deny the existence of any other form of energy in the human body than that emanating from known physicochemical processes. To consider the nature of the heart's code and how cellular memories may be made from this code, the choice between vitalism and mechanism is unnecessary if we are willing to concede that questioning everything does not mean anything might be possible. No one can deny the mechanistic qualities of the human system. Every day, scientists are exposing more of the mysteries of the biomechanical properties of life. To be so skeptical as to deny even the possibility of a vital energy force like an "L" energy, however, is to lack the necessary skepticism of one's own skepticism that is essential to learning.

While the heart's code may be carried within the known forms of energy, it may also be possible that this code and the cellular memories it creates are manifestations of the vital force that has eluded researchers for centuries. I am not certain that such a force exists or, if it does, that the heart and cells use it to do their work. However, I am skeptical enough of the limits of a totally mechanistic view to be sufficiently uncertain to consider the existence of a life force that medicine cannot yet see.

FROG POWER

Eighteenth century biologist Luigi Galvani was one of the early "L" energy vitalists. Like many persons of his time, he was convinced that there was a unique, mystical force that brought the human system to life. To test his ideas, he suspended the severed legs of a frog from a brass hook connected to iron rods in order to see if they would show any signs of this vital energy when separated from their body. When he observed that the legs twitched in the presence of an electrical storm or even when static electricity was discharged some distance away, he was sure that he had finally discovered the elusive "L" energy. Galvani had wrongly attributed the electromagnetic power behind the movement of the bodiless legs to what he called "animal magnetism." To collect and compound this life force, he tried to make an "organ battery" out of a pile of hundreds of what he thought were vitally energized frog legs. As has happened so often in the history of science, Galvani's mistake eventually resulted in discoveries that led to an understanding of electrical energy and the eventual development of a real "galvanic" battery.

To this day, there is no conclusive evidence that the type of "L" energy I propose could be conveyed by the heart and stored in the cells. Even by modern science's own standards, however, lack of conclusive evidence of a proposition is not proof of its falseness. This chapter explores the possibilities of the "L" energy that may relate to the way the heart thinks and the cells remember.

A FIFTH FORM OF ENERGY?

Energy is the ability to do work. It is the force that moves things, including atoms, molecules, cellular processes, consciousness, and bodies of all shapes and sizes, from planets to toes. It moves systems because it contains the information that tells systems how to move. Measuring energy has become a very precise science, but interpreting what energy actually is challenges even the most brilliant physicists.[2] The difficulty in understanding the true nature of energy and how an invisible process can contain information that affects every system in the cosmos may be one reason why the various traditional or alternative medicines that place such emphasis on this kind of energy have not found their way into mainstream modern medicine. Nonetheless, the fact that the heart pumps biochemical nutrients to every cell in our body means that it is also pumping or circulating patterns of energy containing the information that tells every object in the body how to do its job.

All of the four general categories of energy that science currently accepts—gravity, electromagnetic energy, strong and weak nuclear energy—are processes that have at least some forms of easily measurable effects on the world in which they operate. In a sense, however, even these four known forms of energy are "vitalistic" in that how they convey their information is implied from measurements of the effects of the kind of work they do. Gravity holds you in your chair as you read this book, but you can not see or touch it. We know and feel the effects of electromagnetic energy, but we can only see it in its indirect manifestations accessible to our physical senses. Strong and weak nuclear energy are even more theoretical and confounding in their natures. The possibility of a fifth force should not be ruled out because of our current inability to directly measure it with our current instrumentation or to understand the nature of its encoded information.

ENERGY KEEPS US TOGETHER

The basic unit of all life, the cell, exists only because it is held together by energy. The atoms and molecules that make up a cell also exist because their various parts are held together by bonds of energy. Surgeon Sherwin Nuland, who describes himself as mechanistic in his orientation and not at all a proponent of the existence of a vital spiritual energy, writes, "It is energy . . . that keeps a human being in one piece."[3] The cardio-energetics hypothesis that energy and information are interchangeable may mean that even the four categories of energy science is willing to accept contain a code that represents who we are. If who we are is at least in part a representation of our soul, then all types of energy are "vital" forms of the life force.

The magnificence of the energy of the human system impresses even the scientifically rigorous Dr. Nuland. He is convinced that the wisdom of the body is traceable to known biochemical processes, yet he writes, "The unheard din of living is the symphony before which the chorale of the spirit soars in song."[4] It also seemed to impress the much more vitalistic or vital force-believing Ralph Waldo Emerson when he wrote, "One moment of a man's life is a fact so stupendous as to take the lustre out of all fiction."

IN SEARCH OF THE SOUL

Vitalists have always thought that the soul is associated with having its own unique energy, a fifth force that may sometimes accompany but also transcends gravity, electromagneticism, and strong and weak nuclear energy. It has been seen as what author James Hillman refers to as a sense of calling from within, what he calls a type of central, guiding force and what we know in our "heart of hearts" we must do and be, and why we are here in the first place.[5] Victorian scholar E. B. Tylor traced the word "soul" as referring to a mostly invisible physical power or force.[6] The romantic poet

Keats referred to a sense of "calling from the heart," and Michelangelo said he saw an image radiating from the heart of the person he was sculpting. The list of great minds aware of the subtle energetic power is long, urging us to continue to look for an animating force of the human spirit that expresses our soul and connects it with all other souls.

Webster's dictionary defines the soul as the immaterial essence or substance, the animating principle or actuating cause of life, a definition that resembles the vitalist's definition of a vital force.[7] I have found hundreds of references to the brain and heart in the major medical texts, but not one reference to the soul and certainly none to its vital "L" energy. One group of brilliant scientists, however, base their entire approach to understanding the cosmos on the presence and nature of a "fifth force," or subtle "L" energetic intelligence, which is invisible to our mechanical instruments but infinitely pervasive in its influence. These energy scientists are the quantum physicists who have learned that they cannot do their experiments or begin to understand quarks and stars or particles and waves without referring to a subtle and often tricky "fifth force."

NONLOCAL ENERGY

One reason "L" energy may be so difficult to study is that it may be what scientists call "nonlocal," meaning that it exists not just in one place at one time but everywhere all the time. Its nonlocal nature seems so beyond what we have come to expect of the better known forms of energy that scientists dealing with "L" energy can only set up their experiments in such a way as to invite the fifth force to just "do what it will" and be ready to watch and learn. What makes things even more difficult for quantum physicists, or so-called "new physicists," is that the very act of their watching seems to result in their own "L" energy influencing their experiments.

Based on the often paradoxical findings from the field of quantum physics, the science of how the tiniest particles and their mysteriously unpredictable energy operate, it has been learned that objects on opposite sides of the universe seem energetically connected with one another. Faster than the speed of light, a change in one of a pair these objects is instantaneously replicated in its info-energy-sharing partner. The quantum physics principle of nonlocality says that, in the minuscule buzzing quantum world of which our body's cells are a part, there are no barriers, time is relative, that mass, energy, and information are one and the same, that objects once connected forever retain the info-energetic memory of that connection, and the separateness of any kind in the world, human or otherwise, is mere illusion.

Although it may seem impossible to our brain, "L" energy's influence means that space and time are the brain's approximation of reality and its own unique version of reality. Quantum physics suggests that we are all a part of and contributors to a subtle energy field that operates by the rule of timeless connection and not the mechanical limits of miles and walls. Nonlocality refers to the energetic intelligence field of which all that is or has ever been or will be is forever a part. While lovers speak in such terms as together forever, being inseparable, and feeling energetically connected, many scientists are intimidated by the discourse about subtle energy that seems to be the language of love rather than objective scientific discourse. While most of us seem to know in our heart that space and time are not limits to love, prayer, and caring, our brain insists on its privatizing of its existence and prefers to deal with forms of energy its technology can measure.

TOGETHER FOREVER

To understand the impact of a nonlocal, invisible form of info-energy that the brain finds very difficult to accept, consider the results of an experiment done in 1993 under the direction of the United States Army Intelligence and Security Command (INSCOM).[8] White blood cells (leukocytes) scraped from the mouth of a volunteer were centrifuged and placed in a test tube. A probe from a recording polygraph—a lie (or emotion) detector—was then inserted in the tube. The donor of the cheek cells was seated in a room separate from his donated cells and shown a television program with many violent scenes. When the volunteer watched scenes of fighting and killing, the probe from the polygraph detected extreme excitation in the mouth cells even though they were in a room down the hall. Subsequent repeats of this experiment with donor and cells separated up to fifty miles and up to two days after donation of the cells showed the same results. The donated cells remained energetically and nonlocally connected with their donor and seemed to "remember" where they came from.

If this connective energy can be verified in more such studies, it is possible that what we call "paranormal" events are "normal" and that our recent reliance on the brain's way of thinking and its urgent, pragmatic, selfish, rational, cardio-insensitive approach to life are the exception that we are making to the first rule of human consciousness—we are all vitally connected energetically. More than seventy studies on intercessory prayer have shown the same nonlocal energetic connection effects as detected in the cheek cell experiment. One example of such a study was conducted by Dr. Randolph Byrd in San Francisco. It showed that patients undergoing heart surgery who were prayed for by groups scattered around the world did significantly better in their recovery than those who were not prayed for by these groups.[9] Some form of healing info-energy seemed at work, and distance and time made no difference.

We go to school to learn to "use our head," but what if all of us were required to use our heart to sense the subtle "L" energy all around us? Perhaps, as psychic researcher Stephen Schwartz speculates, if we were sent mandatorily through twelve years of schooling in literacy in subtle energy instead of learning only analytical brain-oriented approaches to living, we would grow up believing that alertness to, and behaving in accordance with, awareness of a subtle energy connecting all of us "heart to heart" is normal and not such a rare thing and that a brain-dependent orientation is what is "paranormal."[10]

THE PEAR PROGRAM

Throughout this book, I will be referring to the more than twenty years of research on subtle energy connection conducted at the Princeton Engineering Anomalies Research program at Princeton University. The results of ongoing studies at Princeton, perhaps more so than any other established research center, give at least preliminary evidence of the possibility of some type of vital fifth force such as the "L" energy. I have read their research reports and in early 1997 had the opportunity to visit the PEAR program, to speak with the researchers there, and to be a participant in a few simple experiments that illustrated their approach to the study of subtle energy connections.

In a cluster of dimly lit rooms in the basement of the engineering building on the Princeton University campus in New Jersey, a team of highly skeptical, careful scientists using the most uncompromising scientific protocols have conducted more than one million trials assessing the impact of "L" energy.[11] Established in 1979 by Robert G. Jahn, Ph.D., dean of the School of Engineering and Applied Science, the PEAR program's purpose is to pursue rigorous scientific study of the interaction of human consciousness with sensitive physical devices, systems, and processes. Volunteers, called operators, are asked to sit down near a machine designed to generate random numbers. This means that, just like flipping a coin, the machine turns out large sets of zeros and ones that, over a period of time, should show no trend toward either zero or one. The volunteers were asked to consciously attempt to alter the output of the numbers from the machine. The operators are not psychics and are not given any instructions or special training other than being told to try to influence the machine toward more ones or more zeroes or, in some cases, to act as what the PEAR staff calls "percipients": persons who, using some as-yet undefined sense, try to extract details from a remote scene at a location often hundreds of miles away from the PEAR laboratory. Beyond any reasonable scientific doubt, the PEAR laboratory team has documented small but statistically significant differences in the way the machines "behaved," in terms of the numbers they generated, when operators were present and trying, in some way, to influence the machines. The team also documented evidence that percipients could accurately describe scenes they had never been to or seen themselves.

It is startling to observe random numbers generated by a machine become less random and move in a positive or negative direction in compliance with the intent of the operator or to hear remarkably accurate descriptions of remote locations by persons sitting hundreds of miles from the location of these scenes. It is also amazing to watch a pendulum's pattern or a computer image altering in accordance with a person's intent, a drum beating a new rhythm in keeping with the rhythm selected by an operator, a robot made to look like a frog (I called it Galvani) summoned to an operator merely by the influence of the subtle energy of the person energetically calling the frog. The PEAR staff reports that the odds of chance explaining such occurrences are one in one billion.

To begin to try to explain their amazing results and how it could be that some form of subtle info-energetic connection seemed to exist between a person and machine, the PEAR research team refer to quantum concepts. The principles of complementarity (meaning the action in one system can affect the actions of another system on a quantum energetic level, free of the limits of time and space) and wave mechanical resonance (matter and energy exchanging manifestations as vibrating waves and particles) can begin to explain what they have discovered, but they say they are very far from not only answers to what is going on but also from knowing exactly what questions to ask.

Most scientists insist that quantum concepts such as nonlocality, complementarity, and wave/particle resonance do not apply to human consciousness. They assert that ideas such as Hiesenberg's Uncertainty Principle, a quantum fact of life that asserts that if we choose to measure one quantity (e.g, the position of an electron), we inevitably alter the system itself and therefore can't be certain about its other quantities (e.g., how fast the electron is moving), are only a manifestation of the interaction of particles that constitute a quantum mechanical weirdness. This strangeness, they say, has nothing to do with the consciousness of the observer. They ignore the fact, however, that the observer and his or her consciousness are also made up of info-energy that is not exempt from effects of quantum principles. Some scientists, including the staff at the PEAR program, are not as certain about the Uncertainty Principle's limitations.

DISCOVERING LOVE POWER

Since I began my work in the area of the heart's code more than ten years ago, I have been using the letter "L" to represent the vital life force that may come from and be circulated by our heart. Although I did not know it until I visited the PEAR program, the staff there often refers to the subtle energy they are dealing with as "L" energy. They report their data indicates that two persons in a loving bond working on the same experiment together do not simply combine what the PEAR staff calls their "individual subtle energy signatures," as shown by changes in the various measurements of the equipment. Instead, there seems to be a "coupled" subtle energy effect that is a unique blend of each co-operator's unique energy signature. While two men or two women working as a team tended to have stronger energy influences on the machines and to be more accurate as a team than a single percipient in describing remote locations, the strongest energy-connection effects were achieved by male/female pairs who reported that they were "bonded," connected heart to heart in a love bond.[12]

While they are the most rigorous of practioners of the scientific method, Drs. Robert G. Jahn and Brenda Dunne of the PEAR program refer to the "love" power of resonating energy bonds. They point out that the recipe for the strongest "L" energy influence as revealed in their laboratory "is also the recipe for any form of love: the surrender of self-centered interests of the partners in favor of the pair."[13] Male/female loving bonds may manifest the strongest joined "L" energy because they comprise an example of what author Arnold Lettieri, Jr., Ph.D., also at the

PEAR program, identifies as "two primordial aspects; 'substantiality' [our particle "stuff," singular, individualistic "male" nature] and 'relationality' [our more "female process," interactive energy wave nature]." (brackets mine)[14] It appears that "L" energy relates to being able to transcend our xenophobic proneness to cellular separateness as well as remembering our substantive and relational natures and combining the brain's more objective, rational code with the heart's more subjective, intuitive code.

THE VANILLA YOGURT TECHNIQUE

The PEAR program may be revealing another aspect of the heart's code by showing that "L" energy connection does not require hard thinking, strong focus, and intense effort. In fact, such mental effort seems to get in the way of subtle energy connection. The type A, hard-driving orientation does not seem to be the way to vitally connect with another person or thing. Thinking hard about subtle energy seems to lessen its influence, while just being seems to make its influence stronger.

During my recent visit to Princeton University, I had lunch with Dr. Brenda Dunne and the research staff at the PEAR laboratory. I spoke with Dr. Dunne about what I identified as a "subtle energy spurt" effect I noticed in my heart transplant recipients. Many of them seemed at first to connect profoundly with various aspects of their donor's personality, then seemed to lose or deny that sense of connection, and then regain it later if they stopped denying their energetic connection or stopped trying too hard to make that connection. It seemed that the cellular memories of their donor were best connected with by not trying and just letting it happen. A fifty-two-year-old female heart transplant recipient described this subtle energy spurt phenomenon. Referring to the PEAR researchers' own successful documentation of some form of "L" energy connection, she said, "Don't expect this cellular memory thing to knock your socks off. It just sort of happens if you let it. If you try too hard, I don't think it happens or at least you don't sense the connection. I feel my donor's presence most when I just sit down, shut up, and let the energy flow."

I asked Dr. Dunne, who manages the laboratory at PEAR, about this patient and others who seemed to experience a U-shaped curve of subtle energy connection that went from being strong initially, to a severe decrease, and then back to connection. She related a story that helped me understand what I was seeing.

"It seems that the less you try to connect with the [random number generating] machines, the more successful you are," she said. "At first, most people get the effect, however small. Then it almost always reduces significantly. If they try harder and harder, they become frustrated and the effect remains elusive. If they just let it happen, relax, have fun, and gently encourage and tease the machine into cooperating, the effect returns and is often even more pronounced. One of the most successful women at connecting with the machine simply sat next to it, decided in which direction she wanted the random numbers to begin to change, ate a snack of vanilla yogurt, and read." Dr. Dunne added jokingly, "I almost thought it was the vanilla yogurt that caused it!"

While much remains to be learned about the nature of "L" energy, preliminary indications from the PEAR program and the experiences of my heart transplant patients seem to indicate the following five steps may be involved in becoming aware of the fifth force that is the heart's code. Each of these steps is similar to practices suggested by healers and shamans of ancient and indigenous peoples and it also helps protect and heal the physical heart itself, according to the fields that are contributing to a better understanding of the heart (such as psychoneuroimmunology, health psychology, and cardiac psychology).

1. Be Patient. Be still, tolerant, enduring, and open enough to be available to become sensitive to "L" energy. Realize that, while the brain's way is to "just do it," the heart's way is to "let it be." Think in terms similar to a heart transplant recipient's body systems, which must learn how to be patient enough with their new hearts to let them fit into a new system so that rejection does not occur. Like the operators and percipients at Princeton, remember the U-shaped curve of energy connection, and that it usually occurs very easily and suddenly at first until the brain resumes control and tries to force the issue. By relaxing, having fun, treating the world with respect and caring, and perhaps having a little vanilla yogurt or indulging in any other enjoyable distraction from the brain's constant "trying," the connection is most likely to happen again and again.

2. Be Connected. Try to "unite" more than "control," and to do "our thing" rather than "your own thing." Think like the systems of heart transplant recipients, which have to be able to allow the body to connect with the new cells it is receiving. Like quantum physicists do, be open-minded, accepting, and creatively alert enough to recognize and be open to the influences of as yet immeasurable forces that may result in strange, meaningful coincidences and life's little accidents that could contain lessons about your place in the cosmos. Open your heart to the vague, subtle energy influences that may seem to attract or repel you to and from other people, places, and things. It may be that sensing the code of the heart in the form of its "L" energy is more a matter of becoming more fully aware of a connection that already exists than trying to make a new connection. Remember the uniquely powerful "loving bond" energy connection effect noted in the PEAR program and the impact of that shared energy signature on other persons, places, and things. It is not individuals but systems that connect, so try to be more alert to being a system within a system that is a part of what is happening, rather than an individual observer looking for what happened. Be as open to subtle energy surprises and paradoxes as a quantum physicist must be if she is to discover more about the mysteries of life.

3. Be Pleasant. Go along! Like a heart transplant recipient must do, learn to get along with your heart. In the PEAR program, those persons who talked nicely to the machines and tried to connect pleasantly with them tended to be more successful in influencing them than those who became angry and yelled at them. Like an organ donor, give the gift of life and treat those around you like energy transplant recipients. Send out an agreeable, tolerant energy that energizes those around you and draws people to you. The brain tends to be defensive, negative, and prone to hostility, but the heart's nature is to be agreeable, congenial, and harmonious. To connect with our heart, we have to be more like our heart.

4. Be Humble. Realize that your idea of "self" is your brain's illusion of separateness. We are all connected and mutually dependent as participants in a universal system. Ignore the brain's selfish prodding and try to override its individualistic force, the "cellular xenophobia" we all have, which is an evolutional cellular memory. Our cells may contain memories of a quantum paradise, a less selfish and more profoundly pleasurably connected time. By being less territorial, self-assertive, and demanding, and rejoicing in all the gifts that God the Absolute, or a Higher Power, has given, the memory of paradise lost can override our fear of "otherness." Cardio-energetic connection is trying to have the heart we might want to receive if we were to be a heart transplant recipient.

5. Be Gentle. Take it easy, take your time, and take what comes. Follow the Polynesian hula principle suggested by an Hawaiian named Boy Kanahe: "When things don't work out right, take 'em to the left." Remember the epitaph of the person who works too hard too often is "Got everything done; died anyway." Like the operators in the PEAR experiment, try less to control and more to let the force of natural connection happen. As an organ transplant recipient must do to survive, we have to shut down our instinctive immuno-tendency to "reject" and make the effort to more tenderly and lovingly allow our life to unfold. Using our heart to moderate and instruct the brilliant brain with its wisdom, we have to start learning to want what we have instead trying to have what we want.

THE EYE'S BLACK HOLE

"Look me in the eye and say that." "Look at me eye to eye." "I can see it in your eyes." "You're giving me the evil eye." All of these phrases may hold another clue about how "L" energy may work. Physiologists know that large pupils are a sign of attention, arousal, interest, fear, rage, and love. When we are sexually aroused or physically threatened, our pupils dilate.[15] When we are confronted with a pleasant stimulus such as a beautiful flower or lovely child, our pupils become large black pools.[16] This is one way the heart uses the brain to help it drink in its energy. When the heart is energetically opening up, either to absorb the beauty of a positive info-energetic event or to become more alert and contemplative of a more negative energy around it, the pupils enlarge to help absorb that energy.

The black color of the pupil results from an energy convergence and the total absorption of all of the energy waves of the color spectrum. When you look into another person's eyes at their black pupil, you are looking at what has become of you in their eyes. When someone "lays eyes on you," that person is also putting energy into you, sending a dose of infra-red energy from the heart of the many vessels in their retina. It may be a kind of info-energetic telegram that most of us are experiencing when we say, "I felt someone looking at me."

When two lovers gaze into one another's eyes, they info-energetically connect. Each absorbs the energy coming from the other's eyes and all of the waves of color energy that "is" the image of each lover dissolves into the black pupil pool of the other. Like cosmic black holes that suck in all the energy around them, the black hole in the middle of the eye is where energy passes to the retina, to the occipital area of the brain; pulsates as info-energy from the heart throughout the body system; and is ultimately stored as a cellular memory imprint, or info-energetic love map, left within in every cell in the body.

Since energy, including light energy, carries information and you are constantly sending out energy, you are forever in an act of info-energetic intercourse that recreates who and how you are. In accordance with the "systemic memory" hypothesis proposed by Drs. Schwartz and Russek, we are constantly engaged in a reverberating info-energetic dance. Our energy is collected by another energy system, our energy alters the pattern and resonation of energy in that system, that system sends out its newly modified form of energy that has now become stored as a part of our energy, and on and on and on with every beat of our heart.

"L" ENERGY AND THE GRATEFUL DEAD

Another and unlikely source of more information about "L" energy was provided by the rock group the Grateful Dead. More than twenty-five years ago at a series of six concerts in Port Chester, New York, this well-known group of musicians conducted their own version of a scientific study of a subtle, nonlocal energy. They wanted to see if thousands of people could convey images of slides projected on a screen to a person miles away at Maimonides Hospital in Brooklyn.[17] They asked independent judges, people who did not know of the "concert consciousness experiment," to rate the concertgoers' "L" energy target's dream report. These judges said that the reports of the concertgoers' "target" dreamer were more similar to the content of the slides shown at the concert than the dream reports of another person not designated to receive the Grateful Dead's concertgoers' images. While some other studies have failed to replicate the Grateful Dead research, other versions of such energy-sending and receiving studies, such as the PEAR studies, have shown a similar subtle, fragile, but statistically significant energy connection effect.[18]

THE HEART OF EINSTEIN'S FORMULA

Albert Einstein showed us that matter (M) is an expression of energy (E); cardio-energetics suggests that energy (E) is interchangeable with information (I). That matter, energy, and information may all be the same quantum stuff is a starting point for understanding how the heart might be a cellular mass that is at the same time an info-energetic wave and buzzing bundles of particles.

Some physicians are beginning to recognize the M=E=I effect and the role of subtle info-energy in health and healing. Dr. Richard Gerber's pioneering book in this area, titled *Vibrational Medicine,* points out that the animating life force is an energy that is currently unaddressed by today's Newtonian mechanistic thinking. He writes, "The spiritual dimension is the energetic basis of all life, because it is the energy of spirit which animates the physical framework."[19]

There is no doubt that molecular interactions, such as enzymes and neuropeptides, are also involved in cellular memory and that there is subtle energy involved in the way these substances do their work. As Einstein's formula predicts, the cellular "matter" (M) of enzymes and neuropeptides is a specialized, subtle form of energy (E), and that energy also contains information (I). Nobel Prize–winning physicist David Bohm summarizes this "M=E=I" formula when he writes that there is a limitless amount of information enfolded into the structure of the universe and we are a manifestation of that energy.[20] Every body event, whether the workings of our enzymes, neuropeptides, hormones, blood, or skin, is an info-energetic event.

THE PHANTOM LEAF AND HOW WATER REMEMBERS

As another example of the permanent tracings of subtle energy, consider the "phantom leaf effect." Electrophotographic pictures of a leaf with its top half cut off and destroyed reveal that the remaining leaf fragment contains a precise image of the detached part of the leaf even though that part has been discarded and destroyed. Apparently, its "energy" is remembered by the leaf that is left. While skeptical scientists assert this "remembered image" must be due to moisture remaining and leaving some type of imprint on the photo plate, other researchers have shown this not to be the case.[21] The implication of the Phantom Leaf Effect is that some type of organizing energy field is present and systemically remembered.[22] In limited work with plants at the PEAR program, people not only energetically connected with plants but various forms of vegetation seem to be able to exert influence on the randomness of various mechanical devices. By setting a plant next to a random number generating machine, the presence of that plant seems to alter the numbers produced.

Greek philosopher Thales said that everything is water and that water is the basic element in all life. In Hawaii, water (or "wai") is the ultimate source of "mana" (or energy). "Wai wai" means being wealthy with plenty of energy, and as you have read, "pu'uwai," the Hawaiian word for heart, means "lump of water," or life energy. Water covers two thirds of our planet and constitutes 99 percent of the body's molecules. Researchers have discovered that water, like everything in the cosmos, contains, receives, and sends subtle energy and has it own form of "liquid memory."

Dr. Bernard Grad at McGill University in Montreal wanted to find out if psychic healers had real energetic effects upon their patients or simply had "charisma" that influenced the emotional outlook of their patients. To study this "subtle healing energy," he substituted plant subjects for human patients to exclude the effect of "belief." To create a "sick plant patient," Grad soaked barley seeds in salty water to retard their growth. He then had a healer hold a sealed container of salt water which was to be used for germinating the seeds. Grad found that the seeds placed in the healer-treated water sprouted more often than those in the regular saline group. Grad also had depressed patients hold containers of water. When barley seeds were placed in the sad patients' water containers, the seeds showed a suppressed rate of growth.[23] Numerous other studies have confirmed this "energy to information to matter" energetic transaction.

I do not present the above research because of its relevance to psychic healing, or even its apparent relevance to homeopathy and its use of healing dosages of substances that seem to express their essence in the water in which they are placed. I present this research because of the significance of these findings in illustrating the subtle energetic properties in "brainless" things such as leaves and water. These natural elements have no way to be fooled. If even these simple substances can be "charged' with and then "remember" subtle info-energy, then certainly human cells can do the same.

FEATURES OF THE FIFTH FORCE
Based on the research on "L" energy that you have read about so far, here are twenty preliminary characteristics of "L" energy.[24] With each proposed characteristic, I have included comments from transplant patients and healers that illustrate and seem to substantiate these characteristics.

1. "L" energy travels faster than the speed of light. At more than 186,000 miles per second, it radiates out everywhere within and from you, accounting for the "nonlocal" effects of occurrences such as telepathy, remote healing, and the power of intercessory prayer.

"L" energy's effects are limitless. We may be able to sense it radiating from someone we care about even if that person is a thousand miles away. A heart transplant recipient described the limitless speed of "L" energy connection when he reported, "I know I was completely out, but before and after my surgery, I could feel her. I mean, waiting there, I could feel my wife's energy come to me from the waiting room. It even seemed to come to me when she was at home and I was still in the hospital."

2. "L" energy is nonlocal or free of the limits of space and time as we know them. It is everywhere at the same time, meaning that tuning in to this energy is not as much a matter of "sending or receiving" as "connecting."

As indicated in the PEAR research, "L" energy seems to surround us much like the air we breathe. Along with everyone else, we seem to be immersed in it. It is less something we "send" and "receive" than something we "are." The pervasiveness of "L" energy was identified by a heart transplant recipient who said, "When I say I can feel the energy of my donor I mean it's like I am her and she is me. The energy doesn't seem to be coming from anywhere, it just is. I'm not getting or receiving it. It just seems that I am it."

3. "L" energy passes unchanged through any known substance and nothing shields or deflects it.

There seems to be no known barrier to "L" energy. Unlike other forms energy, "L" energy does not travel in the sense that it goes from one place to another. Since it is everywhere all of the time, nothing provides a shield against its influence. The subtle power of "L" energy was described by a transplant nurse. She reported, "I could feel the energy of the ex-planted heart through its metal container. As soon as they brought it into the operating room, I could feel it."

4. "L" energy is often accompanied by an electromagnetic field and the other of the four known forms of energy (gravity and weak and strong nuclear energy) but is different from all of these forms of energy in its power, measurability, conduction, speed, and reception.

It may be that "L" energy is so pervasive that it is found within all of the known forms of energy or that all of these energies are various manifestations of "L" energy. This mixing of energy influences is indicated in the comments of a transplant surgeon. He said, "I know that the energy of some patients causes my machines to work better or smoother. Somehow, some patients just seem to connect with the machines better than others and some even seem to screw up the machines with their energy."

5. The heart is uniquely composed of "L" energy and communicates and conveys it in its own form but also "piggybacked" on the electromagnetic field (EMF) created by the heart. The heart's EMF is five thousand times more powerful than the electromagnetic field created by the brain and, in addition to its immense power, has subtle, nonlocal effects that travel within these forms of energy. Superconducting quantum interference devices, magnetocardiograms, and magnetoencephologorams that measure magnetic fields outside the body show that the heart generates over fifty thousand femtoteslas (a measure of EMF) compared to less than ten femtoteslas recorded from the brain.[25]

It is possible that the heart, because of its immense energy potential, is the primary center of "L" energy conduction. The role of the heart as "L" energy central was described by the wife of a heart transplant recipient. She said, "As soon as I went to his room after he got his new heart, I could feel myself drawn to him. I felt so much energy coming from his heart that it was like a magnet. It made my own heart flutter."

6. "L" energy fills all of space in the form of bundles of vibrating energy that can manifest themselves as either particles or waves that contain the information transmitted within, and to, all persons and things.[26]

We often think of matter as one thing and energy as something else, but, as stated before, the quantum fact is that energy and matter are manifestations of the same info-energetic stuff. Matter, energy, and information may combine to be communicated as "L" energy. What quantum physicists call the "wave-particle" duality principle associated with "L" energy was described by a heart transplant donor (a participant in a "domino transplant" in which she received a healthy heart and lung from a deceased donor and her still-healthy heart was given to another patient; this way, her new lungs, connected to their original heart, are less likely to fail.) She said, "I think there was a time there when I was dead. It did not feel like I was gone but actually like I was never more connected with everything and everyone. I think I went from body stuff to body energy for awhile and then back again. It's like heaven was not a place you go but a process you fall back into that makes you remember that you have always been connected with everything and everyone. Now, sometimes I feel like I can still sense my heart, wherever it is. I think it's because the energy that was my heart is still in me and connected with the stuff that is my heart in another body."

7. "L" energy is often conducted effectively by denser materials but seems to be refracted by more solid or metal objects and absorbed faster and better by organic material such as humans, animals, and plants.

While "L" energy is nonlocal and everywhere all the time, it still seems to sometimes also function by some of the rules that affect the other forms of energy. It seems to more easily permeate living tissue and cells and seems to radiate more strongly from things that are alive. This vital essence of "L" energy was described by a fellow member of the Hygeian Heart Club mentioned in the introduction. He said, "When they brought the plastic plants to my room, I could feel nothing from them. They didn't want any live plants because my immune system might react negatively or I might get an infection from them or the soil or something. When they finally let me get real live plants, I could feel the energy in my room. They really gave me an energy boost."

8. "L" energy is not only nonlocal (everywhere) but also negentropic (does not fall apart and disappear), formative (creative and not destructive), and organizing (integrative and not divisive) in its effects, the exact opposite of the effects from Newton's Second Law of Thermodynamics and the entropy it predicts—that everything is gradually falling apart.

"L" energy does not seem to diminish over time. While all of the other known forms of energy seem to follow most of the Newtonian laws of physics, including burning things up and burning itself out over time, "L" energy seems to be a creative, connecting energy. Instead of burning things out, it seems to hold them together. It seems to be one of the strongest integrating, connecting forces in the universe. One of my heart transplant recipients described the positive, constructive impact of "L" energy this way: "My new heart has not only saved my life, it has created a whole new life within me. I feel pulled together in one new being, stronger, and more powerful."

9. Changes in "L" energy precede physical or observable biophysical changes.

When we say we are "getting a sense" that something is about to happen, we may be tuning in to "L" energy and the coded message it carries. A heart transplant nurse reported her "L" energy sense of imminence. She said, "I can tell when things are going to go well and when they are going to go bad in surgery. Even while the surgeons are working and everything looks fine, there's a time just before things go wrong when, just like you can sense a storm coming, I feel the energy change."

10. "L" energy is the energy related to quantum occurrences, meaning that it operates by the principles of nonlocality, relativity, and freedom from Newtonian principles of linear time and space. When we are tuned in to our "L" energy, we can experience a sense of freedom from time and space constraints.

Our bodies may look like "stuff" but they're mostly space. Because our molecules are buzzing around with plenty of space surrounding them, and since that space may be filled with "L" energy, and since every one of our 75 trillion cells is also mostly energy, we can experience the sense of freedom from our body and the constraints of the outside world when we are tuning into our subtle energy. This personal experience of the nature of "L" energy was described by a heart transplant recipient who said, "My whole sense of time has changed with my new heart. Maybe it's because of my fear that time was running out, but now I am less concerned about what time it is. I am much more in the now than looking to the future."

11. Although it is not typically revealed to the see/touch world, "L" energy occasionally reveals itself in various observable ways, such as spirals, a cloud surrounding the body (aura), glowing, etheric webs, etc.

Scientific doubts about the existence of "L" energy may derive in part from the various unusual descriptions of it. Seeing angels, strange glows, lights, haloes, and auras may indeed be evidence of a manifestation of "L" energy, but such descriptions can seem so bizarre as to put off those who struggle to accept the hypothesis of a vital life force. An example of one such report was given by a heart donor's mother. She said, "When they said my son was dead and only being kept alive by a machine, I could still see his energy. It was like a soft cloud all around him and mostly around his chest. It came from him like a mist. When I saw him after they took his heart, I couldn't see the energy anymore. His body was there, but he wasn't. I think his essence or whatever you want to call it went with his heart and it is in someone else now."

12. While it is likely that "L" energy's nonlocality means that it is everywhere, there sometimes seem to be tracings of its presence that make it look as if it is flowing back and forth from one person and object to another.

One of the most influential aspects of "L" energy is its power to connect systems. Sometimes, particularly when two persons are in a loving bond, their "L" energy may even become visible, particularly to those who themselves are loving. This flowing connection of "L" energy was described by my own intensive care nurse, Betsy, following my bone marrow transplant. She said, "I could see a connection between you and your wife. I could actually see what looked like a white, glowing web connecting you and your wife. Even when you were sleeping, I would see the connection and I would see you settle down and your vitals balance when your wife was near you."

13. A principle related to nonlocality is called Bell's theorem. This is a quantum physics law that says that once connected, objects affect one another forever no matter where or when they are. Following the principle of Bell's theorem, "L" energy seems to be "sticky" in the sense that an invisible stream of energy will always connect any two objects that have been connected in any way in the past.

This "stickiness" or permanent connection nature of "L" energy is one of the most prominent features in the reports from heart transplant recipients. One example is from a twenty-six-year-old recipient, who said, "I will be connected with my donor forever. Not a day goes by when I do not feel him. It's like people I have met and really loved. No matter where they are, as soon as I think of them I can feel them in my heart like they are with me."

14. Of all the forms of energy, "L" energy is the one best and longest known and written about forms. It is described in ancient occult and spiritual documents as the intrinsic vital force of all creation.

While modern science emphasizes the importance of controlled studies, there is also a form of validity in the consistency and sincere endurance of reports from ancient cultures regarding the existence of a subtle life force. One of my Hawaiian teachers, a kahuna (or healer), said, "All healers know of the energy you are talking about. Our ancestors and their ancestors knew and taught of it. They called it "mana" coming from the "na'au," or from your gut, and the pu'uwai, your heart. It is as real as the ocean, as powerful as the wind, and as infinite as the night sky."

15. Two of the oldest established forms of medicine, Chinese and Japanese medicine, are based on subtle energy, which is called "Qui" or "Chi" in China and "Ki" in Japan.

Two of the longest tested and most relied upon forms of healing, Chinese and Japanese medicine, have always based their approach on the existence of a vital life force. One family practitioner described the importance of not ignoring the energetic focus of these two systems. He said, "Modern medicine is struggling with the fact that the form of energy the Chinese have known for centuries may in fact exist. Our mechanistic denial system is leaking. Every doctor and nurse has felt some version of it, we use techniques that seem to employ some form of it, and every patient I have talked with seems to know something about it. Anyone who has ever been sick knows how it feels when it is blocked or disrupted."

16. So pervasive is "L" energy that indigenous peoples and ancient religious systems have given it over one hundred different names and base their healing systems on it. In India and Tibet, this energy is called "prana." Polynesians call it "mana," and the Sufis called it "baraka." Jews in the cabalistic tradition call it "yesod," the Iroquois call it "orendam," the Ituraea pygmies call it "megbe," and Christians call it the "Holy Spirit."

Not only Chinese and Japanese medicines but almost all forms of medicine other than modern biomedicine have recognized and named a subtle "L" energy they say is crucial to health and healing. Another Hawaiian kahuna described the universality of "L" energy: "Not only our ancestors but all ancestors everywhere knew well the powers of mana. They all gave it a name. Why would so many wise people so many places have a name for something that did not exist?.[27]

17. Many modern psychologists have dealt with and named "L" energy. They have used names such as "the fifth force" and "X" energy. Psychologist Wilhelm Riech called it "organum," Sigmund Freud called it "libido," Franz Anton Mesner (like biologist Luigi Galvani) called it "animal magnetism." Karl von Reichenbach called it "odic forcem." Psychologists in Russia used to call it "biplasma."

In dealing with emotional development and distress, almost every form of psychotherapy has offered its own version of "L" energy that serves as a motivating life force. One hypnotherapist described her version of "L" energy, saying, "I just call it "H" energy. There are many explanations for hypnotism. Many say it is a form of consciousness dissociation or, more recently, what they call neodissociation, or a kind of splitting of consciousness with other aspects still functioning. I think it involves tuning in to another form of energy we share together."

18. The heart may convey "L" energy along with its electrical activity. While the normal frequency range of the electrical activity in the brain is between 0 and 100 cycles per second (CPS), most of the brain's electrical activity hovers between 0 and 30 CPS. The heart's normal frequency is 250 CPS. Since "L" energy can travel within other forms of energy, the heart may be the most powerful sender and receiver of that energy.

Most of our current measures of the functioning of the heart are primarily electrical in nature. Since "L" energy may be an as yet immeasurable component of that cardio-electrical energy, the heart again emerges as a candidate to be the primary "L" energy mechanism in the body. A nurse technician who spent her days administering electrocardiograms reported her sense of this "L" energy amidst the electrical impulses she was measuring. She said, "I can take an ECG of one patient and get completely different vibes from him than another patient even though their electrocardiographs look exactly the same. I wouldn't tell the cardiologist, but I do think there is another tracing hidden within the ECG that our eyes can't see."

19. One of the oldest sources of healing lessons, yoga literature, refers to centers of "L" energy as "chakras," from the Sanskrit word for wheel, describing spinning vortices of energy.[28]

More physical therapists and other health-care workers who deal primarily with rehabilitation are speaking about "blocked levels of energy" and "subtle energy disruptions." One physical therapist, who used yoga in her own practice described her view of "L" energy, saying, "There is no surprise for me in this talk of 'L' energy. I think the whole world is suffering from some kind of subtle energy dysfunction. The fourth chakra is the heart chakra, and it is key to our energetic connection with all of the other chakras, the earth, and with everything and everyone." (The seven chakras, or energy centers, of the body are explained in detail in chapter 11.)

20. While many persons in the bioscience community do not recognize "L" energy, many report its influence and attempt to incorporate its power in their healing.

One example of a respected medical professional who has studied "L" energy is Dr. Shafica Karagulla, a neurologist and psychiatrist. She refers to HSP or "higher sense perception" as a sensitivity to "L" energy. Dr. Karagulla interviewed dozens of physicians who reported sensing this energy and concludes, "When many reliable individuals independently report the same kind of phenomenon, it is time science took cognizance of it."[29]

COMING UNDER THE SPELL

The French magus Eliphas Levi described "L" or subtle life energy as the "imagination of nature . . . the great Arcanum of Magic." He was referring to the mystical, enchanted, pervasive, but elusive nature of "L" energy. Emily Dickinson wrote, "Life is a spell so exquisite that everything conspires to break it." In effect, the busy brain keeps breaking the enchanted spell cast by our heart and the memories it sends. Subtle "L" energy is always within us, however, and we can become more aware of it not by trying harder but by slowing and quieting down to, as fifteenth-century philosopher Marsilio Ficino suggested, turn toward the mystery of our own nature the way a sunflower turns toward the sun.[30]

Nurse and energy healer Julie Motz has assisted in many transplant surgeries at Columbia-Presbyterian Medical Center. She describes her experiences with the influences of "L" energy. She writes, "The idea that information is a form of energy, and that the heart uses energy to communicate with and receive communication from the rest of the body as well as communicating and receiving communication from outside the body, correlates with experiences I have had during heart transplant surgery."[31] She speculates that each form of energy has its own unique emotional equivalent, suggesting that gravity can make us feel heavy with anger and lighter when the anger leaves, electromagnetic energy can make us feel electrified with fear, strong nuclear energy radiates pain through our body, and weak nuclear energy may be experienced as feelings of love.

Energy cardiology and cardio-energetics provide a starting point for scientists such as those above to meet with healers, kahuna, shamans, heart transplant patients, and all of those who seek to be re-enchanted by the energy of their heart and lessons of their cellular memories. As long as the division remains between bioscience and energy medicines, the brain will continue to break the enchanted spell of our heart.

The heart is not easily dissuaded from its mission of balancing the brain and body interaction. The next chapter describes this most powerful, mysterious, muscular pump that seems to pump not only the biochemical nutrients that keep us alive but perhaps the spiritual energy that represents our soul.

The Changing Portrait
of the Heart

"The heart of creatures is the foundation of life, the Prince of all, the Sun of their microcosm, on which all vegetation does depend, from whence all vigor and strength does flow."

— WILLIAM HARVEY, M.D., 1628

LESSONS FROM ONE HUNDRED MONKEYS

In the late 1970s on the outer islands of Japan, the Japanese government maintained small colonies of monkeys in order to study their habits. A young female monkey named Ima discovered how to clean dirt from sweet potatoes by dunking and washing them in a stream. She taught this skill one at a time to several other monkeys and, suddenly, after one hundred monkeys had learned Ima's potato-washing technique, every monkey in the entire colony was observed as being able to use her skill without any direct interaction with her or any of her students. Biologist Lyall Watson described this spontaneous "monkey oneness" as the "hundredth monkey phenomenon" and reported that Ima's skill spread quickly to other islands and to the mainland even though the potato-washing monkeys had never been sent there. He wrote that Ima's skill "seems to have jumped natural barriers [time and space]."[1]

Heart cells also seem to have the ability to jump the same barriers transcended by Ima's skill. Place one throbbing heart cell in a laboratory dish next to another heart cell and they will beat in their solitary rhythms. Place several heart cells together in a dish without any physical contact between one another and with no synapse connecting them and they suddenly fall into a rhythmic unison, a rhythm that is distinct from the rhythm of each individual cell. This is another manifestation of the heart's subtle energetic code.

The brain resonates with bioelectrical energy, the circulatory system hums with the pressure of surging blood, and the heart sits in the center of the body pumping not only the blood needed to nurture the body but the biochemical messages from the brain that make us conscious beings. It may be that, because of the immense info-energy that is circulated by the heart, the soul is also nurtured by the information continued in the heart's code.

THE POWER OF THE THIRD THING

Plato wrote, "Two things alone cannot be satisfactorily united without a third; for there must be some bond between them drawing them together."[2] The heart may serve as a powerful third thing, the info-energetic mysterious "and" in the "brain and body" relationship. To Aristotle, the heart was the seat of the soul. While Hippocrates and his contemporary Plato taught that the brain was the center of our human essence, all three of these great thinkers agreed that life depends on some innate quality or subtle energy situated in the heart, something they called "animal heat." Cardio-energetics suggests that the heart joins with the brain and the body to form the physical manifestation of the soul and that this remarkable organ is much more than is described in physician William Harvey's four-hundred-year-old declaration that "the blood in the animal body moves around in a circle . . . and the action or function of the heart is to accomplish this pumping."

Physically, the heart is an amazingly powerful and tireless muscle, called the myocardium, located in the center of the chest. It is actually two pumps situated side by side and divided by a wall called the septum. In a cardiovascular version of yin and yang, each side has its own unique kind of energy and job to do. Each has an upper collecting chamber (atrium) and a lower ejecting chamber (ventricle). The left-side pump is the most powerful, sending blood through thousands of miles of vessels under sufficient pressure to shoot water almost six feet into the air. The right-side pump propels blood primarily to and from the lungs under just enough pressure to shoot water about a foot into the air. Life begins when this systolic/diastolic, systemic/pulmonary rhythm begins, and with this alternating stress and strain of circulatory pressure come the immense amounts of info-energy that constitute the heart's code.

While all of the body's cells are made up of an enveloping membrane called the cell wall, a nucleus that contains the cell's DNA (or genetic code) that tells it what to do, and cytoplasm containing thousands of structures that do the work that makes life possible, heart cells do something other cells in the body can't do: They pulsate. Every one of the billions of heart cells throbs along with other heart cells, constantly communicating between one another by what seems to be a process related to "L" energy. Brain cells called neurons communicate via biochemical impulses received through dendrites as sent by axons. They exchange electrochemical energy across the synapse, a sparkplug-like gap that exists between brain cells. Heart cells also communicate biochemically, but unlike brain or any other body cells, they also seem able to exchange life information by using a subtle and as yet immeasurable vital force.

THE LOGIC OF THE LIFE SYSTEM

Author Joseph Pearce writes, "Two closely bonded people often share information across time-space, to which we attach occultic labels of various sorts, while all the time it is only our true biology, the logic of our life system, the language of the heart."[3] How the heart cells communicate with one another may offer clues as to one way we and all systems also communicate and connect with one another.

Our billions of heart cells may be able to combine to form a quantum energy generator that operates not only by mechanical pumping rules but by the laws of the quantum world such as nonlocality, thus instantaneously organizing the info-energetic connection that constitutes all systems in the universe. The heart may be capable of resonating a nonlocal "field" of intelligence throughout every one of the trillions of cells in our body, using them as info-energetic storage pods and temporary holding areas for the kind of information that makes us who and how we are. To assume that the "L" energy passing through our cells is not remembered in some form by these cells is to assume that, unlike any other living system, cells have a special info-energetic amnesia.

PUMPING ENERGY

The brain may contain more cellular connections than there are stars in the Milky Way, but it is nowhere near as energetic as the heart. By bioscience's own measurements, the heart is five thousand times more electromagnetically powerful than the brain.[4] By the twenty-fifth day of life, when a woman may not even know she is pregnant, the embryonic heart has already formed and started to beat. While we may debate the meaning, complexity, and spiritual significance of this early form of life, there can be no debate as to when the heart announces its presence so we can hear and feel the beginnings of the heart's code. Some form of subtle, nonlocal energy we cannot yet measure causes a tiny clump of cells to begin to beat together in the rhythm of life that will resonate within us until our death. In the first few days after the heart begins to beat, it is already pumping blood manufactured in the liver throughout the fetus, and along with this measurable substance comes an immense amount of as yet immeasurable life information.[5]

To say that the heart's energy is subtle is not to say that its physical manifestations are not powerful. Unlike any other muscle in the body and unless it is afflicted with disease, the heart muscle does not seem to weaken with age. The heart's physical strength surpasses all known mechanical pumps the brain has been able to construct. It is never still and, even if a patient is declared "brain dead," the heart can continue to beat on its own. Through a process no scientists can yet fully explain, a heart removed from its body still remembers how to beat. I have seen a dying heart quivering for several minutes in its valiant, lonely struggle to stay alive after it has been disconnected from its brain.

The heart beats approximately one hundred thousand times a day and forty million times a year. For more than seventy years, it supplies the pumping capacity for nearly three billion cardiac pulsations and propels more than two gallons of blood per minute through the body. The heart transports about one hundred gallons of blood per hour though a vascular system that, if extended, could be wrapped around the earth two and one half times, and each fiber of that system is crammed full of the info-energy traveling through it, helping that "L" energy to broadcast energy everywhere like a huge vascular antenna.[6] One heart transplant recipient summed up the info-energetic power of the heart when she said, "I never thought much about it before, but there is an immense amount of news about life being broadcast twenty-four hours a day from my internal CNN—my cardiac news network."[7]

SAFE IN SOUND

If you sit very still, listen very carefully, and focus on the center of your body, you may be able to feel and hear a cellular memory. You may be able to sense the most familiar and reassuring sound in the world in the form of the "lub dub, lub dub" beating from your chest as an echo of your mother's heart still resounding within you, a permanent cellular memory of what author Diane Ackerman describes as "the womb . . . an envelope of rhythmic warmth, and the mother's heartbeat a steady clarion of safety."[8] This ultimate cellular imprint is the acoustical portrait of our mother as played by our heart's comforting cadence until the day we die. When you pay attention to the code your heart is beating out, you are tapping in to an "L" energy legacy left within your cells not only by your mother but by all of your ancestors' souls.

Research shows that a recorded heartbeat played in a nursery for newborns reduces their crying by almost 55 percent. Puppy and kitten owners often place a ticking clock next to their new pet to comfort it through the night. Seeking a restful sleep, insomniacs buy "sound machines" that mimic a beating heart. We often say that the world is so hectic that we cannot hear ourselves think, but the real problem is that our brain is thinking so hard we can't hear our heart think, so we are unable to tune in to our cellular memories of the natural healthy rhythm of life.

HOW THE HEART STARTS

No one knows for sure how a clump of fetal heart cells a few weeks old "decide" to suddenly and spontaneously begin to beat together. It is suspected that the mother's heart energy conveyed in primal sound waves contains the information that is the code that jump-starts our life. Once the heart starts, it beats until we die or require an approximation of our heart's natural code in the form of an electronic jolt to bring our heart back to life. When we silence our brain, quiet our body, and become still enough to feel the beat of our heart, we may be able to remember more profoundly the thrill of being alive.

While our brain's urgent defensiveness often causes us to behave as what poet William Blake refers to as "armed crustaceans eternally on the alert," the gentle, steady beating of our heart soothes us, makes us feel loving and loved, and assures us and those who love us that our soul is still here as expressed in the spiritual energy resonating through our heart. The silenced heart is our greatest dread for ourselves and those we love, and regardless of legalistic definitions, death is ultimately the loss of the rhythm of the heart. Whenever I become too busy, too impatient, and too cynical in my daily living, I stop and remember to listen and feel for my heart. I attend to it before it has to demand my attention by gripping me by my chest. During business meetings, on airplanes, or standing in a long, slow line, I place my index finger and thumb together on my left hand and feel the energetic thumping of my heart's code that reminds me to lead life and not be led by it.

SENSUOUS RHYTHMS

We are constantly provided with memories of our heart's code by those who seem intensely cardio-sensitive. Some of our greatest poems are written in an iambic pentameter that resembles the steady, slow beat of a restful, secure heart. Our most soothing music usually beats from about 70 to 80 tones per minute, replicating the natural rhythm of a healthy heart. The quiet ticking of an old grandfather clock settles us, the swaying movements of a dancer are bodily expressions of life's natural rhythm, vibrations felt from the heavy alternating gate of a huge animal connect us with the primal resonating nature of life, and the rocking movements of two lovers embracing can make our own heart jump with joyful recognition of the passion of living. More recently, it is possible that those who receive a new heart may become cardio-sensitive and also be able to teach us about the heart's code.

Cardio-sensitive Hawaiian singer and ukulele virtuoso Moe Keale, expressing the Polynesian concepts of "na'au" (gut feelings) and the sensitivity of the pu'uwai (heart) described earlier, says, "Music is not something you just hear with your ears. It's something you hear with your pu'uwai— heart."[9] An American Indian shaman told psychologist Carl Jung that white men, with their wrinkled faces and constant anger, were so cruel and murderous because they thought with their heads. Whole, healthy people, he said, "think in their hearts."[10] There are countless other examples of cardio-sensitive and "L" energy-aware wise sages and healers throughout the ages claiming that the true seat of the soul is in the heart, and now modern science is beginning to suggest that they may have had it spiritually right all along.

THE CONSCIOUS PUMP

To construct a complete biography of the heart, it is necessary to see how the heart actually functions as a conscious entity. Just as recent research on the brain changed our perceptions of how we think about life, what we are now beginning to learn about the heart will forever alter how we feel about living together and, in the process, drastically change science, medicine, and spirituality in the next century.

Since physician Lester Sontag first reported in the late 1940s that the mother's heartbeat affects the infant's heartbeat in utero, concepts regarding the nature of the heart have been changing radically to keep up with new insights about the heart as the primary organizer and communicator of the energy of our life.[11] Summarizing the current research on the possibility of a sentient heart, author Joseph Chilton Pearce writes, "Our heart plays a major if fragile role in our overall consciousness."[12] The fragility to which he refers may be the more subtle nature of "L" energy and the fact that the heart tends to be much less brash than the brain in the manner in which it influences our life.

The central thesis of cardio-energetics, that the heart and not the brain is where our most basic thoughts, feelings, fears, and dreams are gently but profoundly mediated, is becoming increasingly supported by the Platonic science that initially denied this Aristotelian possibility. Consider some of the recent findings from research in the new field of neurocardiology, the study of the heart as a neurological, endocrine, and immune organ.

- Neurotransmitters found in the brain have also been identified in the heart, establishing a direct neurochemical and electrochemical communicational link between the heart and the brain beyond the purely neurological connections known to exist between the brain and the heart.
- The heart, through hormones, neurotransmitters, and what scientists call subtle quantum energies and I call "L" info-energy, exerts at least as much control over the brain as the brain exerts over the heart.[13]
- Drs. John and Beatrice Lacey of the National Institute of Mental Health report that there is direct evidence that the heart neurohormonally calls for a constant environmental update from the brain in order to organize the energy of the body.[14]
- When the muscular walls of the heart's atria (the upper chambers of the heart) contract, the heart produces a hormone that profoundly affects

every major organ of the body including the brain. Called Atrial Naturetic Factor (ANF), sometimes called peptide, this neurohormone communicates not only with the brain but directly with the immune system, the hypothalamus (which helps mediate our emotional state), and the pineal gland (which regulates the production of melatonin that is related to our sleep/wake cycle, aging processes, and general energy level).[15] The ANF from the heart also influences the thalamus and pituitary gland in the limbic or emotional part of our brain, an important center of our memory, learning, and emotions.[16]

As research from neurocardiology continues, it is becoming clearer that the central role of the heart in our consciousness is much more than metaphor and that, as happened with the brain, continuing research will reveal complexities of a conscious heart that our brain cannot yet imagine.

BEYOND THE SOGGY COMPUTER

A little more than a decade ago, the brain was seen as a powerful neuro-electronic computer and described in terms of analogies to advanced communications systems. As the complexities of the brain were explored, it became clear that it was much more than the body's computer and electronic relay center. It began to be seen as a "soggy" computer and more a neurochemical gland than a phone switching station. As scientists free themselves from their materialistic view of the brain and begin to look more at its info-energetic nature, the brain is beginning to look more like an energetic manifestation and holographic info-energetic system, parts of which can be found throughout the body and within every cell. Now that scientists are beginning to also look at the heart in info-energetic terms, much the same sequence of new understandings of the complexities of the brain will take place for the heart.

What makes the heart unique in its role in our body is its tone and its rhythmicity. Unlike any other organ including the brain, we can hear, feel, and constantly sense the workings of our heart. It constantly and powerfully oscillates with the information we need to live and love. With every beat, we can literally feel the heart working as it communicates its info-energy to every cell in our body and other bodies. Like the brain, the heart influences the entire body, but unlike the brain, it constantly provides a resonating reminder that we are sending and receiving the information of our soul.

NATURE'S HEART

Our heart seems to share its code with all systems in the universe. Poets and scientists know that we pulsate with energy and that this rhythm and pulsation are intrinsic to all life. Scientists can observe bacterial "biorhythms" as they look at their tiny cilia pulsating under their microscopes. There are alternating cycles of photosynthesis and responses in plants, and the soil constantly changes and shifts its composition to its own natural rhythm. If you learn to tap into the heart's code, you will be tapping in to the code that is the life force of all systems. As a result, you will be able to sense the steady heartbeat of the forests, flowers, and rocks.

Our body operates in a circadian rhythm, and our body biochemistry has its own cyclical rhythmicity.[17] Since all life is both biorhythmic and info-energetically rhythmic, and scientists know that rhythmic energy contains information, every oscillation of our heart represents the resonance of nature's code within us. Author Ernest Bennett describes this phenomenon as continuing contests of opposites including birth and death, give and take, night and day, summer and winter, work and play, love and hate. Each of these contests of opposites are represented in the systolic/diastolic contractions of the heart.

A PSYCHOLOGY OF THE HEART

Clinical interest in the interactions between psychology and the heart has increased over the last several years. While research and clinical work in the psychosocial aspects of heart disease has gone on for decades, cardiac psychology as a distinct field was first proposed in 1996 by cardiologist Dr. Robert Allan and health psychologist Dr. Stephen Scheidt. It is the branch of health psychology that identifies psychological and social risk factors for the development of cardiovascular disease, the psychological repercussions of cardiac illness, and lifestyle changes that can prevent or minimize serious medical and psychological complications stemming from heart disease.[18]

Cardiac psychology does not yet deal with the heart itself as a thinking, feeling organ. Instead, it focuses on the psychosocial effects on the health of the heart. Historically, however, the recognition of a profound spiritual or energetic interaction between the psyche and soma, which is part of what modern cardiac psychology studies, can be traced back to the ancient Far East. Emperor Juagn Ti (267–297 B.C.) observed, "When the minds of the people are closed and wisdom is locked out they remain tied to disease."[19] This statement is one of the first ancient recognitions of the lethal covenant between the selfish brain and its body that can, without the intervention of the kind of spiritual wisdom the heart's code may be able to bring to our daily life, enslave the body and drive it beyond its limits.

The modern version of cardiac psychology has roots all the way back to 1628 when the discoverer of the circulatory system, William Harvey, wrote that "a mental disturbance provoking pain, excessive joy, hope or anxiety extends to the heart, where it affects temper."[20] This point of view is reflected in my cardio-energetics hypothesis that our heart, not just our brain, can react directly to the stress of life.

In 1897, the father of modern internal medicine, Sir William Osler, wrote about atherosclerosis, or hardening and clogging of the arteries, as "the Nemesis through which nature exacts retributional justice for the transgressions of her laws."[21] Osler described the typical atherosclerotic patient as "a keen and ambitious man, the indicator of whose engine is always at 'full speed ahead'." Osler was describing the undisciplined brain governing a "heartless" body and was years ahead in his anticipation of the "type A" busy-body being driven through life by a brain unresponsive to the subtle energy code of the heart.[22]

In the twentieth century, research into the type A behavior patterns forecasted by Dr. Osler was published. The heart disease risk factors of a rushed and hostile life were identified by two San Francisco cardiologists, Drs. M. Friedman and R. H. Rosenman. Since their pioneering work in 1959, there has been a proliferation of research related to the social psychology of the heart, which culminated in the establishment of the field of cardiac psychology.[23] Thanks to this work, there is now considerable evidence that looking to the psychology of the heart not only helps improve the quality and length of life for cardiac patients but may provide a new psychology of daily living for all of us.[24]

Not until the proposal of a field of energy cardiology and the concept of the heart as conscious organ has the full spectrum of the role of the heart in our life been realized.[25] Heart disease prevention programs focusing on psychological components have been shown to be effective in reducing the risk of heart attack and even reversing preexisting heart disease.[26] Cardio-energetics puts energy cardiology and cardiac psychology together to form a new paradigm of well-being that extends lifestyle change to include spiritual balance and soul awareness.

If the heart thinks, feels, and communicates, and if we can tap into its code and recover its wisdom and the memories it helps store within our cells, we have the possibility of an entirely new way to view health and healing. For the first time since modern biomedicine's brain fixation, we have an additional way to understand life's mysteries beyond the range of Western science's explanatory system, which is limited to the five basic senses used exclusively by the brain.

Energy cardiology and cardio-energetics help explain the one mystery modern medicine has never been able to solve. They provide a theory of how trillions of highly specialized cells can function as an organized, responsive, interactive, remembering, loving whole. They suggest that the subtle energy of the heart and the cellular memories this energy creates are the missing pieces of the most sacred puzzle—what is life and what is it for?

A CARDIO-ENERGETIC PORTRAIT OF THE HEART

Based on the research summarized above, here is a cardio-energetic portrait of the heart.

1. The heart is our most powerful organ. There is no subtleness about the immense physical power of the heart. The brain's power pales by comparison. The heart is the largest generator of electromagnetic energy in our body and produces, sends, and receives a broad spectrum of other types and frequencies of energy occurring over time.[27]

2. The heart responds directly to the environment. It can be demonstrated that the heart reacts to electromagnetic energy outside the body. It contracts when an electromagnet is placed near it.[28] The heart also reacts neurohormonally to the outside world not only in response to the brain but sometimes without the brain's awareness.

3. The heart is a conductor of the energy of the body's cells. The energy from the heart, while strong, does not have to be strong to influence cellular functioning. The subtle form of energy emitted, conducted, and received by the heart is sufficient to cause significant changes in the cells of the body that may be described as info-energetic cellular memories.[29]

4. The heart is a dynamic system. The heart, like all living systems, is an open, fluctuating, interacting system. As quantum physics teaches about all systems, it expresses itself as energy, matter, and information, and it is as much wave of energy as particle of matter.[30]

5. *The heart is the body's primary organizing force.* The heart holds us together. It is the maker of the gestalt that we call "me" and the catalyst for Mind that is our experience of "us." It uses its info-energy to connect our brain and body and works in coordination with the brain but is not directed by it. Unless we remain numb to the code of the heart, neglect it, and leave the lethal covenant between a selfish, survivalist brain and hyper-responsive body unchallenged, the heart can serve its natural role as the major organizer, integrator, and balancer of the body's vital energy and can play a unique and major role in the coordinating of our cells' memories of what it means to be healthy.[31]

6. *The heart resonates with information-containing energy.* Energy, matter, and information are one and the same. Wherever any one of these three characteristics of nature is present, the other two are also "there" in some form whether we see them or not. Whenever we send or receive energy, we also are communicating information. When the heart beats out its energy, it sends information and affects the "matter" within us and outside of us. Energy going into matter is the information that becomes memory. No matter how subtle and as yet unmeasurable, memory exists within matter in the form of energy, and the heart may be able to communicate that memory.[32]

7. *The heart is the body system's core.* Because of the heart's central location in our body and the extensive connection it has to all of the cells within our body, its energy transmission becomes highly influential for our body and all of the bodies around us. The heart is constantly pumping energy and information to, from, and within every cell in our body.[33]

8. *The heart "speaks" and sends information.* We can learn to decipher the heart's code by silencing the brain, quieting ourselves, focusing on our heart, and sensing what it has to say and what memories it may bring forth from the cells that store it. The heart has its own form of wisdom, different from that of the rational brain but every bit as important to our living, loving, working, and healing.[34]

9. *All hearts exchange information with other hearts and brains.* Cardiac energy patterns have dynamic interactive effects. When one heart sends energy to another, that energy becomes a part of the receiving heart's memory. When the receiving heart becomes a sending heart, the energy it sends

is no longer just its own. It blends its energy with the memory of the vibrations of the energy it has received. This resonating process continues infinitely, meaning that with every beat of our heart, we continue to create the info-energetic vibrations that become our collective soul.[35]

10. Transplanted hearts come with their own info-energetic cellular memories. Since the first animal heart transplants in 1959, through the first human heart transplants that began in 1967, to 1984 when heart transplantation began to offer hope for a long and healthy life for those whose own hearts failed, a new respect for the unique nature and power of the heart has been emerging. The subtle effects on personality and consciousness reported by certain heart transplant recipients are beginning to provide new clues about the nature of the heart's code.[36]

The transplant of new hearts to save the life of a different body provides experiments in energy cardiology and cardio-energetics that could never be performed otherwise. Once we are aware of the heart's centrality in our consciousness, we can examine the reports from those who have most intimately and profoundly experienced the power of the heart's code to learn more about the wisdom of the heart. From those who have literally had a change of heart, we can discover lessons about tapping into our own heart's code and insights into making and recovering our own cellular memories so we may have a change of heart about how we live our own life.

If it is possible that there is vital "L" energy and that the heart is its primary center, then cells may be able to make memories out of the info-energy circulated by the heart. Evidence of this possibility exists in the form of the remarkable accounts from heart transplant recipients about receiving cellular memories from their donor. Before I discuss the mechanisms that may be involved in cellular memories, the next chapter presents some of the stories from those persons I call the first "astronauts of the soul," those willing to allow the challenge of their new heart to take them to the far reaches of the human spirit.

Receiving the Most Precious Gift

"There is no such thing as a miracle which violates natural law. There are only occurrences which violate our limited knowledge of natural law."

— *ST. AUGUSTINE*

GLENDA'S STORY

"Oh my God, David, no!," cried Glenda when she saw the bright lights headed straight for their car. As the squeal of the tires burning to grip the road became one with her own shrill shriek of helpless terror, she knew that she had lost her husband forever. Moments before the car came crashing through their windshield, the couple had argued over something silly and had been sitting in resentful silence. They had had these little emotional scuffles before, but unlike in the past when they had had skirmishes, this time there would be no opportunity to apologize and reconfirm their love.

Years later, Glenda sat with me in the dimly lit hospital chapel. At her request, I had arranged a meeting between her and the young man whose life had been saved by the gift of her husband's heart. The heart recipient and his mother were almost a half hour late for the meeting, and I was ready to ask Glenda to leave. The issue of recipients meeting donor families is a very sensitive one, and I understood why the man might have changed his mind.

As I stood and took Glenda's hand, she said quietly, "Oh no, we have to wait. He's here in the hospital. I felt him come about thirty minutes ago. I felt my husband's presence. Please wait with me."

Glenda is a practicing family physician. She is well-versed in bioscience and, as I do, admires the rigor and healthy skepticism of modern science. Now, however, the power of something that transcends what science calls common sense was tugging at her heart. "David's heart is here," she added. "I can't believe I'm saying that to you, but I feel it. His recipient is here in this hospital." At that moment, the door opened and the young man and his mother walked hurriedly down the center aisle of the chapel. "Sorry we're late," said the young man with a heavy Spanish accent. "We got here a half hour ago but we couldn't find the chapel."

After introductions and awkward attempts at humor about a "heart-to-heart" meeting between the young wife and her husband's heart, the usually shy Glenda blurted out, "This embarrasses me as much as it must embarrass you, but can I put my hand on your chest and feel his . . . I mean your heart?"

The young man looked at me and then his mother, put his hand to his chest, and finally nodded his head. As Glenda reached forward, he unbuttoned his shirt, took her hand, and gently placed it against his naked chest. What happened next transcends our current view of the brain, body, heart, and mind, but it has happened in various forms in the lives of those people and their family members who have experienced the awesome force of a life system of one person's being transplanted into another.

Glenda's hand began to tremble and tears rolled down her cheek. She closed her eyes and whispered, "I love you David. Everything is copacetic." She removed her hand, hugged the young man to her chest, and all of us wiped tears from our eyes. Glenda and the young man sat down and, silhouetted against the background of the stained-glass window of the chapel, held hands in silence.

Speaking in her heavy Spanish accent, the young man's mother told me, "My son uses that word 'copacetic' all the time now. He never used it before he got his new heart, but after his surgery, it was the first thing he said to me when he could talk. I didn't know what it means. He said everything was copacetic. It is not a word I know in Spanish." Glenda overheard us, her eyes widened, she turned toward us and said, "That word was our signal that everything was OK. Every time we argued and made up, we would both say that everything was copacetic."

Our discussion about a magic word that seemed to reveal a code of the heart within him stimulated the young man to share story after story of changes he experienced following his transplant. Described by his mother as a former vegetarian and very health-conscious, he said he now craves meat and fatty foods. A former lover of heavy metal music, he said he now loves fifties rock-and-roll. He reported recurrent dreams of bright lights coming straight for him. Glenda responded almost matter-of-factly that her husband loved meat, was a junk food addict, had played in a Motown/ rock-and-roll band while in medical school, and that she too dreams of the lights of that fateful night.

GIVING THE GIFT OF LIFE

Dr. Sherwin B. Nuland, in his compassionate and fascinating book *The Wisdom of the Body,* traces transplantation from the Iliad to the modern operating room. He describes the primitive work of seventeenth-century Hindu surgeons making new noses from their patients' own skin, the strange doings of eighteenth-century Scottish surgeon John Hunter's trans- plantation of a human tooth into the comb of a rooster and testicles from one chicken into another, and the remarkable lifesaving work of Drs. Nor- man Shumnway and Richard Lower's first description of how to hook one person's heart into another person's body.[1] Surgeons now have the process of heart transplantation down to an organizational masterpiece. Because of drugs such as cyclosporine, azathioprine, and antilymphocytic globulin (a new heart drug used in cases of severe rejection by the immune system) they are only limited in the hearts they can transplant primarily by their availability and size (the donor heart must be the right size for the recipi- ent).

Availability of transplantable organs is one of the crises of our time. While more than two thousand heart transplants are done in the United States each year, some persons still consider the entire process of organ transplantation to be experimental. In fact, the techniques involved are now highly refined and have greatly increased patient survival and chances for a longer and better quality of life. Eighty percent of heart transplant recipients are alive and well a year after their operations and 70 percent are in good shape five years after surgery. Despite these facts, about fifty thou- sand people a year whose life could be saved by the gift of new heart will never get one. Many thousands of people die waiting for a new heart or other lifesaving transplant, yet more than twenty thousand potential do- nors are allowed to die each year with their unneeded organs unused—the ultimate gift that was never given. It is my sincere wish that this book's discussion of the remarkable possibilities of the "L" energy of the heart will encourage you to consider sharing that energy through organ donation. Almost all of us are potential donors of some type of life-giving tissue and, recognizing that fact, many European countries now have a "presumed consent" policy. Such a policy allows doctors to assume, unless the family objects, that a legally dead accident victim has consented to donation.

WHERE THERE'S FIRE, THERE'S SMOKE

What no transplant surgeon can yet explain completely is how a new heart has the subtle energy to start its own spontaneous beat. While feedback from the body influences heart rhythm, the heart provides its own rhythm and, once placed in a new body, the surgical team usually waits and watches as it quivers and shakes until it finds its own pace with no help at all from the new brain it will now help keep alive. Learning to reduce the body's rejection to new tissue was one major barrier to transplantation that was largely overcome. The other obstacle turned out not to be a problem at all, a manifestation of biomedicine's brain bias. It had been assumed that the brain, which medicine sees as ultimately in charge of everything, made the heart beat and that the heart's rhythm was exclusively maintained by the outside influences of nerves traced back to the brain. In fact, the heart has its own "nervous system" and does not need the brain to tell it what to do.

When I asked a transplant surgeon about the spontaneous starting of a heart after its implantation, he responded, "I know you want me to say it's some mysterious kind of energy, but it's not. It's a self-generated stimulus arising in the SA node. That's all it is." The SA node, or sinoatrial node, is the heart's internal pacemaker. It is a tiny patch of tissue in the back wall near the right top of the heart's upper collecting chamber (called the atrium). It serves as the center of what cardiologists call the "cardiac conduction system," a complex set of bundles of fibers relaying info-energy within and from the heart. It is one of the most powerful, highly evolved info-energetic systems in the world, and when I asked the surgeon what constituted the "self" that he said "generates" the stimulus, he laughed and answered, "Look. It's just a form of bioelectrical discharge." "Some form of energy, then?" I asked. "Well, of course there's energy involved, but it's just a neurochemical event." This surgeon mistakes the intense "fire" of the neurochemistry of transplant for the more subtle "smoke" of the subtle energy that accompanies it. He forgets the fundamental principle of cardio-energetics: Wherever there's energy, there's information.

THE ENERGY OF A NEW HEART

The most recent published report from a bioscientist that seems to confirm some of my findings regarding the heart's code comes from Dr. Sherwin Nuland, whose book I referred to above. Dr. Nuland followed a patient through the entire heart transplant procedure. The words of the patient he followed reflect that a new heart has an impact beyond that of physical organ replacement. For example, there is the often angry resistance, strong denial, and sardonic humor that masks acknowledgment of the energetic impact of the new organ. When Dr. Nuland asked the patient what it felt like to live with another person's heart in his chest, he answered, "When I catch myself thinking about it, I try to forget about it. You know—I think, What is it? A female? A Male? Black? Orange? White?"

The sudden, spontaneous clicking-in of a subtle connection with "L" energy, as noted in the PEAR studies mentioned earlier in this book, and through the process of "just being" rather than "doing," is reflected in the patient's response to Dr. Nuland's question as to what he wanted his heart to be. He answered, "I even get upset talking to you about it. When I talk about it, I get paranoid. . . . I can be sitting here feeling fine and all of a sudden something clicks and I get nervous and everything starts going. Something in my body changes, as if somebody pushed a button. I talked to another transplant patient—he's in his fifth year—and he says it still happens to him."[2]

Dr. Nuland's patient's wife confirms the "hypnotic" or "hidden observer" quality of the energetic connection that "just happens" to occur between recipient and the new heart. Dr. Nuland writes that the wife said "her husband occasionally seems to go into a trance, sometimes for hours at a time. He seems to be thinking about nothing, she said, but his mind is really trying to escape those thoughts about whose heart he is carrying."[3]

Like the young Spanish boy who carried Glenda's husband's heart and the other cardio-sensitives whose stories you are reading, Dr. Nuland's case study offers additional support for the possibility of the existence of a unique subtle code of the heart. Dr. Nuland himself reports concern that the patient's attitude about his heart might negatively influence his recovery and that his "psychic form of xenophobia" might cause a rejection of his heart. Cardio-energetics suggests that it is this same issue of the brain's illusion of our separateness that threatens all of our survival and that some heart transplant recipients may be acting out the drama of confronting and defeating the illusion of otherness.

Dr. Nuland's patient, whom he describes as not by nature a highly reflective, uncontrolling, open person, reflects this struggle to deal with the imposed requirement to overcome what Dr. Nuland calls "the ancient xenophobia we have learned from every cell that has ever existed on earth." Seeming to struggle with his bigotry and discomfort with the issue of whether he had received the heart of a person from another race, Dr. Nuland's patient says, "you know, they tell you it doesn't make any difference what kind of heart you get. And I'm sitting there thinking, I don't believe that. . . . These people have different stuff in their body."

BELIEVING IN YOUR HEART

When I listen to the tapes of my interviews with heart and heart-lung transplant recipients and the donor families, I am still taken aback by what they've shared with me. My brain tells me to dismiss these stories as symptoms instead of signals, as emotional reactions to the trauma of transplant, the effects of the cocktail of medications used to depress the immune system's rejection of the new organ. Maybe the patients are acting out a role in keeping with their own image of their donor, or maybe they have a prior existing psychopathology exacerbated by long illness and the process of transplantation. Many patients not receiving a transplant but who are also on strong medications report unusual feelings, thoughts, and fantasies as well, so perhaps it is just the toxic nature of medications and the severity of life-threatening illness that is creating a trauma-induced, transitory, semi-psychotic state.

Something in my own heart seems to keep telling me, however, that something very important is taking place, as revealed by the consistency and sincerity of stories of cellular memory retrieval told by some heart transplant recipients. Something tells me that the sensitivity, humbleness, and integrity of the cardio-sensitive heart recipients requires us to at least listen to their reports with respect and enlightened skepticism. If we do not, these brave persons may become even more reluctant to share their experiences than most of them already are.

While my clinical work and my own personal experience as a cancer patient has taught me that most very sick nontransplant patients experience often drastic changes in thoughts and imagery, I also know that these changes do not correlate with those of another person who has donated a part of his or her body so that another person may live. Perhaps the medications given to those of us who have been close to death can cause various levels of delusion, but they may also act like a psychotropic drug, lowering the threshold for perception of the subtle energy that constitutes cellular memories, which exist in all of us. Perhaps the trauma of life-threatening illness promotes insights that only seem to those who have not yet had their turn to confront their mortality to be strange manifestations of mental pathology rather than spiritual brilliance. Perhaps receipt of the most powerful info-energetic organ in the body is a surgically induced nearer-to-life experience that any of us could experience if we would focus as intensely on our own heart as someone who receives a new heart is forced to do. As physicist Dr. H. E. Puthoff writes, "That the heart is involved in energetic, and hence informational, processes, cannot be denied. There is more to this tale to be told."[4]

LESSONS FROM WHITE CROWS

Dr. William Kuhn, a researcher in the area of transplantation, writes, "Adjustment to the rigors of the heart transplant protocol requires a degree of personality strength, resilience, and adequacy of coping skills which some patients simply do not possess."[5] The cardio-sensitives, those few heart transplant recipients and their families who do possess the spiritual strength to overcome the innate cellular xenophobia we all share, are what psychologist William James referred to as the "white crows." He wrote, "If you wish to upset the laws that all crows are black, it is enough if you prove one single crow to be white."[6] Like those who experience a medical miracle and survive "always fatal" illness, the cardio-sensitives who transcend their energetic xenophobia to allow in the cellular memories of their donors can be the white crows of bioscience that can teach us all how to fly together. If only one of their many stories is accurate, then we know that there is much more going on in transplantation than a tissue implantation and much more to life and death than biochemistry.

As remarkable as the reports from heart transplant recipients are, they are nothing more than interesting and entertaining anecdotes if they represent experiences that can only be had by receiving a new heart. At the very least, these stories can serve as teaching parables pointing the way for our own spiritual reconnection and for overcoming our evolutionary cellular suspiciousness that, when it is expressed on a higher systems level, results in so much alienation and conflict.

BEWARE OF COUNTERFEITERS

Wherever there is gold there are counterfeiters, so there is a real danger that the dramatic accounts of cellular memory will become the stuff of New Age psychology or media hype. There is the possibility that those looking so desperately for meaning in life or for support for their own "new movement" or alternative approaches to healing may try to use the stories of heart transplant patients to substantiate their unrealistic claims. There is also the danger that, because these stories speak so strongly to the issue of our energetic connection with one another, some may shy away from the lifesaving process of transplantation for fear, as expressed by Dr. Nuland's patients, of getting another person's "soul stuff" placed within them. As a bone-marrow transplant recipient myself, I too fear these possibilities and am as saddened by the efforts of those who would use our experiences in a sensational manner as much as I am disappointed by scientists and doctors who dismiss our experiences without a fair hearing. As a scientist, I regret that the possibility that the great potential for health, happiness, and healing that may be derived from seriously looking at the meaning of these accounts may be lost because of our own bioscience's bias against those events that challenge our current Newtonian-Cartesian view of the world.

One of the Hygeian Heart Club members, a sensitive, loving nurse who had worked for years on an oncology unit and became an energy healer two years after her transplant, expressed her view of the different rules of life to be learned through the experiences of transplant patients. She said, "I had a new heart with new energy and memories physically placed in me. That really gets your brain's attention about 'otherness' and 'individuality.' Unless you let your brain deny the whole thing and make it into something that happens in an auto-parts store, there's no denying the force of your individuality fighting against the fact of your connection with another person's heart. I assure you that the rejection you will get when you write about this comes from the same fear and anger we transplant recipients feel when we think about what and who has happened to us. It comes over you like a trance when you least expect it, and you feel that you have to just start to go with it or quickly dismiss it. There's no middle ground. You may want to deny it and you even get mad and afraid about it, but I think it helps us to realize that anyone can think and feel the same things we are even if they didn't get a new heart. It's just that we can't hide from it so easily. It's like we are experiencing a forced spiritual integration. Those who don't get a heart transplant are just going to have to make the choice to integrate on their own. In some ways, that's much more difficult."

THE RULE, NOT THE EXCEPTION

While the more profound examples of heart recipient awareness of the heart's code are impressive, research shows that experiencing some feelings about the donor, the donor heart, and sensations of a subtle energy from the donor are the rule, not the exception.[7] While the stories are not always as dramatic as the ones told by the cardio-sensitives, I have never spoken to a transplant recipient who did not have a story to tell, no matter how humorous, sardonic, and laden with denial and anger at the deeper meaning of their transplant that seems to sometimes involuntarily just "click in."

After my recent appearance on national television in support of a heart transplant recipient who was discussing changes in her personality following her surgery, I received a letter from a board certified psychologist. He expressed his skepticism and discomfort and challenged me to share my data. At the end of his letter, he shared that he had received a new kidney and, despite his profound dislike of spicy foods, now craves tacos and burritos and has taken a class to learn to speak Spanish. He ends his letter reporting that, "By the way, I just found out my donor was a young Hispanic man."

The forced course in energy connection such as the one reported above may be so threatening to the brain's sense of self and its total control of the body that it can employ its strongest forms of denial. When the new organ is the heart, the most info-energetically powerful organ in the body, it may be less willing than less energetic and nonoscillating organs to submit to the old brain's domination. While some organs can be donated without donor death, the guilt and shame of waiting eagerly for someone they do not know to meet a sudden death in order to get their heart can be overwhelming, leading to even more denial.

Another source of strong denial is that fact that even the most cynical and brain-driven person may still view his or her own heart as the focus of love and source of personality, thoughts, and feelings, resulting in a fear of loss of self with the taking of the old heart.[8] Researchers are acknowledging Dr. James Rauch's statement, "Transplant professionals generally agree that psychological rejection of the heart is sometimes associated with physiological rejection."[9] The denial of heart transplant patients may help them through one of the most difficult of all life experiences, but denial by doctors and scientists of the importance of studying and learning about the heart's code and the cellular memories it negotiates goes beyond being narrow-brained. It is also bad science, insensitive medicine, and it indicates an inadequate and incomplete understanding of the depth and extent of the rejection phenomenon.

ENDURING THE ULTIMATE INSULT

The new heart, attached as it is to the vessels but not directly to the new brain as the old heart was, may be less willing to be dominated by its new brain. As a result, the brain suffers the ultimate narcissistic insult and works hard to deny the explosion of subtle energy and forced sense of connectedness imposed upon it.

My interviews of transplant recipients reveal that the insecure and threatened brain may fear the new heart.[10] It can cause a heart recipient to become concerned that the body will take on the sexual behavior, preferences, or even the gender orientation of the anonymous donor, or become promiscuous, or completely lose the sex drive. It can convey concerns that, because most hearts come from those who have met sudden, often violent deaths, it is being forced to welcome a restless spirit that was unprepared to leave its body. It may be concerned that new religious feelings and beliefs the exact opposite of prior ones will dominate long-held convictions. Dr. Richard Frierson and his associates have screened dozens of heart transplant candidates and report many such concerns and that their patients also often express some level of fear that they will assume the characteristics of the deceased donor. They describe one of their patients who was concerned about killing himself after he received a new heart when he learned that his heart had come from a person who had committed suicide.

THE HEART OR MY HEART

Dr. Frieson's patients often regarded the heart as if it had a mind of its own and called it "the heart" rather than "my heart." My interviews revealed, however, that the cardio-sensitives tended to refer to their new organ as "my heart," seemingly incorporating and connecting more strongly with it. This association is similar to the phenomenon as noted in the PEAR subjects who, when they referred to "my machine" rather than "the machine," seemed to have the most marked connection with and influence upon the machine.

Some of my patients reported a concern that the heart they received would reject them. One patient said, "I'm ready for a new heart, but I just hope it is ready for me. What if it doesn't like me and we don't get along? What if it refuses to take me?" Dr. Frieson also quotes one of his patients as saying, "I'm afraid my new heart will reject me." This concern of the implanted heart and not the host's body doing the rejection was reported by many of my patients and may be misunderstood by transplant professionals who see rejection only as a one-way issue and due solely to some biochemical reaction of the host rather than donor-host energy incompatibility.

Even the brains of those closest to the transplant recipient can experience the narcissistic insult of transplantation. A heart is not only placed in a new body. It is also placed in a new family and social system, both of which have their own unique energy templates that may or may not be compatible with the energy system of the new heart, as well as the cellular memories implanted not only from the donor but from the donor's family. The donor family has lost the energetic heart of their loved one and thus also may experience a major subtle energy change.

Families, heart-care professionals, and caregivers also fear the consequences of losing or altering the personality of the recipient or of the impact of the new "soul stuff" from a complete stranger. One Hygeian Heart Club heart transplant patient's wife said, "I just hope he didn't get the heart of an ax murderer." Even though she was joking, she later confessed that she had concerns and even fears of "how my husband will act toward me now." Another one of my female patients who had received the heart of a young man expressed concern that her husband would no longer want to make love to her because he may think he "was being homosexual." She later added, "When we dance now, my husband says I always try to lead. I think it's the macho male heart in me making me do that." Concerns such as those expressed by this woman make it essential that the issue of cellular memories and the heart's code be dealt with in a caring, careful, respectful, and even sacred manner that acknowledges the fact that the new heart joins a system, not just one body.

CHOOSING THE PATH OF THE HEAD OR HEART

Dr. Benjamin Bunzel in the Department of Surgery at the University Hospital in Vienna has studied the impact of heart transplant on the personalities of recipients. Agreeing with the physicians and researchers referred to above, he writes, "Heart transplantation is not simply a question of replacing an organ that no longer functions. The heart is often seen as a source of love, emotions, and focus of personality traits."[11] He has investigated the cases of forty-seven heart transplant recipients. His data approximates my own findings regarding a very small but consistent and unique group of cardio-sensitives.

Dr. Bunzel reports that 15 percent of his sample stated that their personality had changed due to what they felt was the life-threatening event of transplantation itself, but they did not attribute their experienced change to their donor. Six percent, or three patients, reported a distinct change of personality due to their new hearts. They added that they felt compelled to change their prior feelings and reactions to accommodate those they sensed as coming from the memories of their donor. Seventy-nine percent said that their personality had not changed in any way at all postoperatively.

As I also saw in my research, Dr. Bunzel noted that these "no-change" patients employed massive defenses and often angry and hostile reactions to questions about the possible receipt of the energy from their donor. They called questions about such a thing "complete nonsense" and ridiculed the idea that their donor could influence their life. They were often eager to change the subject and mocked the question itself. However, Dr. Bunzel reports that even those patients who most vehemently rejected the idea of subtle energy and memories coming from their new heart still, like Dr. Nuland's patient and my patients, indirectly reflected their deep concern about such issues.

THE DANGER OF DENIAL

Denial is clinically defined as conscious or unconscious repudiation of part or all of the total available meaning of an event in order to ally fear, anxiety, or other unpleasant emotional or cognitive effects. It can help patients going through the trauma of transplantation and any patient undergoing serious medical procedures to avoid feelings that may otherwise be almost unbearable to deal with.[12] I used denial myself during my own chemotherapy and whole-body radiation. I knew I was having deadly poison dripped directly into my veins and being burned with enough radiation to kill a man twice my size, but I chose to deny that reality most of the time. When that denial failed me, I spent hours crying and in a cold sweat of terror at what was happening to me. Of concern here, however, is the extreme intensity and persistence of the denial and its occasional "leakage" revealed in the jokes and sarcasm on the part of those who vigorously reject any possibility that something of the donor comes with the donation.

Researchers have consistently found that, compared to other severe medical procedures, there is an atypically high degree of denial in patients receiving a transplanted organ, particularly a new heart.[13] Research also clearly documents that fantasies about the donor, the donor heart, and its influence on the recipient's personality are common and so threatening to the self-concept that denial, escape, and even regression tend to be significantly stronger with heart transplant than any other surgical process. Could it be that such intense denial reflects the intensity of the impact of a new heart's code and, as Shakespeare warned, some of us may protest too much when the sacred nature of our energetic connection is so physically confrontational?

Writing about adjustment to transplant, transplant researcher Dr. Nathan Haan writes, "The person will cope if he can, defend if he must, and fragment if he is forced do so."[14] All three of these patterns were present in Dr. Bunzel's and my patients' adjustments, indicating that what is being denied is not just the impact of an intense and complex surgical procedure but the suddenly imposed insight of our ultimate info-energetic connection that either tears the psyche apart or puts it back together again in a most profound and life-altering way.

"HEART-FELT" REPORTS FROM RECEIVERS

To review and illustrate the nature of the energy connection experienced by transplant recipients, I selected for this chapter five more sample transplant stories from the 140 verbatim reports from my audio tapes. Because I am focusing on the heart's code, I have selected stories from heart transplant recipients, but the various other organ recipient stories also reflect varying degrees of cellular memories. I present the following five stories because, in each case, I was also able to speak with a relative who seemed to confirm each report. To protect the identity of these patients, I have been intentionally vague about the recipient's background.

1. Forty-one-year-old male heart transplant patient (received heart of nineteen-year-old-girl killed when her car was struck by a train).

"I felt it when I woke up. You know how it feels different after a thunderstorm or heavy rain? You know that feeling in the air? That's kind of how it felt. It was like a storm had happened inside me or like I had been struck by lightening. There is a new energy in me. I feel like nineteen again. I'm sure I got a strong young man's heart because sometimes I can feel like a roar or surging power within me that I never felt before. I think he was probably a truck driver or something like that, and he was probably killed by a cement truck or something like that. I feel this sense of speed and raw power in me."

Wife of recipient: "He's a kid again. He used to struggle to breathe and had no stamina at all, but now he's like a teenager. The transplant changed him completely. He keeps talking about power and energy all the time. He says he has had several dreams that he is driving a huge truck or is the engineer of a large steam engine. He is sure that his donor was driving a big truck that hit a bigger truck."

2. Thirty-six-year-old female heart-lung transplant recipient (received the heart and lungs of a twenty-year-old girl who was killed while running across the street to show her fiancé a picture of her new wedding dress).

"At first I didn't even want to think about it at all. I didn't want to think that someone had had my heart before me. I knew they did, of course, but I preferred to think of it as like a new heart made somewhere else and given to me. I got mad when people asked me about how it felt to have someone else's heart inside me. I heard other transplant recipients say it was crazy talk to talk about this stuff, but I couldn't avoid it. Almost every night, I had this dream about her. I know she was young and pretty and very happy. I've always been sort of a somewhat down type of person yet, somehow, I have this new happiness in me I never experienced before. It's strange, because I'm still afraid sometimes that I will die and that the new heart will fail. In some ways I seem to have more of a reason to be afraid now than when I was sick because I was given this great gift from someone who lost her life. I owe it to her to keep living. It feels like, no matter how down I get, a little joy keeps bubbling up from inside me. The medication makes me feel angry and depressed sometimes, but inside I feel this strange kind of happiness, excitement, and joy that I cannot fully explain or put into words. I just want to go around telling everybody about it, but I'm afraid they'll think I've totally lost it."

Sister of recipient: "The one thing about her that we all noticed right away was that she smiles a lot more. She was always a frowner, but now she smiles and laughs even when we don't expect it. It's probably just because she has a new lease on life, but we can see it. She was lucky and seemed to get a very warm heart."

3. Thirty-five-year-old female heart transplant recipient (donor a twenty-four-year-old prostitute killed in a stabbing).

"I never really was all that interested in sex. I never really thought about it much. Don't get me wrong, my husband and I had a sex life, but it was not a big part of our life. Now, I tire my husband out. I want sex every night and I masturbate two to three times a day sometimes. I used to hate X-rated videos, but now I love them. I feel like a slut sometimes and I even do a strip for my husband when I'm in the mood. I would never have done that before my surgery. When I told my psychiatrist about this, she said it was a reaction to my medications and my healthier body. Then I found out that my donor was a young college girl who worked as a topless dancer and in an out-call service. I think I got her sexual drive, and my husband agrees. He says I'm not the woman he married, but he wants to marry me again."

Husband of recipient: "Not that I'm complaining, mind you, but what I have now is a sex kitten. It's not that we do it more, but she wants to talk about sex more and wants to see sexually explicit tapes which I could never talk her into before. When we do have sex, it is different. Not worse or better, just different. She never talked much during sex, but now she practically narrates the whole thing. She uses words I never heard her use before, but it kind of turns me on, so who's complaining? Our worst argument came a few months after her transplant and well before she knew who her donor was. I was joking and at a passionate moment said that she must have gotten the heart of a whore. We didn't talk for weeks."

4. Fifty-two-year-old male heart transplant recipient (donor a seventeen-year-old boy killed by a hit-and-run driver).

"It's two years after my transplant. I still feel sorry for my old heart. It just comes over me sometimes when I least expect it. It served me well and it died so I could live. Sometimes I wish I could have seen it one more time and I wonder what happened to it, but I hate thinking about that too long.

That's hard to deal with. I could never understand it. I loved quiet classical music before my new heart. Now, I put on earphones, crank up the stereo, and play loud rock-and-roll music. I love my wife, but I keep fantasizing about teenage girls. My daughter says I have regressed since my new heart and that I act like a sixteen-year-old."

Daughter of recipient: "It is really embarrassing sometimes. When my friends come over they ask if my dad is going through his second childhood. He's addicted to loud music and my mom says the little boy in him is finally coming out."

5. Forty-seven-year-old female heart transplant recipient (donor a twenty-three-year-old gay man shot to death in a robbery and died from severe wound to lower back).

"For three years I never told anyone about this. It still bothers me. I met the family of my donor and they said their son was a bright young artist and that he was gay. Now I wonder if, when I look at my husband, I am looking at him like a woman would look at him like I used to do, or if I am looking at him like a young gay man would look at him. I'm glad I can finally talk to you about this. And one more thing. His mother said they shot him in the back. After my surgery, I've had shooting pains in my lower back, but I guess that's just the surgery acting up."

Husband of recipient: "I was surprised when one of the first things "X" asked me when we started having sex again after her surgery was whether or not I ever had gay fantasies. She has completely changed how she dresses now. She wears very feminine and revealing clothes where before she wore unisex clothes. Sometimes during the night she will awake suddenly and scream. I used to think she was having a heart attack, but she would point to her back and say it was like a shooting pain right in the middle of her back."

WAR OR PEACE?

Even the most prestigious and pioneering researchers in the field of heart transplant are reexamining their fundamental assumptions about the process of placing new organs in new bodies. Dr. Thomas Starzl, a leader in the study and treatment of the organ rejection phenomenon, now wonders if he and his colleagues had not been going about organ transplantation and dealing with rejection in the wrong way.[15] Doctors typically use pharmaceutical force and try to beat the patient's immune system into submission with drugs until it surrenders and reluctantly accepts the donor organ.

Despite this chemical warfare, the brain's defense system does not easily accept what it sees as invaders to its territory, and rejection continues to be a major obstacle to successful transplantation.

Dr. Starzl now reflects, "The mystery was not about [the body's] rejection, and more about the intermingling of cells and the achievement of a peaceful truce between the patient and the donated organ."[16] [brackets mine] While Dr. Starzl was not talking about cellular memories and the centrality of the heart, he was recognizing the issue of the body as an informational system and the issue of transplantation as much more than just the beating down of one system to cram in another.

Dr. Starzl now asserts that the challenge in transplantation is not to win a war against the body's body defenses but to more gently create a cellular peace by "convincing" the body's defense system that the "intruder" is really "self" and should be "seen" as a welcomed new part of the host's whole system. The new paradigm in transplantation of the future will have to take into account not only the manipulation of a biochemical encouragement of immuno-hospitality but energy cardiology's new fact of the heart's energy and its role in maintaining a harmonious organ concert.

THE CARDIO-SENSITIVE CYCLE

Psychiatrist Pietro Castelnuovo-Tedesco interviewed many of the world's leading heart transplant surgeons.[17] In addition to seventy-three heart and heart-lung transplant recipients and sixty-seven other organ transplant recipients I interviewed for this book, I also interviewed three transplant surgeons, all of whom asked to remain anonymous, stating, "I want to wait until this stuff is verified," "I don't want my colleagues to think I'm nuts," and "I'm afraid I would frighten my patients." I have also interviewed six nurses who assist in heart transplantation, and all but two asked to be anonymous, primarily because they felt the doctors with whom they worked would "be uncomfortable." Dr. Castelnuovo-Tedesco interviewed Drs. Cleveland, Cooley, DeBakey, Hallman, and Rochelle. His interviews were conducted in 1971 and mine were conducted in 1993 and 1995. More than twenty years have passed between Dr. Castelnuovo-Tedesco's and my sets of interviews, but the denial and discomfort with the issues of cardio-energetics remain.

In my interviews of heart transplant recipients, I detected a cycle of adjustment common to almost all of them that not only seemed to be echoed in the words of the surgeons but may reflect the way in which all of us deal with the prospect that our own heart thinks and our own cells have memories. First, there was the fighting stage, a severe anxiety, cynicism, and often anger with their situation. This was followed by a flow stage, a kind of enlightened euphoria and sense of being a pioneer or great adventurer often shown in the form of transplant advocacy and political and spiritual commitment to the issue of transplantation. Next, there was the anguish stage in which grieving and guilt not only for the donor but for the heart they lost took place at various levels and in various ways. There was often severe depression during this part of the cycle of adjustment. Finally, there seemed to be a crossroads in the heart transplantation adjustment process.

One road, and the road most often traveled, was a return to cynicism, intellectualization, and much stronger denial than that prior to or just after the transplant. There was often anger when confronted with ideas about the special nature of the heart. A smaller group, however, chose a different path. The "heart path" was taken by about one of ten of the transplant patients. These patients became intensely interested in the meaning of their heart transplant, interested in the characteristics of their donor, and reported experiencing clear and intense dreams not only about the transplant but about their often very accurate image of their donor. Finally, for many of the heart-path patients who had discussed their feelings regarding the meaning of a new heart and its innate energy, there was a disavowing of their early reports and feelings and an attempt to distance themselves from the issue.

I have worked with hundreds of very sick cancer patients, heart bypass patients, and recipients of new kidneys and livers. I have seldom seen the severity of the new heart adjustment cycle of fighting, flowing, anguish, grieving, guilt, deep denial contrasted with complete personal immersion in the meaning of the organ transplant, and later disavowing by those who had expressed so many deep feelings about the meaning of their new organ. At the very least, the consistency and magnitude of this cycle as experienced by heart transplant recipients may illustrates the special significance of the heart.

SURGEON-TO-SURGEON, HEART-TO-HEART

In my interviews with the surgeons and nurses, and from the interviews conducted by Dr. Castelnuovo-Tedesco, the transplant surgeons in both groups reported that heart transplant patients were, as a group, exceptionally anxious as compared to other transplant patients. While they could die without a liver or healthy kidney just as they could die without a heart, the surgeons reported an extraordinary anxiety in the heart transplant group. For example, Dr. Cooley said, "I think they react differently. . . . Patients have a great deal more fear about the heart."[18] Only Dr. DeBakey disagreed, stating that he felt it inappropriate and fallacious to try to erect a special mystique about heart transplantation. Dr. DeBakey, apparently thinking that physicians have different personal interests and concerns than other people, thought that such talk about the significance of the heart may "appeal to the lay public and press" but is not something physicians should concern themselves with.

Dr. Cooley described the extreme denial of heart transplant recipients with a story about a used car dealer. When Dr. Cooley showed the man his old heart floating in a jar of formaldehyde and asked his patient if he had any particular feelings about looking at his dead heart, the patient commented, "Well, I've owned a lot of cars in my life. Not one of them did I develop an emotional attachment to." The patient saw his heart as only a discarded part that had outlived its usefulness.

All but one of the transplant surgeons and nurses agreed that heart transplant held a very special significance over other forms of transplantation. The dissenter, Dr. DeBakey echoing the used car salesman, said, "The heart is a pump, a magnificent pump, but just a pump."

Even though they often intellectualized, most of the surgeons and nurses did report strong positive, even spiritual, feelings about the nature of their work. In my interviews, perhaps because of their more Hygeian orientation to healing, it was particularly the nurses who spoke of an awe and even euphoria they felt with the whole process. Many had become very active politically in the transplant cause, and two had become "energy healers" because of their experiences in heart transplantation. The response of both Dr. Castelnuovo-Tedesco's and my interviewees showed various degrees of the same transplantation adjustment cycle shown by the patients I interviewed.

THE HEART AS HIDDEN OBSERVER

Research into hypnosis may provide another clue for one way in which the heart exercises its interactions with the brain and body and the nature of cardio-sensitivity. The neodissociation theory of hypnosis suggests that the process of being hypnotized creates a split in consciousness. The theory is that one part of our consciousness accepts suggestions from the hypnotist while another part acts as a "hidden observer," vigilant to what is going on without participating directly in the hypnotic suggestion.

To test the neodissociation theory, hypnotized subjects are asked to put their arms into icy water but are informed that they will feel no pain. Many obey, and when they do, they report none of the discomfort a nonhypnotized subject would immediately report. However, if asked to describe their feelings in writing, they indicate that they did in fact experience intense cold. Hit two pieces of wood near the ear of a hypnotized subject who has been told he is temporarily completely deaf and he will not respond. While he is still under hypnosis, ask him if he heard anything and he will respond "no," his response to the hypnotist's voice indicating that a part of his consciousness was still on the alert. Something inside these hypnotized persons seems to know they were cold while the body ignored it and seems to hear sounds that another part of consciousness did not.[19] Cardio-energetics suggests that the heart may receive the info-energy of these events even as the brain itself yields to the illusion. In effect, the brain becomes hypnotized but the heart does not. As lovers, poets, prophets, and priests have said, it is much easier to fool the brain than the heart.

Perhaps the heart, because of the immense "L" energy with which it deals, acts like a kind of "hidden observer." In my interviews of transplant recipients, the one in ten who seemed to be particularly cardio-sensitive focused on the issues of the heart and seemed to be astute and intense observers of the transplant process. They seemed to be incorporators of their new heart more than passive biological recipients. Although often reluctant and embarrassed, they seemed to need to talk about the meaning of having a new heart and welcomed a scientist, clinician, and fellow transplant recipient willing to listen not only with personal empathy but also with scientific sympathy. They wanted to know more about their donor and to confront and understand the many signals they said they were receiving. The 10 percent of transplant recipients who are cardio-sensitive, or on the "heart path," is about the same percentage of persons who are very receptive to hypnotic suggestion.

PROFILE OF A CARDIO-SENSITIVE

My interviews with seventy-three heart transplant patients indicates that those who go down the path of the heart rather than the head and transcend their natural denial—the group I have called the cardio-sensitives—had a very perceptive hidden observer. They seemed fascinated with the meaning of the transplant even as the brain saw it as a mechanical repair and replacement, and their courage and willingness to "come out" with their feelings about the significance of the heart makes them a set of people from whom we can learn much about the song of our soul.

Based on my many interviews, here are eighteen characteristics of the cardio-sensitives. They are similar to the characteristics of easily hypnotized subjects and similar to the traits reported in the more successfully energetic-connecting "operators" and "percipients" in the PEAR program.

1. *A Feminine Point of View.* All but two of those who reported recovering the cellular memories of their donor were women. Researchers, including psychologist Carol Gilligan, have shown that there are key differences in the way women and men view the world, so it is not surprising that they may see the placement of a new heart in their body differently than men. Gilligan's work suggests that men tend to value independence and be more uncomfortable with dependence, meaning that their denial of connection with their donor may be more profound. Women, on the other hand, tend to be uncomfortable with independence and more highly value interdependence, perhaps resulting in their willingness or ability to confront the psychological and spiritual significance of a new heart.[20] As one transplant nurse told me, "My male patients refer to their new heart as 'it' while the women patients call it 'theirs.' " Gilligan and her colleagues assert that men tend to embrace an ethic of individual rights while women take a more collective orientation based on caring connection.[21] This may explain why women, more easily than most men organ recipients, are more comfortable dealing with the new connection established with a new heart and express more interest in their donor.

2. *Open-Minded.* Most were "accommodators" rather than "assimilators." Psychologist Jean Piaget described the process of "accommodation" as revising existing schemata, our mental models of persons, objects, events, and situations. He defined "assimilation" as interpreting new information in light of and without changing existing schemata.[22] The recipients taking the "heart path" tended to *accommodate* most events that happened to them and did so with the most significant event in their whole life—their receipt of a new heart. Unlike their assimilating male opposites

on the head path, their transplant more significantly altered the way they thought about the levels of connections between human beings and the meaning of life in general.

3. Body Aware. Most were very tuned in to their body and showed a high degree of what psychologist Howard Gardner calls "bodily kines- thetic intelligence."[23] They seemed to have good control of their bodily motions and high capacity to handle objects skillfully. Many were athletes, carpenters, musicians, and dancers.

4. Music Lover. They enjoyed music (often classical), showed a good sense of rhythm, and reacted strongly and emotionally to various sounds and tones. You have read that the body, from its DNA to every cell within it, resonates with a scale of energy and gives off its own unique "pitch." Cardio-energetics suggests that cellular memories are a form of recorded cardio-energetic music recalled in much the same way as a favorite tune seems to suddenly, and sometimes persistently and annoyingly, cycle through our system, defiant of our brain's objections.

5. Highly Creative. Most reported a vivid, active fantasy life prior to their transplant. Many reported that they loved to read and write, enjoyed po- etry or going to plays. When asked if they "were more head or heart," they all responded "heart."

6. Environmentally sensitive. They were hyperalert to their environment. When asked to write down a description of a scene they had just experi- enced, they were extremely accurate down to very fine details compared to the patients who took the path of the head. When asked to describe a room they had just left, they did so with amazing accuracy and detail.

7. Good Visualization Ability. They were easily able to conjure up and share visual images. When asked to describe their donor, they were more than willing to do so and were often surprisingly thorough and accurate.

8. Psychic-Sensitive. They were described by family members or friends as being "psychic" or "very sensitive" to things others are not sensitive to and that they showed this sensitivity long before their illness was diagnosed and their eventual transplant.

9. Dependent. They showed a tendency to be very trusting and depen- dent on others and very sensitive to others' views of them. Many had been in therapy, reported enjoying books about psychology, and had embraced various theories of self-help in prior years.

10. Compulsive. They tended to be compulsive and self-critical. Family members described them as hard workers and as being more impatient with their own imperfections than with those of other people.

11. Unresolved Grief. They had experienced what they described and family members confirmed as a "severe break" in a prior emotional bond. Many reported an especially difficult divorce or the premature loss of a parent, which still plagued them emotionally even after several years had passed. There seemed to be a chronic, mildly depressive nature sometimes masked by self-deprecating humor. For some of my patients, heart transplantation seemed to serve as a metaphorical ritual of "reconnection" that promoted healing a past broken bond.

12. Animal Loving. They loved animals and felt certain that animals were sentient. Most had pets or wished they had pets and said that animals were often more sensitive than many humans.

13. Climate Sensitive. They reported loving nature, talking to plants, enjoying a stroll in the woods, and were emotionally very dependent on climate. Despite their love of nature, however, many had allergies.

14. Involved. They showed a high degree of absorption and creativity in anything they attempted and often said whatever they were doing was fun. Family members said they often got so involved with what they were doing that they lost track of time or forgot to eat or sleep.

15. Dreamer. Long before they had become ill or had a transplant, most reported extensive dreaming, memory for dreams, and interest in the significance of their dreams. Following their transplant, most reported dreaming about their donor.

16. Sensual. Most reported being highly sensual. Spouses and family members confirmed that they were gentle, tender, and enjoyed hugging and hand-holding.

17. Ectomorphic. Most were slender, had narrow faces, tended to be underweight even before their illness and transplant, and—less consistently—had dark eyes.

18. "Flow-er" more than "fighter." Most were able to "go with the flow," as opposed to trying to control situations.

Transplant recipients who were less cardio-sensitive tended to show the exact opposite traits from those described here.[24] They often impatiently described the cardio-sensitives as the "weird group" who were prone to fantasizing, irrational, weak-willed, self-deceiving, and even crazy or abnormal. One of the key lessons to be learned from the characteristics of the cardio-sensitives is that normalcy may not be the only or even best path to well-being and the development of insight into our true essence.

THE WISDOM OF WEIRDNESS

Edgar Allan Poe suggested that it is not yet clear whether a mild form of madness is not the loftiest intelligence and whether much that is glorious and profound may not be exposed to us at the expense of the general intellect. Perhaps our view of intelligence leaves too little room for the aptitude of the heart. Perhaps the heart path represents a different way of interacting with the world than our current brain-dominant approach, a path many of us may want to explore and one that is based more on sensing the energy that resonates within everyone and everything rather than always trying to master and control things, people, and the cosmos.

CHAPTER FIVE

Cellular Memories Are Made of This

"When water turns to ice, does it remember one time it was water?"

— CARL SANDBURG

THE BASIC UNIT OF LIFE

Seventeenth-century philosopher and mathematician Gottfried Leibniz wrote that "there are no souls without bodies." Four hundreds year later, surgeon Sherwin Nuland writes, "it must certainly be true that there is no spirit without cells."[1] While Leibniz was referring to a much more abstract form of energy than the now familiar biochemical energy generated by the 75-trillion-cell human body about which Dr. Nuland was speaking, it appears that most people who try to describe the magnificence of the human systems and their basic cellular units seem unable to resist speaking about these issues in spiritual terms.

Another piece in the puzzle of deciphering the heart's code is understanding the potential for our body's cells not only to do the work of turning the sun's energy into our life-giving energy but also to remember on some level why we are living. This chapter explores the possibility that cells can store and process not only the various energetic codes from the sun and plants but also the info-energy that is the heart's code, a code that may not only be passed on with a transplanted heart but may also be available to all of us who chose to become recipients to the heart's code.

CELLULAR CONTAINERS, CONVERTERS, OR REMEMBERERS?

You may remember having to complete one of the standard requirements in almost every high school biology class: being able to see a cell under a microscope. Most of us recall trying to delicately slip a piece of almost anything onto a slide and then squinting to peek into the microscopic world that is the framework of the universe. If we were lucky, we got to look at living cells. They were the most fascinating because, unlike the strands of hair and various other inanimate objects we placed on slides, living cells didn't just sit there; they actually did something. That every living cell seems to be able to somehow "remember" what it is supposed to do and when, where, and with which other cells it is supposed to do it, is one of the still largely unexplained miracles of life.

Whether or not a cell's memory is only a simple chemical signaling process conveyed through a sack of cellular jellylike fluid called cytoplasm or, on another level, a subtle info-energetic process involving "L" energy, is the question science must address if it is willing to look for memory in places other than in various clusters of brain cells. If we want to learn more about the possibility of a heart's code and the cellular memory it may coordinate and express, we must be willing to study the possibility that cells have more than a biochemical imperative stored within them as a genetically driven energy conversion system. We must be willing to consider the possibility that cells also store the info-energy that represents all of the experiences of a cardio-energetized Mind.

MEMORIES OF A PARAMECIUM

One popular high school laboratory performer that I remember thinking showed at least some level of memory was the single-cell paramecium, a complete living thing in one tiny package. It has no brain, neurons, or synapses, yet every one of them seems to have retained some level of its paramecium heritage. They all remember how to swim, hunt for food, identify and escape their predators, court a mate, and even engage in a rudimentary type of sex. Using their tiny cilia that stick out like paddles from a misshapen canoe, they move about in the microscopic sea of the solution we place them in so they become visible under our microscope. Paramecium may not be able to remember in the way we or our brain usually thinks about memory, but it is possible that they and all living cells have an "L" energy form of memory. Some of the characteristics of cells as described in this chapter, when combined with the theories about subtle energy and the sentient heart as described in the previous two chapters, seem to give at least some credence to that possibility.

THE CELLULAR SYMPHONY

All living things are made of cells. Like trillions of tiny tuning forks resonated together by the energy of the heart, the cells reverberate in a concert of energetic harmony. Cardio-energetics suggests that this cellular symphony, including the billions of brain cells, constitutes a dynamic systemic memory system that is constantly vibrating with other remembering systems to share and create info-energetic memories of their lives.

From the tiniest cell hardly more than a few thousand atomic diameters across to the biggest single cell known—an ostrich egg twenty inches around—every cell is reverberated by the strumming of the energy of our "heart strings"—the powerful energized heart muscle fibers. Energy cardiology might be seen as a kind of musicology of our spiritual song of life, the study of how the heart coordinates not only our individual cellular symphony but plays in duets and major symphonic arrangements with all hearts, persons, places, and things.

Every cell is literally a mini-heart humming with the energy. The ultimate biomedical illusion has been the view that the body is made of solid matter with fluid pumped through it by an unconscious heart and a powerful conscious brain that is the primary controller of the entire system. Energy cardiology suggests, however, that the heart and not just the brain is what holds this system together by a form of spiritual info-energy, in a temporary and ever-changing set of cellular memories we refer to as "the self." This "self" is the dynamic gestalt of information that might be considered the code that constitutes our soul.

As complex as they are, our cells are more space than stuff. Although they are tiny packages made up of energy-conducting walls with various receptors, cytoplasm full of substances that conduct the business of cellular life, and a nucleus that serves as the cell's mini-brain, every cell is also 99.999 percent empty space with subatomic bundles of energy whizzing through it at the speed of light.

You are humming with energy as you read these words, your energy is merging with all the energy around you, and anyone who chooses to try to tune in to your energy may be able to sense it. If you really want to know what the body looks like, look up to the evening sky and see the stars, the cells of cosmic energy scattered in the infinite vacuum of the dark night sky. If you really want to know what the body sounds like, listen to the waves and the wind for the energy they carry. If you really want to know what the body's energy feels like, be aware of a gentle breeze caressing your cheek and sense the information carried in the molecules breathed in and out by every person and thing that has ever lived. If you want to get a glimpse of how your whole body/heart/brain Mind system sounds when it works collectively, listen to a symphony. Compositions by Beethoven might be a good start, because his deafness forced him to tune in to his heart's code rather than rely on his brain's sense of hearing.

The energy of the heart, right down to our DNA, is musical and rhythmic in nature. Geneticist Susumu Ohno at the Beckman Research Institute of the City of Hope in Duarte, California, has translated the four nucleotides on the strands of DNA. He transposed adenine, guanine, cytosine, and thymine to musical notes, encoding "do" for cytosine, "re" and "mi" for adenine, "fa" and "so" to guanine, and "la" and "ti" for thymine. He chose a key and time and, with the help of his musician wife who helped set the duration of each note and a key and timing, the result was a melodic composition. When performed by musicians, listeners compared it to the music of Bach, Brahms, and Chopin. Many listeners were moved to tears.[2] When organ transplant recipients recover the cellular memories of their donor, could they be tuning in to the song of their donor's cells? When Dr. Ohno transcribed one of Chopin's musical passages to a chemical notation, the resulting formula resembled that of the DNA of a human cancer gene. It appears that even cancer cells have a memory for their own tune, one that is playing out of tune, too loud, or too separately from the rest of the cellular orchestra. Ultimately, cancer may turn out to be a severe form of cellular disharmony caused by a section of the cellular symphony that has forgotten how to play with the rest of the group. Energy cardiology suggests that the heart is the conductor that keeps all the cells playing the same score.[3]

QUANTUM HEAVEN

In Western medical terms, cellular energy is primarily due to something called ATP (adenosine triphosphate). ATP is a tiny molecule made from the food and sunlight we take in every day. Ultimately, all of the physical energy of a cell comes from the sun. In every cell, there are about two million ATP molecules vibrating every one ten-thousandth of a second.

Like the synapses in the brain electro-chemically sparking energy messages back and forth, much the same process is occurring within and between every cell in your body right now.

A very powerful, sensitive, centrally located instrument is required to coordinate the immense energy and information generated by the billions of cellular vibrations taking place every second of our life. Multiply two million vibrations of ATP molecules by 75 trillion cells, multiply that number by the 51 to 78 billion cycles per second at which human DNA resonates and conveys its information within each cell, and multiply yet again by the energetic vibrations of the sixty or so neuropeptides that are the biochemical means by which our emotional state is manifested throughout our body. The total number would be a very rough low estimate of the energy surging within you as you read these words.[4] If it is true that information about what we call our soul could be represented as "L" energy riding along within this energy, the heart is at the center of its own galaxy as powerfully complex as any in the cosmos.

Energy cardiology hypothesizes that the heart is the sun of our cellular universe, holding together the whizzing energy described above, in the shape of a soul having a brief "personal" experience on earth. Billions of galaxies were once originally compressed into a space millions of times smaller than the dot at the end of this sentence. With what physicists call the "Big Bang," a massive energy explosion that began the cosmic clock, that dot became an infinite energy field that the principle of nonlocality suggests we are not only a part of but actually "are." Within our cells may linger the memories of the info-energy of the Big Bang. Just as the sun provides the gravity to temporarily hold the planets in a group around it, so the heart is the center of the body's solar system huddling our cells together for a brief cosmic moment before we merge again with quantum heaven: the nonlocal infinite energy field that is everything always.

THE SOUL'S PACKAGE

The cells in our body vary from about .0002 to .0004 inches in diameter, making it possible for all 75 trillion of them to crowd together to make the temporary and ever-changing cellular package that is the physical manifestation of our soul. Like everything in the cosmos, cells are both energetic and material, both stuff and force. Although mostly space, these tiny energy-particle "wavicles" still make up about two thirds of our body weight, making us literally heavy with info-energy. Such a powerful system needs something extremely powerful at its center to hold the system together, and it may be that the heart is made to serve that purpose.

In 1665, long before our advanced microscopes, Robert Hooke used a simple magnifying device to study a piece of cork and saw what he called "many boxes" or "pores or cells." The word "cell" derives from the Latin "cellula," meaning "small chamber," and each chamber has within it hundreds of specialized compartments called organelles sharing a common energetic bond. Because energy is information, it is accurate to say that our cells are also held together by information.

Each of the organelles has a memory of the info-energetic job it is supposed to do, including digestion, disposal of waste, and extraction and conversion of different forms of energy passing through the cell. These various organelles, including ones called Golgi bodies, lysosomes, mitochondria, and the nucleus of the cell itself, each have their own cellular cognitive style or special type of memory for its place in the body's system.

There is a more technical, mechanical process that also accounts for how our cells may remember. When I was a graduate student using microscopes much more powerful than my high school version, I remember my first clear look at the process called mitosis, or cell division (you may remember seeing pictures of this same process in your high school biology class). What I saw resembled a microcosmic square dance of carefully choreographed movements. I saw what looked like a marching band performing intricate patterns to some form of music to which the parts of the cell seemed to be marching. Tiny spindles lined up, strings of chromosomes swayed and moved apart, cytoplasm separated, and two new cells were made from a buzz of organized activity. I could almost feel the energy coming from the intense cellular activity, and I asked my instructor how the cells "knew how to do what they do and how they remember what goes where?" I also remember his laugh as he answered, "They just do. There's no place in a cell for intelligence, if that's what you're asking. They are just tiny bags of cytoplasm."

Research is showing that my teacher may have been wrong. In order to prepare cells for viewing under a microscope, it is necessary to place them in a special fluid that keeps them stable enough to see. Because of the chemical used to allow me to view the inside of a cell, the true structure of a cell was essentially dissolved, and what I was seeing was only a foggy representation of the cell's actual activity. Now that a new fixative is used to look at cells that allows a much clearer and more detailed view of a cell's insides, one can see that they contain a network of structures called "microtubules," possible candidates for a place where a form of cellular memory may occur.

Anesthesiologist Stuart Hameroff, a professor in the Department of Anesthesiology, College of Medicine, at the University of Arizona Health Sciences Center in Tucson, Arizona, suggests that the cell's microtubules are perfectly designed information-processing devices. He suggests that these microtubules serve as a rudimentary nervous and circulatory system for the cell. Made up of hollow tubes latticed with kernel-like hexagons representing information, they serve as the cell's "info-energetic computers."[5] Like most scientists, Dr. Hameroff is interested primarily in brain cells, but all cells have microtubules that may act as a cell's own unique memory storage system.

There is as yet no conclusive evidence that microtubules have memory and compute and process information. Most scientists still assert that simple information is conveyed within a cell not by the info-energetic process I propose but exclusively by chemical signals. Dr. Hameroff argues, however, that it seems unlikely that the kind of information processing shown by a cell's activity can be conveyed as rapidly and accurately as it is through a bag of water or a sack of Jell-O.[6] It may be that cellular memories are not only neurochemical but also take place info-energetically at the level of the cell's microtubules.

CELLULAR CONSCIOUSNESS

Biologist Lynee Margulis describes the way cells function as a type of cellular consciousness, writing that even the simplest one-celled organisms such as protozoa and bacteria have what he calls "a simple consciousness."[7] Flowers, trees, dogs, chickens, quails, and humans all have cells that respond to sound and contain microtubules and other microscopic parts that may combine to constitute some form of cellular memory.

Perhaps you have experienced a form of your own cellular memories today. Perhaps something "in your heart" seemed to try to remind you that there is much more to life than the hectic daily life you lead? Perhaps you have felt a vague longing for "the good old days" when life seemed simpler, happier, more easygoing, and joyful. Even if you never actually had such a life, you may remember something about living more blissfully. When the hysteria of what author Jeremy Rifkin calls our "nanosecond culture" dies down for a few moments, perhaps you have sensed in your heart that you should be living in more healthy balance and returning to "how it used to be" even if it seems that "used to be" is for you "yet to be?"[8] Such vague memories may be the heart's code calling.

If information is carried in the energy of the heart and circulates within the cells, and if energy cannot be destroyed, whatever memories of a life experience anyone has ever had may be able to become our own individual memories. Unlike the more individual and personal information stored by your brain, cellular memories may be experienced as representations of universal, archetypical, infinitely shared memories that represent the collective unconscious. Beneath our stressed and busy life, our heart and the body's cells may have latent memories of a paradise lost, or what author Richard Heinberg calls "our shared paradisal infancy."[9]

No matter how hard we work and how pressured we feel, the subtle longing many of us seem to occasionally feel for a better, more connected, and joyfully blissful life may not just be the brain's own fond memories but also cellular memories experienced from within us as a call from a paradise lost. This lingering spiritual faith "re-Minds" us to let our heart back into the brain/body dialogue to re-create a full brain/heart/body Mind. By listening to our heart for the echoes of the "better," more sane way to live, it can retrieve the cellular memories that draw a map back to paradise.

SLIPS OF THE HEART

Even though we have become the pressured brain-children of an abusive father time, our cells have stored more than the memories of the modern fast-paced world we live in now. The info-energy from those who may have been much less rushed and more connected than we moderns may still influence us as cellular memories, a latent code left within us by our ancestors. Something of the great myth of a paradise lost that permeates every culture is still nipping at the heels of our racing brain and trying to get it to slow down to attend to what our cells remember longingly as a more pleasurable, loving existence.

Sometimes when we least expect it, our heart cries out about what it and its cells remember. Like the Freudian slips of our brain that betray our real thoughts, we can also experience parapraxes of our heart—those moments when we accidentally reveal our cellular memories. We sigh and speak from our heart to no one in particular, asking the brain why it seems to rush us so and make it so difficult to enjoy being fully alive in the present moment.

Philosopher Marsilio Ficino writes, "Those who are in a frenzy utter many wonderful things, which a little later, when their frenzy has abated, they themselves do not really understand, as if they had not spoke them but God had sounded through them as though through trumpets."[10] When we are most overwhelmed by working too hard and entranced by the hypnotic hassles of modern living, our heart may leave its own version of a hypnotic suggestion for a more sensible, blissful, balanced life.

More like a quiet violin than a trumpet, our heart softly utters a vague cellular memory to our brain. It may cause you to say out loud while you are stuck in a traffic jam and late for a meeting, "What is life for anyway?" "What am I doing to myself?" "I've got to be crazy to live like this," and "There's got to more to life than this." Instead of pausing to focus on our heart and responding to its subtle tap on our spiritual shoulder by slowing down and tuning in, our brain impatiently and helplessly shakes its head at what it has come to view as the inescapable necessity of running in the human race.

Our mother's heart and all hearts that have gone before ours have left traces of our safer, more restful paradisal infancy. There are cellular memories within us that can remind us of the importance of "being" and not just "doing," of how to lead a more blissful, heart-felt life, and that, contrary to the powerful protective evolational drive toward individuality contained within our brain, we are all One. To find these memories, we have to understand the difference between the brain's disenchanted short-term memories of the hectic world it has created for itself and the enchanted ancient remembrances of the heart. The brain one-sidedly caters to the evolutionary imperative of our cellular singularity. It neglects the heart's cellular memories also left within us as a loving legacy from those persons, places, and things that have gone before us and who were more enraptured and connected with their chance to live on planet paradise. If the brain is driven by its directive of survival of the fittest, the heart's code may be less a directive than a question, asking if we are fit to survive.

"CHAILS" AND "QUICKENS"

Imagine a quail that cackles and pecks exactly like a chicken and a chicken that sings and tilts its head exactly like a quail. Imagine that this happens because the quail received transplanted cells with the basic memories of "chickenness" and the chicken received transplanted cells with primary memories of "quailness." This is exactly the result of research by Dr. Evan

Balaban of the Neurosciences Institute in La Jolla, California. By extracting nervous system cells from chicken embryos and implanting them among quail embryo cells and vice versa, the result was the transfer of the cellular memories that constitute the habits of one species to another.[11] Even though it itself has never actually "been" one before, the quail "remembers" what it is like to be a chicken and a chicken "recalls" his quailhood. Dr. Balaban's work focuses on how characteristics of cells and related neurochemicals relate to various behaviors. While he does not directly address the "fowl cellular recollections" he is transposing, there are important implications of this type of research for understanding the concept of cellular memory.

WILL HUMANS OINK?

In a process called xenografting, more humans are having animal cells mixed with their own. Primate cells, particularly baboon cells, have been placed in humans for years, and now adult humans are having pig cells transplanted into their brains and pig heart valves sewn into their hearts. Sometime next year, the first pig heart is scheduled to be implanted in a human being. To reduce the severe rejection of animal tissue that is the biochemical reflex of our xenophobic cells' defensive clinging to their individuality, scientists are genetically preparing donor pigs and other animals by introducing human genes to pre-acquaint them with their future host.[12] It is likely that animal organ farms are not far off and that scientists will be harvesting animal organs to suit our human needs.

"We don't need to worry that if you have a porcine cell transplant you'll suddenly begin oinking," said Dr. Tom Murray, chairman of a genetics subcommittee of the National Bio-Ethics Advisory Committee. He added, however, that since we are indeed tampering in this work with the very thing that makes us who we are, "there are big ethical issues."[13] There is more to a pig than its oinking, and no one knows the complete implications of cross-species transplantation and what cellular memories if any could come along with a pig's tissue. While our anthropomorphism causes us to demean animals and use them as if they were put on earth for our pleasure, in our heart we know that animals are a part of the same nonlocal info-energetic system in which we live and as much a part of the making of our cellular memories as we are a part of theirs.

STARFISH, STARS, AND HUMAN CELLS

You have read that energy cardiology is based on "systemic memory," which asserts that the very nature of systems from stars to starfish to human cells is to store and share info-energy, and that memory occurs at all levels of cellular structure.[14] It asserts that information in the form of energy is stored, as it is in all systems, within all cells and molecules. Saying that memory could only be stored in brain cells and not all body cells is to impose a distinction that does not stand up to logic, current scientific evidence, or to our spiritual instincts that seem to make us able to remember in our heart and feel in our bones. If cardio-energetics is even partly right, then Dr. Murray's statement that there are "big ethical issues" involved when we merge cells of various systems is an understatement. There are also major spiritual and moral issues involved.

Whether our brain knows it or not, what has happened to any and all of us is forever within each of us. Dr. Balaban's "chails" and "quickens" represent much more than an interesting experiment by "higher" animals on their "lower" animal ecological associates. They are simple but preliminary examples of one of the most significant and important medical, physiological, psychological, and spiritual issues of the new millennium. All cells contain info-energetic memories, all of us from the simplest to the most complex share common cellular memories, all memories are forms of energy and therefore can never be destroyed, and what the cells remember is the code of the eternal collective soul as represented in this energy we share with everyone and everything.

Whether their cells are physically transplanted within us or not, starfish, the stars, chickens, quails, and pigs are a part of our cellular intelligence and we are a part of theirs. While it is obvious that the complexity and impact of cellular memories differ from a quail to a human, the info-energetic process involved is exactly the same. Every sound, touch, odor, and scene we and everyone and everything encounter becomes who we are by making deposits in our memory bank. The brain may not think so, but the heart knows so.

LISTENING CELLS

While most of our cellular memories take place on the quantum, nonlocal level, "L" energy also comes along with the more observable forms of energy. One example of how a cellular memory is made is related to the way sound energy works. The first embryonic cells are sound sensitive, and by four and one half months in the womb, a baby's auditory system is virtually complete. The mother's heartbeat is a major sound stimulus throughout a child's life in embryonic, fetal, early childhood, and on into and through adult development. Not only embryonic cells but every cell in our body registers and is influenced by the energy reflected in sound waves.[15] Since sound is energy and energy contains information, our cells' natural acoustical ability allows them to remember the tones of our life.

If you stop reading for a few minutes, sit quietly, focus on your heart, and listen, you may be able to "sense" some of the prior sounds of your life. This info-energy stored acoustically by your cells will not come to you through your ears to be processed by your brain. It will seem to "resonate from within you" and seem to play from your heart. You might feel vibrations and may even be able to feel its beat. You may "hear" with your heart a song or music that holds great significance in your life and may be able to hum along with a music the ears cannot hear. You may "hear" the cry of your baby who is now an adult child, the erotic echo of the voice of your lover moaning in ecstasy during an act of sexual intimacy that took place years ago, or the anguished sobs of a young playmate who shared a childhood fear with you in kindergarten. Once you "hear with your heart," you may find these acoustical cellular memories playing much like a jingle or musical phrase that keeps recycling within you throughout the day in the form of a cellular meme. (A "meme" is a small mental representation of cultural information, such as a commercial jingle, car design, clothing fashion, dance step, or simple phrase.)

MOLECULARIZED MEMORIES

From a psychological point of view, the concept of memory is one of the most fascinating aspects of nature. What we call memory seems to be everywhere and in everything, yet it itself is nowhere to be found. A memory is more like a hologram than a one-dimensional mental picture. It is "there" but you can't touch it and every part of it contains representations of the whole.

If you pause now and try to remember the eyes of someone you love, you will immediately also recall the complete image of that person. Search as they might, neuroscientists have been unable to find one major central memory center in the brain for even the most basic of human activities. In every case, our memories are constituted from a complex interaction of associations and translation of forms of energy to images, thoughts, feelings, interpretations.

Even though cardio-energetics sees a "memory" as an info-energetic discharge, a memory is no less "real" than a physical occurrence. One of the most loving suggestions coming from cardio-energetics is to try to "remember" (as our arm is a "member," attached to and a part of our body) and actively attend to making those we love a "member," or more a part of us, before they must become only a memory. Take time every day to be open to the energy those you love give off; let your heart receive that energy, store it, and recall it as often as you can. Look, listen, smell, touch, and feel with your heart those you love as profoundly and deeply as you can while the physical manifestation of their energy is still yours for the feeling. A love-map of everyone we have ever loved may be stored forever within us in a form of info-energy imprint, infinitely reverberating sounds and a set of subtle energetic patterns stored in our cells. The brain can forget, but the heart always remembers, so take time to get your brain to pay more attention to the memories your heart desires to make and to help it store an imprint of your loved ones.

The brain is very busy with its own memory system. It is less sensitive than the heart to the more subtle energetic memories. By putting our heart into remembering those we love every day, we are recovering cellular memories every bit as strongly as a heart transplant recipient recovers the memories of his or her donor. When we are loved, we are receiving an energetic transplant, and when we love, we donate our heart energy. When poets describe love as "giving our heart away," they are cardio-energetically correct.

THE SMELL OF HOME

The most commonly reported "cellular memories" described by heart transplant recipients are new smells and tastes related to those of their donor. Some scientists say such reports are merely related to the side-effects of drugs used to reduce rejection or other biomedical phenomena affecting the senses. Cardio-energetics, however, suggests that the donor-recipient correlation in these memories indicates that there is an "inside effect" and not just a "side effect" that is occurring. It is possible that the info-energy of any experience, including an odor, sound, and flavor, is stored on some level within all of the body's cells including the heart, and that these memories may come along with the cells of a transplanted heart.

"L" energy may be able to transmit not only its own subtle version of information about our life but also the various components of our senses that provide the various tones, odors, and tastes that allow for its magnificent artistry.

Our sense of smell is our oldest sense, followed by our sense of taste. If our ancestors could not smell a predator or taste what could poison them, we would not be here now. It may be because our sense of smell and taste are so old, so basic, and so fundamental to our humanhood that memories on this level are the most easily retrieved by heart recipients from the cells of their donor.

What we sense as a smell is really the energy given off by a substance that stimulates the neural receptors in our nose. When we breathe in, we inhale molecules and the info-energy within them through our nose and up through the opening in the palate at the back of our throat. From there, the molecular memory packets make direct contact with our brain. Olfactory neurons, each of which is replaced every month or two, are tiny hairlike fibers that, like the receptors on all body cells, have receptors specially made to respond to specific smell molecules. Unlike all other neural fibers, the axons of your nose extend directly into your brain to an olfactory area and the region that is involved in our most basic emotional memories, including the hippocampus ("Oh, I remember that smell!) and the amygdala ("And I remember it makes me sick!").[16] Because the brain is in direct contact with the smell molecules and because its smell-sensing area is also the brain's primary emotional area, smell molecules become what we call an "odor" that elicits and becomes some of our most primal memories. On this oldest and most basic human sense level, an object transmits its info-energetic code, is turned into a cellular memory, and we not only sense our environment but become it.

Here is one example of an olfactory cellular memory. "When I smell turkey cooking, I feel at home. I remember Grandma and sometimes I start to cry. I remember her cooking our Christmas turkey, the presents she gave us, and I can see her smiling and smacking Grandpa's hand when he tried to sneak a sample before it was ready. And when I look at my pictures of Grandma, I can almost smell the odor of turkey cooking and it warms my heart."

I have not found that my heart transplant recipients actually experience a change in their "sense" of smell or taste. What they do report are changes in odor (smell interpretation) and flavor (the meaning we give to our senses of taste). Memories are much more than brain-cell stimulation and reactions of our basic five senses. They are how our heart senses, interprets, understands, and experiences our world. Everything we have ever tasted, smelled, touched, heard, or seen is recirculated within us as info-energy by our heart, and the heart's cells themselves pick up energetic memories of these events. It is not surprising then that, on at least some level, with a new heart comes a whole new set of memories.

THE TASTE OF LOVE

Our sense of taste (gustation) results from the stimulation of special receptors in the mouth. My transplant recipients still report the same four primary taste qualities of sweet, salty, sour, and bitter, but some of them report that how these four qualities of a substance are combined, interpreted, smelled, felt, and look change after they receive their new heart. They experience a change in "flavor," that is, in the way the basic taste senses are combined into a gustational memory.[17]

Here's an example of a "taste cellular memory" from one of the cardio-sensitives. "It's really strange, but when I'm cleaning house or just sitting around reading, all of a sudden this unusual taste comes to my mouth. It's very hard to describe, but it's very distinctive. I can taste something and all of a sudden I start thinking about my donor, who he or she is, and how they lived. After a while, the taste goes away and so do the thoughts, but the taste always seems to come first."

Instead of dismissing the cellular memories of heart transplant patients as less important because they are "only" changes in taste and flavor, we should consider the fact that these changes reflect a primal connection and very basic recall of memories from these energy-stimulated systems as activated and deeply encoded in their donors' cells. Just as a mother knows well the unique taste and smell of her own child, our most basic senses carry cellular memories within them that translate to our emotions.

MANY MEMORIES

Despite the fact that memory has been accepted as a concept for centuries, direct study of memory as a human function did not begin in earnest until the 1960s. Cognitive psychologists now study memory through what they call an information-processing approach, meaning how the brain thinks about its world.[18] Cardio-energetics speaks in connective terms such as shared energy, information, reverberation, and vibration, but cognitive psychologists speak in computer terms such as encoding, storage, and retrieval.

Psychologists see memory as taking place in a neuro-cellular system somehow represented in a complex matrix somewhere within the brain. While this is a convenient way of discussing memory, it is another example of what happens when the brain studies itself and claims for itself almost any function to which it turns its attention. Author Ambrose Bierce cynically described bioscience's brain bias when he defined the word "mind" as a "mysterious form of matter secreted by the brain." He identified its primary function as "the endeavor to ascertain its own nature, the futility of the attempt being due to the fact that it has nothing but itself to know itself with." When memory is seen purely and exclusively as taking place only in the neurons of the brain, cellular memories reported by heart transplant recipients seem absurd. When it is acknowledged that all cells have a form of shared info-energetic memory and that the heart also thinks, feels, and remembers, the recall of memories from heart donors and systemic cellular memories become possible.

Bierce may have been more insightful than satirical by referring to a "mysterious form of matter secreted by the brain." He may have unknowingly been describing the info-energy contained in the neuropeptides and other substances found in the brain that have now also been discovered all over the body. Bierce was wrong, however, when he said that the brain has only itself to know itself with. The brain also has a heart to help it make up its brain/heart/body Mind and to help it recover a much more meaningful and wider range of memories. If the brain is allowed to forget that it has a heart, and ignores its energy memory system to focus only on itself, we will never have a fully developed theory of memory that takes into account the complex nature of the info-energy posited by energy cardiology.[19]

THE THREE MEMORIES PLUS ONE

In order to distinguish "cellular memories" from modern psychology's view of memories, it is helpful to understand the currently accepted Western psychology theory of memory called the "Modal Model." According to this model, only three distinct memory systems exist.

As proposed by psychologists Richard Atkinson and Robert Shiffren, one type of memory is called "sensory memory."[20] This type of memory serves as a temporary storage system for basic information brought in from our basic five senses. For example, when someone waves a flashlight in a dark room, we perceive trails of light behind it called "icons." This "iconic memory" also exists for sounds, odors, and flavors that linger in our memory long after their physical source is removed. According to this theory, our eyes, ears, and other physical senses have their own unique, individual forms of limited sensory memory. As you have read, however, even our most basic sensory memory is a process of converting the molecules of matter to the "waves" of energy that contain information. Cardio-insensitive heart transplant patients who are reluctant to consider the possibility of cellular memories often report memories of their donor in the form of "iconic" flashes of involuntary, spontaneous associations to their donor.

The second mode of memory is short-term memory, or "STM." This is a system that holds small amounts of information for brief periods of time—usually four to seven seconds. Research in human time perception shows that what we consciously define as a "present moment" is also about four to seven seconds, or what scientists call a "quantum period."[21] "Quantum period" time frame of reference is the period used for retaining phone numbers for immediate redialing. A "quantum period" seems limited by the rule of the "magical number seven plus or minus two."[22] In other words, our STM is limited to seven items or brain-bits of information at one time, so it is no coincidence that phone companies restrict their basic numbers to seven digits and Snow White only had to remember the names of seven dwarfs. Less cardio-sensitive heart transplant recipients often report such brief quantum moment spurts of association with their donor in the form of what they feel to be unexplainable images, daydreams, and brief and often distracting new thoughts and fantasies.

The third "mode" of memory identified by psychologists is long-term memory that can hold vast amounts of information for long periods of time. Whether the recall of heart donor memories is a simple iconic after-image memory that clears over time (sensory and perceptual), a brief association as quickly forgotten as a meaningless phone number (simple recall), or a lasting mental imprint (remembering something or someone by "heart") may in part be due to the type of memory system employed.

FLASHBULB MEMORIES

One category of long-term memory is called "flashbulb memory," referring to major life events that leave a lingering "afterimage" or mental impression. Most of us can recall exactly where we were at the time of a major historical event. Because of the brain's built-in negativity and pessimism, it seems that this is particularly true for traumatic events. While these flash-bulb memories are easy to retrieve, they are not necessarily accurate.[23] When subjects were asked to recall a tragic event such as the assassination of President John Kennedy, Martin Luther King, or the *Challenger* space shuttle explosion, the details they reported associated with the event, such as a robin flying by just when they heard the bad news, later proved to be in error.[24]

Another difficulty with long-term memory is that the very act of trying (racking one's "brain") to recall an event can enhance the sense of having experienced it, whether or not it actually happened.[25] It is possible that, by being asked to tune in to cellular memories of a donor of an organ, a patient can create a set of false memories. Although it is not always possible to do so, in those cases of my heart transplant recipients' recovery of cellular memories of their donor, the details they provided could be confirmed by donor families.

Although long-term memory of tragic events may be flawed and trying to remember something can cause false memories, long-term memory can also be one of the most impressive of human endeavors. Author George Marek gives an example of a bassoonist in conductor Arturo Toscanini's orchestra approaching the great maestro to inform him that the lowest note on his bassoon was broken. Toscanini thought for a moment and then replied, "It is all right; that note does not occur in tonight's concert."[26] The maestro was able to scan through every movement of every piece of the songs on the program to determine the absence of one note among the thousands. It seems likely that the cardio-sensitive heart recipients are capable of such impressive recall.

As crucial as sensory and short-term memory are to daily survival and as impressive as long-term memory may be in our life, cardio-energetics suggests that there is an even more profound fourth memory system that incorporates all three of these processes and yet transcends them. It suggests that memory is not limited to the two body systems most scientists are willing to agree have a memory—the nervous system and immune system. In addition to the immune system's cell's memories and nervous system's sensory, short- and long-term memory, cardio-energetics proposes a "spiritual" or info-energetic memory made especially to store "fifth force," or "L" energy, events.

You have read that energy cardiology views energy and information as ubiquitous processes in nature that are inseparably tied to the existence of all objects, people, and systems.[27] It says that we not only store words, images, and events in the brain but also store the information contained in the energy of every person, place, or thing. This is the essence of our most profound cellular memory, the sensations and feelings of events and persons no longer present, and cardio-energetics shows how the heart, because of its central role as our primary "L" energy body, is our primary cellular memory maker and recoverer.

THE ANGEL IN YOUR CHEST

Charles Siebert is a medical writer who has contributed many insightful, sensitive, and scientifically accurate articles concerning various health issues. In preparation for his *New York Times Magazine* story about one woman's heart transplant experience, he had the opportunity to attend a Valentine's Day party held for more than one hundred heart transplant recipients. Almost every recipient reported "spiritual memories," or feelings of the energy of their donor. Siebert writes, "All the people I met at the party spoke in the same reverent tones about the angel in their chests, about this gift, this responsibility they now bear, and the little prayer they say to the other person inside them. It was as if they were part of some strange new cult, the tribe of the transplanted."[28]

No one forgets that they have another person's heart in their chest, and Siebert acknowledges that no matter how hard we try to see the heart as "just a pump," every heart transplant recipient seemed to "re-inform themselves with a larger spiritual significance."[29] Re-informing oneself with the larger spiritual significance of our existence is a good cardio-energetics definition of cellular memory.

Unlike recipients of other donor tissues, every heart transplant patient I have interviewed, cardio-sensitive or not, and no matter how many years past their transplant, still talks to their new heart in some way and reports some form of spiritual imprint of their donor. One patient identified by Siebert, a fifty-three-year-old woman, one year post-transplant, said of her donor, "I had a talk with her the night after my surgery. I said, 'I hope you're not a sleepwalker.' " The memory of their donor seems there for the having for every person who receives the most precious gift, and from their example and experiences all of us can learn to recover our own forms of cellular memories from the many energetic donors who have come into our lives.

SOME OTHER POSSIBLE SOURCES FOR CELLULAR MEMORIES

Heart mediated "L" energy stored within the body's cells is not the only possible explanation for the process underlying what I am calling "cellular memories." Here are a few of the current alternative explanations regarding how info-energy may be conveyed from one person to another in the organ transplant process.

The "Little Brain in the Heart" Theory: Recent research in neurocardiology shows that the heart has its own intrinsic nervous system. It has recently been discovered that "intrinsic cardiac adrenergic" (ICA) cells in the heart synthesize and release catecholamines—neurochemicals such as dopamine and other substances previously thought to exist only in the brain. Perhaps this type of cardio-nervous system accounts for cellular memory.

Neuropeptide Theory: There are strings of amino acids called neuropeptides that float throughout the body and convey information by attaching themselves where they find a "lock," or cellular receptor, suited to their code. When lock and key match, the door is open for the info-energy of our emotions to be released. These sixty or more known neuropeptides stimulate an electrical charge in neurons, creating an info-energy template (a memory). Neuropeptides have also been found in the heart, so this could explain some forms of cellular memories reported by heart transplant recipients.[30]

The Magnetic Field Theory: Cells in the heart have a unique magnetic property and respond to and interact with magnetic fields. There may be an as yet undiscovered electromagnetic connection between the brain and heart expressed in a form of energy that contains some level of cellular memories.

Electrophysiological Theory: Groundbreaking creative research regarding the power of the heart and its role in our emotional, physical, and spiritual health has been going on for years at the Institute of HeartMath in Boulder Creek, California. Researchers there have used a process called "power spectral density analysis" of heart-rate variability and shown that "autonomic sympathovagal regulation"—focusing quietly and attentively on the heart—can help the heart relax and send a more balanced energy through the body, which results in enhanced immune function and may facilitate sensitivity to systemically stored energetic memories.[31]

Unprepared Spirit Theory: I have interviewed four "healers" who described themselves as "spiritual mediums" or "channelers." They speculated that the energy connection I have reported between heart recipient and donor is due to the presence of a the donor's spirit that has not yet moved on to "another plane" or "infinity." They said that it was possible that, since donated hearts usually come from young people who have experienced a terrible and unexpected sudden end to their physical lives, their spirits were not ready to "move on" and therefore continue to express themselves through the heart recipient.

The Surprised Heart Theory: As an extension of the "unprepared spirit" theory of cellular memories, two of the "spiritual mediums" I interviewed suggested another explanation for cellular memories. They said that, because of the suddenness of the death of most donors, the donor's spirit may not yet have realized that its body is actually dead. The transplanted heart keeps acting as if it were in its former body, not realizing its original owner is gone.

Morphic Resonance Theory: English scientist Rupert Sheldrake does not accept the "cellular memory" or "heart's energy" theory as an explanation for the reports of donor recall from heart transplant recipients. He says he sees no way cells could "remember" and suggests instead that the recipient is tuning in to what he calls "morphic fields," or "invisible infinite nonlocal organizing fields" that connect everything and everyone in ways we do not yet understand. It is possible that a new heart and healthier heart allows the recipient to better tune in to these fields.[32]

Reincarnation Theory: At a meeting of "psychic healers," I talked with three presenters at that meeting who felt that my ideas about cardio-energetics were wrong. They felt that what I was hearing from the heart transplant patients was simply evidence of some form of infinite continuation and connection between the souls of the living and the dead and that the recipient was a vehicle for the traveling soul of the donor that was reappearing in the recipient.

Hospital Grapevine Theory: Many nurses I have spoken to about cardio-energetics suggest that what I am calling "cellular memory" is really a manifestation of messages picked up by the recipient about the donor from discussions by various health-care staff who have worked with the recipient. Some nurses suggested this may even occur "telepathically" and beyond the recognition of staff and patient.

Psychometry Theory: At meetings of psychic healers, I have been told that physical objects can absorb the energy of the persons who have been near them. Some "psychics" suggested that the heart of the donor is an "object" that is imbued with the psychic energy of the donor much as a ring or other object can carry the energy of the owner. Biologist Lyall Watson suggested that physical items with which we are in intimate contact can indeed take on our emotional fingerprints and store our thoughts and feelings. If plants and inanimate objects can store our feelings and thoughts, it is possible that our body organs, which are most intimately connected to us, also contain our emotional imprints.

The Acorn Theory: Author James Hillman suggests that a central and guiding force rests within all of us formed by a spiritual image that calls us to our life destiny. It is possible that the transplanted heart is a not-so-tiny acorn implanted in new terrain to burst forth its info-energy in the form of a new calling from the soul of the recipient.

The "Manifestation of Nonlocal Consciousness" Theory: Physician Larry Dossey doubts that the heart is some form of "character-recording device" that gets put in a new body and plays its messages much like a phone answering machine. He, like many scientists willing to explore the issue of nonlocal subtle energy connections, is concerned about the credibility and acceptability to modern science of "energy healers" and others in alternative and complimentary medicine who speak of "sending" and "receiving" some form of mystical energy. He suggests that like all of us, heart donor and recipient are united nonlocally by a shared consciousness and that the intensity of the transplant experience may serve to magnify and focus the reality of that nonlocal connection.[33]

The "Lowered Recall Threshold" Theory: Some transplant surgeons suggest that reports of associations to donor experiences provided by some heart transplant recipients is due to the strong medications used to reduce rejection. It is also possible that these drugs act as psychotropic stimulants that lower the perceptual threshold of the patient, allowing them to recall all kinds of memories they would otherwise have forgotten, and that transplant recipients are really recalling their own memories of their own life experiences.

The above explanations for the retrieval of the info-energy stored as cellular memories by heart transplant recipients (and other organ recipients to a lesser degree) do not exclude the Systemic Memory Hypothesis offered by Drs. Linda Russek and Gary Schwartz that I suggest explains much of the nature of cellular memories and the existence of the heart's code that helps make them. I suspect that each of the above explanations has its own merit and validity and, like the blind men touching an elephant, the proponents of each theory are in touch with various aspects of the same subtle energy phenomenon.

Instead of exclusively following the brain's way of thinking and trying to determine "which" if any of the above explanations of cellular memory are "right," the way of the heart is to consider "how" all of them might interact to explain how cells may collectively remember who and how we are. By being open to the possibility that cells remember, and that these memories may be deeply registered as a template of our soul, we may be able to understand more about what we often call "our basic temperament."

The Temperamental Heart

"Tell me, where is fancy bred, in the heart or in the head."

—*SHAKESPEARE,* THE MERCHANT OF VENICE,

ACT 3, SCENE 2

SHARING THE SAME HEART

In very rare circumstances, it is possible for a heart transplant recipient to talk with the person whose heart they received. Through a process called domino transplantation, a patient with failing lungs receives a combination of a new heart and lungs from someone who has died, and donates his healthy heart to another person. (Because the heart and lungs function as one unit, and to reduce the chances of rejection, a heart-lung transplant is the preferred approach for some patients.) When I met two men who had taken part in this process, I learned much about how cellular memories and the "L" energy of the heart may play an important role in basic temperament, one's natural disposition or style of interacting with the world.

Two years ago, while lecturing at an international organ recipients' meeting, I met two men who had shared the same heart. A man I will call Jim had nearly died from cystic fibrosis, an uncommon hereditary disease in which the glands in the lining of the lung's bronchial tubes malfunction. While the lungs of a cystic fibrosis patient can deteriorate, their heart sometimes remains strong, so Jim received a healthy heart and lungs from a donor, and donated his healthy heart to a man named Fred. Fred had suffered a severe infection of his heart muscle and was brought back from the brink of death at the last moment by the gift of Jim's heart. Based on their conversation, it seemed that at least to some degree, Fred had not only received Jim's heart but also a large portion of Jim's personality.

I had read about a similar case just months before, and was amazed when I had the chance to meet with Jim and his wife, Sandra, and Fred and his wife, Karen, two couples who had experienced the impact domino transplantation firsthand.[1] Based on my previous interviews with heart transplant recipients, I was not surprised when Fred told Jim that the new food cravings he had experienced since getting Jim's heart had persisted and that Jim verified that these had been his own preferences before his transplant. I was startled, however, when the two men and their wives talked at length about a much more important and enduring phenomenon regarding the possibility of a heart's code, the transplantation of temperament.

Jim, Fred, and their wives all agreed that there were significant changes in the dispositions of both men following their transplants. Since Fred now had Jim's heart, Jim and his wife could confirm that Fred's new personality traits did in fact seem to correspond strongly with Jim's prior temperament. "My Fred got a personality transplant," said his wife Karen. While it's true that the rare and anecdotal nature of this meeting between two men who had lived part of their lives with the same heart does not constitute conclusive evidence of transfer of temperament in the form of cellular memory, it does offer additional evidence of the need for more understanding of the role the heart and cells play beyond life maintenance.

HOT AND COLD RUNNING HEARTS

"Fred has always been the most easygoing, laid back, cool-headed, carefree man I have ever known," said Fred's wife, Karen. "He was never like most of the other men waiting for transplants that we met in the hospital whose type A behavior seemed to have damaged their hearts. But now I'd say Fred's a real go-getter, even an A plus. He's moving all the time, and although he almost never did before, he loses his temper much more easily. I'd say he's gone from a cool head to a hot head."

"It looks like your husband got my Jim's hot heart," laughed Jim's wife, Sandra. "Even though he had trouble breathing and was sick a lot, Jim has always been like a buzz saw cutting through life. He would blow up at anybody who got in his way, drove his car like it was a weapon, and hardly ever had time for anything but work. Now, I hardly know him anymore. Not that I'm complaining. He is just much cooler and calmer. He does seem to get depressed much more and very suddenly without explanation. Of all things, he sends me flowers almost every month. He used to say flowers were a waste of good money, but now I think he likes them more than I do. At least you guys know where Fred's heart came from. I'd sure like to know whose heart Jim got and I'd like to shake his family's hand."

"I don't want to embarrass you, Sandra," said Karen in a suddenly softer voice. "Nobody would believe it, but for months Fred would say the name Sandy when we made love. I could have killed him. He said I was hearing things and he still denies it, but when he was really passionate, he used to say Sandy."

With a red face, Sandra leaned toward Karen and whispered, "Jim always calls me Sandra, but in bed he calls me Sandy." As Jim blushed and took his wife's hand, Sandra added, "In fact, since the transplant he never says my name at all, but he is much more romantic and much less macho. I'd say he donated his type A heart and got a type B version."

My audio tape ran out as the stories of what seemed to be evidence of a temperament transplant went on and on. Years after that meeting, I was able to trace the donor of Jim's heart and meet with her family. As Sandra now knows, her husband, Jim, received the heart of a young woman from New York. Her family said she was prone to depression throughout her life, was shy and soft-spoken, had worked part-time in a flower shop, and had taken her own life in despair over a lost love.

Jim died last year and Fred, as many heart transplant recipients seem to become, is now very reluctant to speak about his feelings regarding Jim's heart. Jim died of a respiratory infection without knowing who his donor was, and Sandra reported that he had remained prone to what she called his "transplanted depression" until the day of his death. Fred's wife, Karen, reported that, even though Fred avoids almost any discussion of his transplant and becomes angry when pushed to explore his feelings about it, she can "see Jim's temperament in Fred more and more."

A SOURCE OF TEMPERAMENT

If energy is information and info-energy is who and how we are, it is possible that, to some degree, the information contained and conveyed within the energy of the heart constitutes a major portion of our temperament. What we tend to call "temperament" may be physical manifestations of an info-energetic constellation of our cellular memories, a projection of the heart's code expressed by the brain and its body.

Can "who we are," our encoded info-energetic temperament, be transplanted? How much of our heart energy is uniquely our own and developed through our life experiences, and how much comes from our parents or seeps into our own heart energetically from other hearts to affect our own temperament? What kind of energy does an angry or a loving temperament resonate within and send from us, and what can all of us learn about the origins of our own temperament and personality from the experiences of the cardio-sensitives who are confronted with a massive info-energy infusion? What are the health implications of temperament, particularly for the heart?

DIFFERENT PEAS FROM THE SAME POD

Psychologists define temperament as the stable individual differences in the quality or intensity of emotional reactions.[2] One of the most careful studies of temperament was conducted by psychologists Arthur Thomas, Stella Chess, and Harold Birch in 1970.[3] They followed the development of children from several weeks old through ten years of age. Using observation, interviews with parents and teachers, and psychological tests, they concluded that children do show individuality in temperament in their first weeks of life independent of their parents' handling.[4]

Ask any parent of more than one child if her children seem to be of different temperaments and you will usually get an affirmative answer. No matter how much we might try to be equal opportunity parents, children from the same parents still seem to behave differently. They seem to give off a different energy, react more or less intensely to stimulation, and seem to be "easy" or "more difficult" to deal with. No matter how similar in intellectual brightness and how many common family gestures and ways of speaking they may share, they also seem to manifest their own unique way of being in the world that I suggest are the public display of their preformed cellular memories.

One of my patients, a thirty-two-year-old mother, described the impact of temperamental differences between siblings. She said, "My two boys look like two peas in a pod, but I think they must have come from two different pods. They are one year apart in age and miles apart in temperament. We raised them the same way, but they just seem to be preprogrammed differently."

COMPONENTS OF TEMPERAMENT

The dimensions of temperament identified in the Thomas, Chess, and Birch study included what most of us consider the key components of our personality: general activity level, rhythmicity of biological functions such as eating and sleeping, the ease and comfort with approaching strangers, tendency to be withdrawn or shy, adaptability to change, threshold of reactivity, intensity of reactivity to stimulation, quality of dominant mood, distractibility, attention span, and persistence.[5]

Three general types of temperament emerged from their study. One temperament was described as the "easy child" orientation, not unlike that shown before his transplantation by the calm and laid-back Fred. The "easy child" temperament constituted 40 percent of the group studied and included characteristics such as a generally pleasant mood, spontaneity, high adaptability, dealing easily with people, and an established regular pattern of sleeping and eating.

A second group identified was the "difficult child" temperament, not unlike that of the more type A Jim. This group constituted about 10 percent of the sample and tended toward agitation and unpleasantness, high reactivity to new situations and people, intense and quick emotional reactions, and irregularity of sleeping and eating patterns.

A third group of about 5 percent had the temperament of the "slow-to-warm-up child" who tended to be more withdrawn, slow to adapt to change, and often negative in mood. The remaining 35 percent were too inconsistent in their characteristics to be categorized. Thomas, Chess, and Birch found that these three categories of temperament, what might be seen as soft-hearted, hard-hearted, and sad-hearted codes, persisted for most children regardless of parental upbringing and life experiences. Temperament, then, may in part be a type of encoded info-energy circulated within a person by the heart and stored within in the cellular memory system from the moment of conception.

WHEN "BAD" KIDS HAPPEN TO GOOD PARENTS

Identical twins present a natural experiment when it comes to understanding the possibility of cellular memories manifested as temperamental patterns (personality) and the possibility of subtle, nonlocal energy connection. If identical twins reared apart differ behaviorally, psychologically, or physically in significant ways, then nurturing and parental behavior would seem to be more important than inherited cellular memories. If, however, the twins remain identical in behavior after being separated at birth, there is evidence that encoded temperament and "L" energy connection may play a role in who and how we are.

In the late 1970s I was formulating my ideas and conducting interviews regarding the heart's code and cellular memories. I was sure that we are not born as philosopher John Locke's version of psychological blank slates. I was convinced that, in addition to the biochemical and genetic codes within us, we are also manifestations of and connected by uniquely subtle "L" energy signatures that help create our temperament irrespective of how we are raised.

My clinical work revealed not only that my transplant patients were experiencing various degrees of personality changes but that many adopted children and adults reported varying degrees of recollections regarding their biological mother; that many adoptive families struggle with basic temperamental, energetic differences between themselves and their adopted child that their most well-intended and intensive efforts seem unable to resolve; that from the moment the newborn peeks her head from the canal, mothers sense and report basic differences in their babies; and that the best, hardest working, and most caring of parents often can have the most miserably moody of children while the most neglectful and unhappy parents can be blessed with the most loving, cooperative child. It was clear that what my patients were telling me did not jibe with the still widely accepted view that it is the interaction of the parents' molding of the child along with the strong influence of genetic coding that is the sole determinant in personality development. I had a lot of prior training in the crucial role genes and parental influence play on the personality development of the child, particularly the role of the mother. Nevertheless, I was learning that it is quite likely that, in addition to being born with a DNA code that is refined to a comparatively small extent through parent influence and environmental modifications, we are also born with a cellular-stored info-energetic template. No matter what our parents, school, or society does to or for us, this template keeps getting drummed through us by our heart and nonlocally across space and time from heart to heart.

While doing my early interviews regarding cellular memories, I was chief of a psychiatric clinic in the Department of Psychiatry at Sinai Hospital in Detroit and an adjunct assistant professor in the Department of Psychiatry and Behavioral Neurosciences at the Wayne State University School of Medicine. The chairman, faculty of the medical school, the entire staff of my department and my own staff, and most of my colleagues were psychoanalytically and biochemically trained. They were convinced that parental genetic code, and perhaps more importantly parental upbringing, were everything when it came to personality development. My views about a thinking heart, "L" energy, and cellular memory were met not only with severe skepticism, but with often angry attacks and unwillingness to accept what they referred to as "a throwback to medieval physiology." When I spoke of the cellular memories from donors that seem to be indicated in the reports of early transplant recipients, and that their temperament or personality seem to be altered in general correlation with those of their donor, my few early reports were relegated to the usual scientific dumping ground for the unexplained—chance. I was tiring of the attacks, doubting my own thinking, and considering going along with the traditional emphasis on nurture over nature and the scientific position that subtle energy templates and cellular memory were pure science fiction. Then I read an article in the prestigious scientific journal *Smithsonian* and a related article in the equally respected journal *Science* that described the "Jim Twins." Based on that article, I realized I wasn't the only person discovering these kinds of findings and felt encouraged to go on with my research.

LESSONS FROM THE "JIM TWINS"

In 1979, identical twins Jim Springer and Jim Lewis were reunited at age thirty-nine after being separated at birth and placed in different homes in Ohio.[6] Here are just some of the remarkable similarities between these identical twins that lends support to the influence and manifestation of temperamental cellular memories and nonlocal energetic connection.[7]

- Both twins had been named James by their adoptive family.
- They had each been married twice, the first time to women named Linda and the second time to wives named Betty.
- They each named one of their sons James Alan.
- They each had owned a dog they named Toy.

• They both reported a preference for Miller Lite beer, chain-smoked Salem cigarettes, and drove Chevrolets.

• They each enjoyed the hobby of carpentry, which they practiced in similar basement workshops, making similar things.

• They both disliked baseball and said they were stock-car racing buffs.

• They had each served as sheriff's deputies in their respective communities.

• They each severely chewed their fingernails.

• Each was reported by their spouses to be very demonstrative in their affection and to constantly be leaving love notes around the house.

• They had voted identically in three prior presidential elections.

• Both said they were present oriented rather than past or future oriented.

• Both had taken several vacations to the same beach area in Florida.

• Their blood pressure, weight, pulse rates, and sleep patterns were nearly identical.

• Both had suffered from hemorrhoids, had put on an extra ten pounds at the same time in their life, had undergone a vasectomy, had identical brain-wave patterns in reaction to stress, and suffered from tension and migraine headaches that usually began in the late afternoons and had begun to occur in their life at age eighteen.

The list documenting the Jims' sameness goes on, but one finding reported in the journals that did not receive much attention fascinated me the most. Though medical tests could not confirm it, each Jim felt that, at about the same time in their lives, they had had a heart attack. They said they had felt something strange and disturbing that bothered them about their heart. Cardio-energetics suggests that their hearts, as my own did during my cancer, may have been "aching" to tell them something.

While the Jims seem to show great similarity on the major components of temperament, there is much we do not understand that represents a very unique and permanent bond that manifests itself between separated identical twins. That a bond exists beyond the known measurable energies has long been reflected in the concern with the seemingly magical connections between twins described in myth.[8] The lesson from twins for cardio-energetics, however, is that if the Jims could remain so profoundly energetically connected despite their separation, any of us may be able to become more aware of our potential for connection beyond time and space. Identical twins, like cardio-sensitive heart transplant recipients, may give evidence of an energetic connection that any of us may be able to experience if can learn to tap into the heart's code. While few of us may have the strong impetus of having had the same maternal heart creating bonding cellular memories, we may all be heart "L" energy transplant recipients and donors through the constant exchange of subtle info-energy. We may all be, to some as yet to be determined extent, info-energetic twins bonded together heart to heart by the same nonlocal energy that flowed between the Jim twins.

There is another lesson from studies of identical twins raised apart that has significance for cardio-energetics. Twin researchers now know that identical twins reared apart are *more* identical than twins raised together.[9] Free of the struggle to differentiate and create an individually unique identity, which is experienced by many identical twins reared together, the info-energetic bond that exists between all identical twins may be free to play itself out when the brain is not incessantly focused on the "me."

TRACES OF A PRENATAL ENERGY BATH

Energy cardiology asserts that a developing fetus is literally bathed in the cardiac energy generated by the mother's heart. If the heart's energy can travel nonlocally between hearts, cardio-energetic influences from the father and others close to the mother may also contribute to a lesser extent to a temperament template established very early in the child's development.[10]

Physicians often consider the energy recorded by the mother's electrocardiogram to be a distracting artifact to be overcome in the study of the developing child. Energy cardiology suggests that this "artifact" may instead be a fact of life that reveals a symbiotic sharing of cardiac energy and an info-energetic exchange between mother and child that contributes strongly to the neonatal info-energy that becomes the child's temperament. In effect, every child is born with an "inner elder" that lives within her for her entire existence.

OPEN-HEART PSYCHOLOGY

Columbia-Presbyterian Medical Center nurse and energy healer Julie Motz has helped hundreds of heart patients through their surgery and rehabilitation. She confirms the speculations of energy cardiology regarding the possibility of temperamental imprints carried within the heart and passed on to the child. She reports that she has worked with many patients who seem to be carrying the energy of their mothers' heart inside their own hearts.[11] She speculates that, if there is a distortion or constriction of the energy of the mother's heart, particularly in the form of grief or sorrow, this distortion can weaken the fetus' heart and may manifest itself later in the form of cardiac disease. She reports that some of her patients report feeling the weight of the mother's heart within their own.

Motz employs a technique commonly used in movement therapy to test the cardio-energetics hypothesis that the heart can communicate with other hearts and that cardio-imprints exert lasting influence on our lives. She asks cardiac patients to move one of their arms as if the movement were energized and originated from their own hearts. She then asks her patients to try to sense the energy stored in their cells by their mother's or father's heart and to move their arm from that orientation. Motz reports, "What is so striking about this exercise is that the movement representing the heart patients' own hearts," which she says is usually rigid and re-stricted, "invariably corresponds to the constricted, limited heart of one of their parents who may suffer from heart disease."[12]

I have found the same general results as Motz in my own work with heart patients at Sinai and Beaumont Hospitals in Detroit, Michigan. I asked my patients scheduled for open-heart surgery if they would try a little open-heart psychology and try to "tune in" to their heart's code by sensing it and drawing a picture of it. Most patients easily do this and they often draw what appears as bloated, distorted, solid-looking hearts and color them black or brown. When I asked them to draw their mother's or father's heart, invariably one of the parental hearts looks almost exactly like their own. There seems to be some association that is maintained heart to heart between child and parent.

In my work with heart patients, I have never had one patient who could not tell me how both of their parents' hearts "felt to them" in their present life. While they may not always use the word "energy" or trace their temperament directly to their heart, they report that they feel that a part of their temperament is the direct result of their mother's, and to a lesser extent, their father's, temperament.

THE CHILD AS MOTHER TO THE WOMAN

When I ask biologically related families to draw a "heart portrait" in which all of the hearts of everyone in the home are depicted, all of the hearts appear somewhat similar in size, color, and shape. When I ask stepfamilies to draw a "cardio-portrait," the hearts appear more dissimilar than similar in shape and color, with the children's drawing of their heart resembling more that of their biological parent. The heart drawn by adopted children often appears quite different from the hearts drawn by the rest of the family. While these findings could also be attributed to the general emotional dynamics within families, it is also possible that some heart-to-heart relationship is involved.

The fetus' heart also influences the heart of the mother and less so the father. The possibility of "L" energy radiated from the embryo may help explain the creation of an energetic dialogue and information feedback system that contributes to the creation of not only the temperament of the child but changes in temperament of the mother, the father, and the entire family when a new heart emerges among old hearts.

FAMILY LESSON FROM TUNING FORKS

Every new heart added to a family brings with it its own unique contribution to the info-energetic dialogue of the family system. When two tuning forks resonate together, each fork's vibrations becomes a part of the other's memory. Each fork than expresses the memory of its interaction with the other in its next vibration, and when a third fork is added, the vibrational memory making becomes even more complex and continues in what energy cardiology pioneers Drs. Schwartz and Russek call a dynamic memory system. When the heart (what may be seen as the body's tuning fork) resonates and sends out its "L" energy to resonate with all family members' hearts, the family system is being constantly energetically re-created, as influenced by the unique "temperamental tone" contributed by each heart.

If one person is an info-energetic system of 75 trillion cells vibrating as coordinated by the heart, a family of four is 300 trillion cells and four hearts all resonating with the immense energy that makes a family "nuclear." Like individual family members, all families have their own unique collective temperament that is an info-energetic whole that is much more than the sum of its cellular parts. Cardio-energetics sees the intensity of the loving and sometimes hating within families as deriving less from the character of one family member than from a resonating energy system constantly being created by all of its members. The most "troubled" person in the family may be the most "cardio-sensitive," the more alert "tuning fork" among the family forks, and should perhaps be viewed as an instructive "L" energy sensor for the quality and nature of the family energy mix.

The word "temperament" derives from the Latin verb "tempare," meaning to mix. Cardio-energetics suggests that our temperament is an info-energetic mixture of information collected and transmitted within and between all of us to constantly re-create the universal family system. Since the subtle energy mediated by the heart is nonlocal and infinite, each of us is a force within a force, contributing our energy to a quantum energy field without limits. Tuning in to our own heart's energy and understanding its origins, nature, and impact is a way of harmonizing with the cosmic family composed of all persons, places, and things.

THE DISCOVERY OF CARDIO-TEMPERAMENTS

Galen, the brilliant second-century physician, elaborated on the ancient Greek and Roman "temperaments" called the humors—yellow bile, black bile, blood, and phlegm—and how they related to the four fundamental substances in the world—fire, air, earth, and water. He said that the healthy person was characterized by a balance of warm and cool and dry and moist energies. Harvard psychologist Jerome Kagan, in his fascinating book *Galen's Prophecy,* summarizes the research on temperament to indicate that Galen may not have been too far off about the power of temperament to influence our living, working, and loving throughout our life.[13]

Kagan suggests that understanding more about temperament, in addition to the more popular matrogenic (mother-nurturing) issues, can lead us to be more forgiving of the energy we sense coming from those around us and help us all realize that we are by our very nature temperamental beings. Reading our temperamental heart's code is not a way of labeling or blaming but of being able to understand who we are, how we are constantly coming to be, and who we can be as creators and creations of energetic systems. We are all info-energetically codependent within the natural chaotic "dysfunction" of evolving cellular memory-making systems.

Since cardio-energetics asserts that temperament is a manifestation of the encoded energy within us and the information conveyed within us by that energy and stored within our cells, it is important to understand how the heart might contribute to the molding of our info-energy into a whole person. For example, research indicates that there is a relationship between low heart rate and antisocial behavior, that psychopaths have less reactive heart rates than healthy individuals, and that there may be such a thing as warm and cool, and even hot and cold, hearts in terms of the energy within and emitted from the heart.[14]

INHIBITED AND UNINHIBITED HEARTS

Kagan's work with children suggests two temperament groups that reflect differences in inherited physiology, brain structure, and general disposition that relates to what I have referred to as the quality of the "L" or subtle energy heart's code. Kagan called these two groups the inhibited and uninhibited temperaments. He traces differences in these two groups primarily to differences in brain structure and neurochemistry, and his orientation is based on the bioscience view of the brain and a neurochemical perspective rather than issues of an info-energetic heart. He writes, "If inherited differences in brain function contribute to temperamental types, there are two places to look for the variations—anatomy and physiology."[15] Cardio-energetics looks beyond the "stuff" of the body to the energy and information that creates it. If the centrality of the heart is our starting point, then we see that the several differences between inhibited and uninhibited temperaments are manifestations of the info-energy radiated to every cell and stored there in a temperament template in the form of more "open" (or what might be seen as "soft-hearted") temperament or more "closed" (or "hard-hearted") temperament.

Kagan studied over six hundred four-month-old children with the object of determining temperamental differences. He found that about one in five infants reacts to stimulation with highly vigorous motor activity and distress. These children end up being more inhibited as they get older. They seemed to have a very sensitive, "softer," more easily "penetrated," hyper-heart that is highly reactive to outside stimulation. About two of every five of Kagan's children had a relaxed, minimally distressed reaction to stimulation, that is, they had what may be seen as a more hardened, hypo-heart, one that is less environmentally reactive, and they grow up to be less inhibited than the other group (hence, "uninhibited"). Cardio-energetics suggests that these are two distinctly different heart codes and that they are expressions of early-established cellular memories that, like the Jim twins, we carry with us forever no matter where we are.

If health is not only physical balance but energetic balance, then a healthy heart might be one that is not too hypo, or hard (uninhibited), or too hyper, or soft (inhibited). Kagan found the following differences in the two groups:

• Soft-hearted (inhibited) children tended to be shyer, quieter, and more reluctant to initiate spontaneous comments with people they didn't know.

• Soft-hearted children smiled less than the hard-hearted (uninhibited) children, particularly with unfamiliar people. They seemed more psychologically vulnerable, reserved, and less "hardened" to social risk taking.

• Soft-hearted children took a much longer time to relax after stress and took longer to adjust to a new situation. Just as with hyperactive children, their hearts did not easily calm and small things seemed to bother them more and longer than they did the hard-hearted (uninhibited) group.

• Soft-hearted children grew up to be more easily upset adults who suffered impaired memory and were distracted after being stressed. The more hard-hearted children grew to be adults who rolled more easily with the punches.

• Soft-hearted children became young adults who were much less comfortable taking risks and more likely to be hurt emotionally when risk taking led to negative consequences. They seem to know on some level that they have an energetically hypersensitive heart and, as if trying not to awaken a sleeping monster, are reluctant to do anything that might arouse it.

• Soft-hearted children had many more phobias and fears than the more hard hearted. From a cardio-energetic perspective their "softer cells" seemed more easily to quiver and be shaken by external events than the more "solid cells" of the hypo-hearted.

• Soft-hearted children became adults who experienced larger heart-rate accelerations when under stress than their hard-hearted opposites. It seems as if the hyper-hearted (inhibited) group were reluctant to "set their heart racing off" than the hypo-hearted whose hearts were less easily "moved." Soft-hearted adults somehow sensed that their hypersensitive heart could more easily be broken than the hearts of their more hard-hearted and less inhibited cohorts.

• Soft-hearted children experience faster and larger pupil dilation when under stress (indicating a lower threshold of agitation of their sympathovagal nervous system). Based on the hypothesis of a heart's code, they seemed to have a low threshold for fear and to be more sensitive, reactive, and emotionally delicate than the more uninhibited hard-hearted group.

• Almost always vigilant and on defensive alert for agitation of their hyper-reactive heart, the soft-hearted (inhibited) group, as if in a chronic state of flinching, experienced more muscle tension than the hard-hearted (uninhibited) group.

• The soft-hearted (inhibited) group tended to physically appear "softer" and more fragile than their "tougher" looking cousins. They tended toward an ectomorphic, thin, more fragile body type and were more likely to have blue eyes and a narrow, more drawn face. The more hard-hearted, uninhibited group tended to look a little tougher by social standards, having a more muscular, mesomorphic body type, dark or brown eyes, and a more round, fuller face.

The inhibited soft-hearted pattern is similar to the "irritable heart reaction" identified by some cardiac psychologists.[16] Using videotaped clinical examination, cardiologists Meyer Friedman and his associates examined what they call TABP, or type A behavior pattern."[17] They noted the same drawn, tense facial appearance of the inhibited hypo-hearted people described above and detected facial tension, hyper-reactivity to stimuli, time urgency, quick heart-rate acceleration, and the same muscle tension identified in Kagan's inhibited children. This suggests a correlation between encoded "soft-heartedness" and a cellular vulnerability to various forms of heart disease. Further study of this relationship by cardio-energetics may reveal that the more hard-hearted also have their own unique cellular vulnerability to various diseases.

FINDING THE "INNER ELDER"

Sigmund Freud saw the unconscious as one's own unique darkened storehouse of repressed sexual impulses. Cardio-energetics proposes that, because much of who and how we are is pre-coded from the heart of our mother and others, our unconscious is really our set of cellular memories that constitute aspects of our life not yet lived—a written but not yet completely played internal cellular symphony, or perhaps the heart's code not yet completely deciphered. Our cardio-unconsciousness may be the cellular memories that manifest as our "soft- or hard-hearted" code, more apparent to others than to ourselves. If this is true, our health and general well-being may depend on tuning in to our temperament template, including the dark side of who we are. It will require that we learn to listen to and read the full spectrum of the energy of our heart by learning to focus and sense it, assess it with instruments like the H*E*A*R*T* questionnaire presented in chapter 1, determine if we tend to be cool- or warmhearted, and develop a more enlightened connection with the energy stored in the hearts of those around us. It will require that, as we consider our unconscious inner elder and his or her as yet unlived life, we ask ourselves, "When am I going to get around to you?"

THE SHADOW OF ANGRY ENERGY

Our inner elder, composed of our encoded cellular memories, has anger energy as well as love energy. Most of the more angry energy is sent to our heart by a selfish brain that is motivated primarily by what I call the four Fs: fighting, fleeing, food, and fornicating (sex). If we deny the dark side of our "L" energy, it will influence us without our awareness, causing us to pull away, angrily overreact, and view the world with hostility and cynicism. If there is angry energy stored within our heart left there from another heart or hearts, or by our own or other brains, it can flow within us, wreaking havoc on our heart and the hearts of those around us.

Unless we clearly read it, confess it, and understand its origins, darkside energy can destroy our life by casting a shadow over how we work and love that others can often see and feel more easily than we do.[18] Based on what we have learned about cardio-temperament, it may be wise to consider the possibility that the heart attracts what it secretly harbors and, when we complain about our life, we are complaining about who and how we ourselves really are in our heart.

PLATELET BULLETS

Anger energy causes perturbations of the heart. It makes it beat more rapidly, increasing the risk of damage to the inner lining of our arteries. Blood sent spurting by an agitated heart shoots platelet bullets through our arteries, scraping and nicking their walls and creating pockets for the deposit of vessel-blocking plaque. Dark-side anger energy from a combative, cynical brain causes an increase in stress hormones to prepare us to fight for what the brain considers its own territory. These hormones can cause fat cells in our body to release fat into the blood, causing even more clogging of our arteries and, in effect, depriving the lethal alliance between the brain and its body of the mediating wisdom of a calmer, less combative heart. The excess stress hormones from anger energy causes our platelets to become much more sticky and to huddle and hide defensively together in the stress scuffs caused by the surging blood. When our platelets group together, they tend to release even more plaque.

"Dark side" energy relates to the ABCs of a cold and hostile heart: anger, belligerence, and cynicism. Perhaps because of its comparative numbness, the heart coded to be less reactive may require more intense emotional energy as stimulation in order to initiate its response than does a more reactively coded heart. The information contained in dark energy is much more a code of conflict and competition than one of caring and connection. My work with patients in my clinic, and the work of other researchers,[19] indicates a formula for predicting the generating of the dark-side energy of anger:

H (HOSTILITY) = T (THE THOUGHT) × F (THE FEELING) × A (THE ACTION)

Put another way, the formula for hostility begins with cynical thought or cognition on the part of the brain, characterized by its evolutionary pessimism, disgust, and unrelenting skepticism regarding the motives of others, accompanied by the brain's selfish view of what it sees as "justice." This factor is multiplied by the emotional state of anger, characterized by the brain's lower and more primitive survivalist levels telling your body that its territory is being violated, or that it is being taken advantage of and/or being robbed of its precious time. The cynical anger is multiplied by aggressive behavior as the body is conscripted into a war with the world and a demeanor of verbal and/or physical threats, or actual assaults, against anyone or anything the brain sees as a threat to its survival, whether these threats are real or not.

PUTTING ON AN ANGRY FACE

Research from cardiac psychology indicates that the heart can put on a very angry face.[20] If you have ever looked directly into the face of a person who is very angry or even on the verge of getting angry, you have probably noticed the universal look of disgust, agitation, and repugnance that can cause your own heart to accelerate. This same angry face is shown in every culture studied, and it is one of the most obvious signs of the lethal covenant between a highly reactive brain and the body it is preparing for attack. Here are some of the features of a heart wearing its anger on your face.

• You can see the dark side of "L" energy on the face of a person when the whites of the eyes around the iris are made larger by the pulling back of the small muscles surrounding the eye. This is due to the tenseness and stress of anger. It's as if the brain is amazed at the arrogance of another brain trying to barge in on its territory.

• You can see the bulging muscles around the upper jaw near the ears, as if the brain were preparing the body to bite what it sees as an enemy.

• You can see a flaring of the nostrils as the emotionally hijacked brain gasps for more oxygen to use for fighting.

• You can note bulging cheeks just in front of the ears and a chin jutting out.

• You can detect tiny droplets of sweat, particularly on the upper lip as the brain heats up its body.

• You may see thin lips drawn into a tight, rigid smirk designed by the brain as anger camouflage. If you look with your heart, you may sense that this cynical smile is a relic of joy unrealized, an approximation of a happy smile in the form of pseudo-happiness, hiding a deep, dark energy and designed by the brain to fool its opponents into a false sense of comfort.

• You may see a discoloration or dark, yellow-brown tone to the lower and sometimes the upper eyelids of a chronically angry person. This is due to deposits of melanin reflective of a chronic state of stress alert that prevents melanin's normal metabolism.

• You may see deep, thin wrinkles appearing in the face of a chronically angry person as permanently engraved emotional war paint, most noticeable to the left side of the mouth. These wrinkles are caused by the brain's chronic expression of disgust. This "disgust dimple" is caused by the emotional right side of the brain pulling up the small muscles on the left side of the face in a frown of frustration. The more soft-hearted among us can more easily feel the negative energy expressed in the look of loathing described above.

Cardiac psychology is documenting that unchecked, unconfessed, dark-side angry energy displayed in the angry face is significantly detrimental to the health of the heart itself. The devastating effects of lack of "lighter" love energy has been documented by cardiologist James Lynch.[21] He describes the heart's reactivity to the lack of gentle, caring connection. Another cardiologist, Dean Ornish, has shown that significant changes in lifestyle, including a less angry, hostile interaction with others, can actually reverse heart disease and unclog arteries without surgery. He writes, "I am becoming increasingly convinced that heart disease is a metaphor as well as an anatomical illness. In poetry, art, and literature, the heart is often portrayed as the organ most affected by our emotions, and I think there is some truth to that."[22]

Psychologist Dr. Beverly Rubik, director of the Center for Frontier Sciences at Temple University, writes, "Some other type of energy even more subtle than electromagnetism but not yet identified by science also may be involved in healing."[23] If we are to heal ourselves, our families, and our planet, we will need to consider not only a more rational approach to dealing with our dark-side energy but also to become aware that each of us carries within us a cardio-predisposition toward either the light or dark side of life. Being aware of that disposition can help us more gently confess our anger to ourselves and to those who care about us rather than submit to our brain's urgent expression or defensively unrealistic suppression of it, both approaches that place our health and the health of those around us in jeopardy.

WORDS OF LOVE

Cofounders of the field of energy cardiology Drs. Linda Russek and Gary Schwartz have documented that one reflection of a strongly love-encoded heart may be the caring, positive words used by medical students to describe their own parents, and that such descriptions may predict a healthier and longer life.[24] They call for further research into the energetic mechanisms that may mediate how parental love and caring contribute to health and illness throughout the life span.

In my work with heart patients, I use a test called the Parental Energy Imprint Test (PEIT) that contains twelve questions about the nature of parental energy that still seems to influence their lives. I have complete responses to this test from 490 patients—363 men and 127 women. I had psychology students unaware of my work in cardio-energetics or the concepts I was testing rate the one-word answers as "good" or "bad" energy words (as you will note, the answer "NO" to items 8 to 12 were, of course, automatic "bad energy" words). Only 29 (less than 6 percent) of the heart patients had 6 or more "good energy" parental words and 223 (almost 46 percent) of these persons with various degrees of heart disease had all "bad energy" words. As an informal "control group." I had my 90 college students (aged 18–23) who categorized the words of the cardiac patients take my test. Forty-seven of these likely heart-healthier students (more than 52 percent) had more than 6 "bad energy" words for their parents and 11 (12 percent) had all "good energy" words. It appears that the seeds of filial discontentment germinate very quickly and that my students may be heart patients in training. Here's a copy of the test.

Parental Energy Imprint Test

1. What one word best describes your feelings about your mother as you were growing up?
2. What one word best describes how you think your mother felt about you as you were growing up?
3. What one word best describes your feelings about your father as you were growing up?
4. What one word best describes how you think your father felt about you as you were growing up?
5. What one word best describes how you felt your father felt about your mother as you were growing up?
6. What one word best describes how you felt your mother felt about your father as you were growing up?
7. What one word best describes the emotional tone of your father and mother's marriage as you were growing up?
8. If you had to say yes or no, would you say you were deprived (not given the basics of life by your parents) as a child?
9. If you had to say yes or no, would you say you were exploited (asked to grow up too soon or do too much as a child by one or both parents because of their own problems) when you were growing up?
10. If you had to say yes or no, would you say you were neglected (not paid enough attention to) as a child when you were growing up?
11. If you had to say yes or no, would you say you were abused (verbally or physically) as a child when you were growing up?
12. If you had to say yes or no, would you want to be seen by your own children just as you now see your own parents?

The above parental energy test is a very general and preliminary reflection of the energy code left in your heart by your parents either at the beginning of your life or during your continued emotional energy encoding as you grew up.

THE VALUE OF A LITTLE MISERY

I do not mean to imply that the dark side of our cardio-energy is not essential to our essence as a person. Psychologist Mihaly Csikszentmihalyi writes that the dark side is crucial for our survival.[25] He states that, had we not had a clear awareness of the realness of the negatives in the cosmos, we would never have been prepared to deal with them.

Scientists are also aware of what they call the opponent process theory. Above the neuronal level of the retina itself, we possess six kinds of cells in our eye that play a role in what we perceive as color. These cells react as teams, reacting to different color energies in the day and night. Opponent process theory says that, because of the cellular interaction, positive and negative afterimages appear.[26] When stimulation to one opponent pair is terminated, the other is automatically activated and an afterimage occurs. This is one reason why you sometimes see green after images of looking at a red object. Every time you look at something, you not only take in the energy of that object but its opposite afterimage as well.

The opponent process theory also applies to our emotional energy. Without exception, if enough time passes, elation will always be followed by the affective afterimage of letdown, and letdown will always be followed by an emotional afterimage of elation. This emotional rebound guarantee should come as bad news for unrealistic optimists and good news for chronic pessimists.

Opponent process theory may be one of the most neglected but important psychological findings regarding our feelings about life.[27] It contains two central assumptions that relate to cardio-energetics. First, emotional reactions to a stimulation will be followed automatically by an opposite or "opponent" reaction. Second, repeat exposures to an emotional stimulus can cause the initial reaction to weaken and the opponent process that follows to be stronger. Built into our nature, then, is a protective compensatory system that promises that, no matter how low we get, we will also get that high, and that the longer we are high or low, the less intense these states become.

The ebb and flow of the subtle energy within also may seek a natural, compensatory, peaceful balance between the light and dark, ups and downs, and hard and soft nature of our info-energy. The physical structure of the heart itself represents a natural opponent process system that illustrates the essential balance of life. Just as the brain has left and right hemispheres that differ in their orientation to life, the heart has its two hemispheres. You read in chapter 3 that the heart is actually two pumps side by side, each with its own atrium or top collecting chamber and a ventricle or bottom sending chamber. The left ventricle has to send blood much further than the right, so it has to be more forceful in its contraction. The right ventricle has only to send blood to the lungs a short distance away, so its contraction is less intense. Just as the brain's left hemisphere tends to be more "hard and coldly logical" and its right more "softly emotional," and both of these sides of our nature must work in balance for our physical and emotional health, so the "hard and soft" energies of the heart integrate into one balanced opponent process energy system. Tapping into the heart's code involves being aware of the importance and impact of both our "systolic" and "diastolic" temperaments.

If we allow ourselves to become too hard- or soft-hearted, we can end up leading an unbalanced life that upsets the balance of our own and others' lives. Energy cardiology researchers at the Institute of HeartMath in California have studied the various patterns of the heart. They search for mathematical representations within the various rhythms and patterns of the heart under various psychological states. Through their advanced technology, they are able to look inside the tracings made on the electrocardiograph to interpret signs of how the heart is emotionally dealing with its world. They refer to a state of cardiac coherence and balance they can measure with their equipment as a state of "amplified peace."[28]

STICKY ENERGY

You read in chapter 2 that one of the characteristics of the heart's "L" or subtle energy is its "sticky" or permanent adhesive nature. The rules of the cosmos teach that, once two systems come in energetic contact, they are forever connected by the infinite cellular memory of their connection. Our cardio-temperament is a manifestation of these memories and the fact that our experiences with our parents and others close to us remain within us. Unless we choose to think that we humans are the only part of the cosmos that does not follow its rules, we too are "stuck" with everyone and everything that has ever happened to us, and others are "stuck" with our energy. We have no choice; we are temperamental creatures.

How would those who know you best describe the nature of your heart? Would they say you are "hot" or "cold" hearted? What would they say is your general temperament when you play, love, and work? How would they say your temperament affects them? How does the temperament of others seem to touch your heart? How and how much different is your cardio-temperament from the person you love the most? How have temperamental differences influenced your love, work, and family life? Being literate in the heart's code can help you be more aware of your social, psychological, and spiritual impact on those you connect with heart to heart.

Part Two

Healing Miracles and Loving Connections

*"What a wonderful life I've had!
I only wish I'd realized it sooner."*

—*COLETTE*

Making Contact with Your Heart

"The real voyage of discovery consists not in seeking new lands but in seeing with new eyes."

— *MARCEL PROUST*

YOUR HEAD OR YOUR HEART?

If forced to chose, would those who know you best say you are a person "of the head" or "of the heart?" Would they describe you as a person who makes decisions almost exclusively based on a rational and analytical consideration of the issues involved or as someone who tends to be more intuitive and instinctive? While the quality and length of our life demands that we learn to constructively use the brain's potential for logical brilliance, we can also learn to share a healthy, less stressed, more loving life by tapping into the heart's code and by realizing that, beyond metaphor, the heart may have its own unique way of thinking and feeling that is no less important than the brain's way of dealing with the world.

You have read that a brain unchecked by its heart can enter into a lethal alliance with its body. In fulfilling its evolutionary imperative of self-advancement and self-survival, it can neglect the spiritual necessity of being aware of the more subtle information that expresses the soul's reason for, and needs within, its physical manifestation. This chapter discusses some possible ways to become more cardio-sensitive and to help the brain be more aware of the availability of a partner that thinks in a different way than it does and with which it may be more creative and connected, and calm its supervision of the body's negotiation through daily living.

LESSONS FROM CARDIO-SENSITIVES

I have been using the term "cardio-sensitives" for the relatively small percentage of people in my seventy-three heart transplant recipient sample who seem able to tap into the subtle "L" or life info-energy that may be the code the heart uses in its unique way of thinking and feeling. While almost all of the seventy-three patients reported some type of association with the energy of their donor, about 10 percent were particularly cardio-sensitive. While this group constitutes the "superstars" among the cardio-sensitives, every patient I interviewed presented some evidence of unique personal changes related to their new heart. In addition to my own patient group, you are reading about stories from other researchers' and clinicians' patients, and from transplant recipients I have met at my many lectures on "L" energy and cellular memories who also seem to be uniquely attuned to their new heart. You read about some of the characteristics of all of these cardio-sensitive people in chapter 4. I noticed, however, that not only these very unique patients but some of their own and their donors' family members seemed to also show cardio-sensitivity. I also observed that these people, too, seemed to show some of the characteristics of PEAR program's percipients and operators who, based on data from Princeton's fifty million experimental trials containing more than three billion bits of information, seemed sensitive to the subtle but significant equivalence of energy and information I refer to as the heart's code.[1] Based on these reports, it seemed that at least a preliminary and tentative list of some traits of a cardio-sensitive was emerging.

To facilitate discussion of cardio-sensitivity and the process of making informational contact with the heart, I put together the preliminary findings about "L" energy, the sentient heart, and cellular memories in order to design a test that might serve as a starting point for further study. With the help of many of my heart transplant patients and those persons they and others identified as being "more of the heart than the head," I designed the Cardio-Sensitivity Inventory (CSI). It in no way represents a direct measure of "L" energy or degree of any special skill. It is a preliminary attempt to begin to understand more about the nature of those who seem well-versed in the language of their heart. I have used the CSI with patients, nurses, residents, and other health-care professionals as a starting point for discussions about possible ways in which the heart may be conveying at least as much spiritual information as it is biochemical nutrition.

Here is a copy of the Cardio-Sensitivity Inventory. Each of the fifty items was taken from my interviews with the cardio-sensitives, as they seemed to reflect to varying degrees and ways some of the components associated with cardio-sensitivity. Each item is stated in the words used by the respondents as indicative of areas they thought worth considering for study. There is no implication that any answer is the correct or better answer. Again, only for purposes of discussion, I provided a very crude scoring system.

The Cardio-Sensitive Inventory (CSI)

Dr. Paul Pearsall, Ho'ala Hou, Inc., 1997

Use the following scale to respond to the questions below. Select the negative or positive number along the following scale that most closely represents where you stand regarding each item.

Almost Never				*—About Half the Time—*					*Almost Always*
–5	*–4*	*–2*	*–1*	*0*	*+1*	*+2*	*+3*	*+4*	*+5*

_____ 1. I think I can influence what happens to people and things just by how and what I think about them.

_____ 2. I think mechanical things can get in "a bad mood" and I talk kindly and gently to my computer and other machines to try to coax them into working better with me.

_____ 3. I have a very strong "sixth sense" and feel like I'm "psychic."

_____ 4. I can tell what a person is going to say before she or he says it.

_____ 5. I am highly suggestible, "go along" easily, and probably could be very easily hypnotized.

_____ 6. People would say I tend to have what society usually sees as a very strong "feminine side."

_____ 7. I go with my "gut" and not "the facts."

_____ 8. I believe people and things give off "vibes," or invisible energy.

_____ 9. I have and trust my very good sense of intuition.

_____ 10. I laugh easily and often.

_____ 11. I cry easily in private or public.

_____ 12. I'm a "dreamer" who spends a lot of time intentionally "not facing reality."

_____ 13. I'm never competitive and would sooner "just play" than "win."

_____ 14. People would say that I'm a very "needy person."

_____ 15. I use the word "we" much more than "I."

_____ 16. I am interested in, read about, and enjoy speaking about spiritual things and those aspects of life one cannot see or touch.

_____ 17. People who know me best would say that I seem a little weird and very different from most people they know.

_____ 18. Even when it comes to simple little things, I can never seem to make up my mind.

_____ 19. I'm absolutely certain that there has to be life on other planets.

_____ 20. I think there is no such thing as a "coincidence" and that everything happens for a predestined reason we may not understand.

_____ 21. I'm a toucher, holder, and hugger.

_____ 22. When the music starts, I'm the first one on the floor to dance.

_____ 23. I'm very good with my hands and enjoy things like painting, carpentry, and sculpting.

_____ 24. I think people can be trusted and are not at all inclined to take advantage of you.

_____ 25. I can see and feel energy flowing between people and things.

_____ 26. I can tell what someone I care about is doing and feeling and exactly where they are even when they are not with me.

_____ 27. I believe in love at first sight.

_____ 28. I'm very easily distracted.

_____ 29. I love to sing or hum along with classical music.

_____ 30. People say I am very innocent and naive.

_____ 31. I prefer to hand-write over typing or working on a computer and I write things like poetry, songs, or letters every week.

_____ 32. I get upset very easily.

_____ 33. I have flashbacks and sometimes seem to go into a trance.

_____ 34. People would say that I am constantly changing my mind.

_____ 35. Animals of all kinds are drawn instantly to me.

_____ 36. Children love me.

_____ 37. I have a "green thumb" and have very good luck with plants and flowers.

_____ 38. I talk with my plants to help them grow.

_____ 39. I have very intense, detailed, long dreams.

_____ 40. I love to share and interpret my dreams.

_____ 41. I have a perfect memory not only about my life but about others' lives.

_____ 42. People would say that I'm a very good listener.

_____ 43. Those who know me the best would say that I am not at all controlling or bossy and a very good follower.

_____ 44. I have a lot of very sad memories that are always with me.

_____ 45. I sometimes feel very depressed for no reason at all.

_____ 46. I am instantly very aware of the "feeling" in a room or house.

_____ 47. My senses of taste, smell, and hearing are all very acute and accurate.

_____ 48. I believe in some form of reincarnation.

_____ 49. I believe in the power of prayer.

_____ 50. I talk out loud to someone who has died.

INTERPRETING YOUR CSI SCORE

_____ 1. Add up the total value of your "+" scores above "0."

_____ 2. Add up the total value of your "–" scores below "0."

TOTAL "+" SCORE MINUS TOTAL "–" SCORE = _____ CSI SCORE

Based on my interviews and the research reported in Part I of this book, it appears that those people whose CDI scores were over 0 but not over 100 were also those who seemed most "cardio-sensitive." They tended not to be significantly biased toward so-called psychic phenomena while still being realistically open and accepting in their willingness to deal with such possibilities as energy connection, cellular memories, and a heart's code. Their stories about energetic connection tended to be verified by their own family members and, in the case of my heart transplant recipients, corroborated by donor family members.

Those persons whose scores were over 100 tended to be more likely to report various forms of what they said were very strong energy or "psychic" connections or experiences in their life or, in the case of transplant recipients, immediately following receipt of their new heart—experiences that were less verifiable. Unlike the 0 to 100 group who were often reluctant to discuss their "L" energy experiences, the over 100 group spoke openly and easily about their experiences and often attributed them to a new life philosophy they had constructed or adopted after these experiences. No such philosophical or psychological life theory change was noted in the 0 to 100 group.

Those people whose scores clustered more toward the negative side tended to dismiss almost any possibility of "L" energy and often expressed anger with those who did report energy connections. As would be expected, I noted in my interviews that the more negative the score, the more anger, denial, and mocking of the possibility of a "vital" energy.

Based on what I have learned from the cardio-sensitives, it appears that there is a process that facilitates some enhanced level of awareness of the information that comes with the energy that is either transplanted with new cells in an organ transplant or, perhaps less profoundly but no less significantly, in anybody, coming into them from all persons, places, and things. This process might be called "cardio-contemplation," quieting the brain and calming the heart sufficiently to become more alert to the signals that may be coming from the heart.

CARDIO-CONTEMPLATION

The word "contemplation" derives from the Greek "tempo" meaning anything marked off, such as a season, period, or time. The Latin word "templum" also comes from the Greek "tempo," and it referred to a place where one came to observe omens. When the Greeks or Romans were inside their "templum," they beheld, pondered, and considered together. "Con" means together or with others, so "cardio-contemplation" means to ponder with our heart about our connection with, and the meaning of, our world.[2] In this case, pondering is less a mental than a spiritual process. Cardio-contemplation is being in a state that allows one to be better able to extract information about the soul from the energy coming from the heart. It is being more sensitive to the subtle energy of life and experiencing it as an "us" and not a "me." It seems to be a way of "being" more than a way of doing something and, as happened for the PEAR operators, being available for the subtle energy connection to occur rather than trying hard to make things happen.

One eight-year-old boy who had received a new heart described the "falling into" rather than "achieving" nature of cardio-sensitivity and cardio-contemplation. He said, "I can feel the other little boy inside me. I didn't at first, but when my immunity was up and they finally let me play with Pierre [the family French poodle] again, I began to call him King. I don't know why. Maybe my donor's dog was called King. Anyway, now I can feel the other boy with me. It's like when you don't know you bumped your knee and then, when you sit down and watch TV or something and you look and see the bruise, that's when you start to feel it and can't ignore it anymore. Even after it gets better or the scab falls off, your leg can always remember where it was hurt."

A WINDOW TO THE COLLECTIVE UNCONSCIOUS

Cardio-contemplation might be seen as one of the ways to connect with what some psychologists, most notably Carl Jung, called the collective unconscious. On some subtle energetic level, all the information gathered by those who have gone before us may still be nonlocally represented in the memory system of every cell of our own body. Being willing to be less cerebrally vigilant and more alert to subtle info-energy being resonated with every beat of the heart may be similar to tuning a radio to the station that contains our collective cellular memory program.

Cardio-contemplation may be a process that allows us to make contact with our soul by tapping into its spiritual energy. It may be a way of recalling our infantile paradise, providing a spiritual glimpse of the way things were before our own brain took charge. It may be one way to find our way back to the way things were supposed to be rather than yielding to the demands the brain's world constantly seem to be placing upon us. It may be a way of establishing an energy connection with the info-energy system that always surrounds us. It may be a way to learn, communicate, and connect the physical experience of one's personality to knowledge contained within the vibrational structure of the brain/heart/body Mind—our shared consciousness.[3]

Cardio-contemplation is similar in some ways to meditation, but unique in its focus on the heart. It is a merging, collective, and connective process that allows us to tune in to the memory of what it feels like to adore being alive. Like the cardio-sensitive heart transplant patients physiologically forced to recognize their connection with the energy they share with another person, any of us might be able to allow free reign for our own "hidden observer," that part of us that is alert and responsive to the thrill of living even when the brain itself is busy and distracted trying to help us make a living.

WAYS OF THE WILL

To understand the process of cardio-contemplation, it is helpful to compare it with the better-known enlightenment or awareness processes such as meditation, visualization, and imagery techniques. The process of meditation usually refers to a group of techniques that induce an altered state of focused attention and heightened awareness.[4] Virtually every spiritual and religious tradition includes some form of meditation, and research shows

that meditative states tend to result in positive physical changes throughout the body, including slower breathing and heart rate, lowered blood
pressure, and relaxation of tense muscles.[5]

While meditation is a complex process, it is generally divided into two
parts—concentration and opening-up techniques.[6] Both of these powerful
approaches to altered states of consciousness tend to rely, to varying degrees, primarily on the path of the head instead of the heart. Concentration
meditations involve focusing attention and awareness on one's breath, a
word, or a phrase. A number, word (mantra), or religious phrase might be
mentally repeated as one breathes deeply. Opening-up techniques involve
a present-centered awareness of the moment, free of judgment and evaluation.[7] Rather than concentrating on an object, sound, activity, or image,
the meditator focuses on the here and now while allowing any distracting
thoughts to simply pass by without regard as clouds across the sky. Both
techniques are essentially ways of substituting sensation for meaning and
they may both in their own unique ways be a means by which "L" energy
may be experienced.[8]

There are two closely related derivations of meditation often used in
holistic healing. Visualization is the process of attempting to instruct the
body directly in healing via imagining, or visualizing, specially chosen images, such as clogged arteries being scrubbed out by brushes or cancer
cells being eaten by sharks.[9] Imagery is less an attempt to "perceive" than
to experience and create thoughts and generate feelings of warmth, caring,
and love. Visualization involves trying to *see* a way to be healthy, while
imagery is trying to connect with the *feeling* of being healthy. Both of these
approaches tend to involve considerable mental or "brain" effort.

The relaxation response as proposed initially by Dr. Herbert Benson[10]
is a means of focusing away from pressured thoughts by attending to
breathing and saying a nonemotional word, such as the number one. It is a
natural body and nervous system response that, like meditation, is a form
of what author Spencer Holst calls a "brilliant silence."[11] Cardio-contemplation may be viewed as engaging another one of our natural responses—
our "resonation response." It is silently pausing to vibrate with all the
energy, feelings, and sensations of the moment, the state described at the
Institute of HeartMath as "amplified peace."

Cardio-contemplation is not just time management or energy "down-
shifting." It is similar to what author Stephen Rechtschaffen calls
"timeshifting,"[12] letting our heart be open to its natural resonation with all

the energies of the present moment and thereby expanding, freezing, or spiritually pausing to allow one's self to be completely immersed in the present quantum moment. Psychologist Mihaly Csikszentmihalyi referred to a similar state he called "flow," meaning being so completely absorbed in what one is doing that all sense of time, space, and self seems to disappear.[13] Pianist Arthur Rubinstein described the power of such momentary timeless pauses when he said, "The notes I play like every pianist. But the pauses, ahhh, the pauses."[14]

Cardio-contemplation involves aspects of all of the above approaches but differs from these approaches in three ways. It tends to be experienced as less private and more connective, more energetically rhythmic than mentally focused and static, and more attentive and receptive to the body's signals rather than distracted from them. It is less visualizing a scene than remembering how to become part of the present scene's energy. In cardio-contemplation, one tunes in to the delicate info-energetic "sensations" that seem to come from the heart rather than a word, sound, breathing, or image that can be experienced as coming from a consciousness somewhere in the brain.

BY WAY OF THE HEART

Physician Alan D. Watkins distinguishes what he calls "mindful intentionality techniques," such as meditation, imagery, visualization, the relaxation response, and positive affirmations, from the process of intentionally shifting *emotional* attention into a positive state by focusing on the heart and deeply and sincerely trying to reexperience past feelings of caring and appreciation stored there.[15] He does not dismiss the value of meditation and other techniques as compared to the heart-focus approach I call cardio-contemplation, but he does differentiate between the head path of mindful intentionality (the ways of the will) and the way of the "emotions" (cardio-sensitivity). He draws a distinction "between the physiological effects of mental, mindful techniques and those of emotional heart-based techniques."[16]

Psychologists use the word "metamood" to refer to being aware of one's own emotions.[17] Cardio-contemplation is a system for developing such awareness not by mental reflection but by emotional focus on the energy center of the body—the heart. As the brain is to intellectual intelligence, so the heart may be to emotional intelligence.

ESTABLISHING CARDIAC COHERENCE

When the meditative and other states described above are studied, researchers often detect changes in brain waves that indicate a more relaxed state. Much the same thing happens to a heart that is in the process of cardio-contemplation. Pioneering work on the state achieved through cardio-contemplation called "cardiac coherence" has been done at the Institute of HeartMath® in Boulder Creek, California, the nonprofit educational corporation mentioned earlier in this book whose motto is "putting the heart back into the people business." Their work shows that cardiac coherence is a balanced, blissful, steady heart energy state, induced by the process I call cardio-contemplation and a similar process they refer to as the "Freeze Frame® Technique." This HeartMath Institute–researched process involves recognition of a specific stressful feeling, making a mental effort to shift focus to sensations coming from the area of the heart instead of the head, recalling a very positive event of the past, and mentally asking the heart for its insights on what might be a better way of dealing with the stressful situation that could induce a state more like that of the past positive event. As if the heart has engaged its natural resonation response, it is reflected on electrocardiograms as a smooth set of gentle curves that reveal the heart's consistent beat-to-beat and between-beat heart rhythms. Cardiac "incoherence" is reflected by inconsistency in the rhythm of the heart, shown as lines on the electrocardiogram that appear as sharp saw-edges.[18, 19]

You have experienced that state of cardio-coherence in your life or you probably would not be alive to read this book. Remember an occasion when time seemed to stand still. Remember a time when, with no effort on your part at all, you seemed to fall into perfect synch with the world around you as if you were vibrating with it and feeling its energy. You may not have been meditating or trying cardio-contemplation and instead may have been knitting, making a floral lei, building a new table, or even eating some vanilla yogurt, but at least for this one moment in time, you lost all sense of self and became "entrained" or synchronized not with the speed of modern life but the natural, gentle, oscillating energies of nature. At such times, you may have contacted the world with your heart. Research at the HeartMath Institute seems to substantiate many of the hypotheses of energy cardiology and cardio-energetics, and it documents relationships between feelings of fondness, appreciation, caring, and pausing to connect with the world with healthier cardiovascular function. As you will read more about in chapter 11, researchers at the institute have also documented how cardiac coherence, or a blissful, peaceful heart, enhances immunity and healing as it creates a synchronized sympathovagal or neurohormonal balance that frees the natural healing instincts of the body to work their miracles.[20]

I have used my own version of the HeartMath Institute's Freeze Frame Technique of cardio-contemplation for more than twenty-five years with my own patients at Sinai Hospital in Detroit, Michigan. As with the Freeze Frame Technique, I asked my patients to emotionally experience feelings coming from the heart rather than trying to mentally recall a visual image of a past positive experience.[21] I asked them to try to differentiate between what psychologist Stephen Rechtschaffen calls "mental" or brain time and more "emotional" or heart time.[22] To illustrate this difference, Dr. Rechtschaffen asks his patients to first think of a red balloon. They usually find this easy to do. He then asks them to feel very sad or very happy. The patients usually report that this is not as easy because "feeling takes time." Cardio-contemplation is taking the time to let the heart feel and to be free from the mental pressures of a brain "entrained," or in synch, more with beeps and buzzes than the chirps of birds and rustling of trees.

Cardio-contemplation is not "thinking" about a new way to deal with stress. It does not involve reducing stress as much as transforming it by falling into a state of resonation with the natural world and other hearts so that stress has less control over the brain/heart/body Mind.[23] It is a state in which cellular memories are freer to emerge, and when they do, my research indicates, their appearance is signaled by the breaking of the lethal brain/body covenant and measured as reduced blood pressure, relaxed muscles, slower, deeper breathing, and a slow, regular, steady heart tracing similar to those reported by the HeartMath Institute.[24, 25]

The last two steps in cardio-contemplation are to try to use the heart to not only retrieve memories of past peaceful states but to store the memories of the present contemplative and more blissful moment as new cellular memories and then to try to send that balanced "L" energy to everyone and everything around you.[26]

Summing up the value of cardiac coherence, researcher Rollin McCraty writes, "We can intentionally generate internal cardiac coherence. This promotes mental clarity as the 'white noise' of incoherent afferent electrical activity (the energetic disruption coming from a stressed brain) is reduced."[27] This is what I call "cardio-contemplation," learning to pay attention to our heart, help it calm down, relating with it as a teacher, and making the brain shut up long enough to let the heart sing. It is a way of avoiding the crisis identified by Oliver Wendell Holmes who wrote, "Alas for those who never sing and die with all their music left in them."

SEVEN HABITS FOR HEARING THE HEART

Philosopher Pierre Teilhard de Chardin wrote, "The ills from which we are suffering have had their seat in the very foundation of human thought." His words reflect the dangers of a world dominated by a heartless brain that seems to say "I am everything" while the often ignored heart says "I am nothing without everyone." Cardio-contemplation's seven orientations discussed below are ways we might be able to have a healthier brain/heart/body Mind help us provide the meaning and balance for the brain's work. By doing so, we may be better able to follow Thoreau's suggestion when he writes, "If you have built castles in the sky, your work need not be lost. Now put the foundation under them."

As a summary of the process of tuning in to our heart's code and the memories it conveys, here is a review of some of the suggestions made throughout this book about how to cardio-contemplate and tune in to the heart's code.

1. Be Still. To tune in to the heart, it is necessary to slow down, sit down, and quiet down. You don't need to assume any particular posture, but it is necessary to be still enough take full notice of being in the present moment instead of getting ready for the next moment or to worrying about a wasted past moment. Thirteenth-century Christian mystic Meister Eckhart said, "There is nothing in all creation so like God as stillness." Stop moving, stop thinking, don't try any particular gimmick or technique, and just be still for a few moments. One way to do this is to take a deep breath and sigh.

2. Lighten Up. Someone once said that the average person thinks he isn't average. Don't take yourself so seriously. You are not nearly as powerful and in control as your brain thinks you are or have to be. Most of the problems, accomplishments, and worries you experience at any given moment are transitory and of very little relevance in the overall scheme of you life. A heart can become heavy both spiritually and in terms of the physiological changes associated with a relentless brain's burdens. Remember the insight of British author G. K. Chesterton who wrote, "Angels fly because they take themselves lightly."

3. Shut Up. Stop talking, and that includes talking to yourself. This is a very difficult step because the brain is constantly gabbing about its four Fs of feeding (or getting more stuff), fighting (or protecting its territory), fleeing (or moving on to somewhere else), and fornicating (or deriving intense and immediate physical pleasure). Try ignoring your brain for a while and just let it talk to itself. Try letting your own "hidden observer," that part of you that is always alert even when the brain is at rest, keep an eye on things while you relax. Doing and saying less is generally good for your mental, spiritual, and physical health. Follow Oscar Wilde's advice when he pointed out, "I do not talk to God so as not to bore him."

4. Resonate. Cardio-contemplation is a form of receptive prayer. It is not asking for something from or talking to a Higher Power but listening to the power within your heart for its profound awareness of your connection with the Creator. Physician Larry Dossey writes, "In its simplest form, prayer is an attitude of the heart—a matter of being, not doing. Prayer is the desire to connect with the Absolute, however it may be conceived. When we experience the need to enact this connection, we are praying."[28]

5. Feel. You share your info-energy and cellular memories with every system in the cosmos. Don't tune out the world around you to tune in to your heart. Instead, be deeply aware and feel with all of your senses your connection with the trees, flowers, water, or any natural system around you.

6. Learn. Cardio-contemplation is learning from and by your heart. When we say we have learned something "by heart," we usually mean we have learned it well and lastingly. As you be still, lighten up, shut up, resonate, and feel, listen for what your heart is telling you about living, loving, and working. Try to store your lessons as cellular memories for later recall at the stressful times in your life.

7. Connect. Try to send your lessons and the balanced "L" energy achieved in a cardio-contemplative state to the world around you and be open to the incoming "L" energy coming from other hearts. Cardio-contemplation is a profound way to become a more complete part and healer of the world.

In order to help you survive, your brain may have to think it is on its own in the world, but your heart knows we are never truly alone. Beyond your busy brain's attention, it seems likely that you are constantly being immersed in the "L" energy coming from your own heart as a message from all the hearts around you. Research shows that it is also likely that other hearts are sending us info-energy right this moment and that we can become more aware of that level of "L" energy interdependence. This is the focus of the next chapter.

CHAPTER EIGHT

Making Contact with Other Hearts

"Everything in this world has a hidden meaning. Men, animals, trees, stars, they are all hieroglyphics."

—*NIKOS KAZANTZAKIS,* ZORBA THE GREEK

LETTING YOUR HEART PRAY

"Hush. Let our hearts pray," said the Hawaiian mother softly. Her family sat hand in hand around the dinner table. Heads bowed and eyes closed, they conducted what Hawaiian families call a "pule 'ohana," meaning to pray together as a family. No words were said, all thoughts and mental distractions were to be ignored, and each child, parent, and grandparent was expected to silence their brain to allow their heart to join in prayer with all of the other family hearts.

As I sat with them, I could feel the energy coming from within the family group. I had been very busy that day, but now I felt gently comforted by the combined healing power of the group. I could feel my heart falling into coherence—a state of serene, sedate composure. Without any signal, everyone simultaneously raised their head, opened their eyes, smiled, and nodded as if to acknowledge that their hearts were finished praying and willing to allow their head to resume control.

There are many forms of prayer, and we often assume that prayer is something we actively do or say in our most private moments. Since the heart thinks and feels, it seems reasonable to assume that it can pray without words. Focusing on one's own heart in cardio-contemplation may be one form of prayer, but joining hearts in shared mental stillness may also be a very powerful way of "corporate prayer." British physicist and theologian John Polkinghorne attributes the apparent power of group prayer to its "laser light power" effect.[1] Laser light is unusually powerful because it is "coherent," meaning that its waves are in complete balance, synchronization, and focus. Joining hearts to allow them to pray together without the brain's interference may combine the cardio-coherent energy of all those present into more coherence, order, and power—in other words, a form of divine "L" energy laser.

HEART-FELT RITUALS

Most of us have some fond memories of family rituals. There seemed to be something soothing and reassuring about doing the same things at the same time in the same way with the same people with whom we share a loving bond. Whenever there is a major event to be recognized, from a celebration of a birthday to a supportive post-funeral buffet, the sharing of food with those we care about seems to be a key part of the observance. Even family squabbling, negative gossip, and an annoying relative can seem to be an essential part of the process. One reason this is the case may be because during such times we become more intensely aware of our heart-to-heart connection with others.

The family ties we refer to may be the bonds of "L" energy that flows between the hearts of each family member. By their very nature, families are less rational than emotional. There seems to be something very powerful that keeps families together even when one or more of them might never be a part of our life if we had to choose them as we do our friends. A family could be defined as a group of people irrationally committed to one another's welfare and held together as an energetic system by commonly shared cellular memories often expressed through their rituals.

The brain's style is one of daily routines that tend to be born out of superstitious self-protection and attempts to maintain control, but the heart's style seems to be more one of imparting dignity and symbolism to the most simple acts of life such as eating together, family bedtime, rising in the morning. Ritual may be the way we fall into a state of mutual cardiac coherence, a form of unstated, regular group prayer that helps all those taking part to recover their cellular memories of their loving connection not only with those present but with ancestors whose pictures and stories may be a part of the ritual. If the cardio-contemplation you read about in chapter 7 allows the heart to sing, family rituals may be one way hearts can sing together.

SHARING CELLULAR MEMORIES

Researchers have shown that heart-to-heart rituals have demonstrable positive effects on the heart and immune system. Researcher and pediatrician Dr. Thomas Boyce and his colleagues have studied the impact of ritual on health. They define ritual as the enactment of the sense that certain central, valued elements of life experience are stable and enduring. This interpretation of family ritual isn't far off from the idea that, some level, in every family ritual, families are sharing cellular memories.[2]

Psychologist Aaron Antonovsky emphasized the importance of a sense of life as being structured, predictable, and explicable, a state he called a "sense of coherence."[3] When the same behaviors are conducted in about the same way by the same people over and over again, it's possible that "L" energy is freed to bond the participating members together. There may well be a universal patterned, manageable, meaningful nature to life that resides within the lessons of our collective soul.

Physician E. W. Jensen writes, "Observable, repetitive behaviors which involve two or more family members and which occur with predictable regularity in the day-to-day and week-to-week life of the family are conducive to child health."[4] Jensen found that those children who do have regular family dinners, sitting at the same table at about the same time in the same chair, tend to have fewer colds and other infections than those who do not have the benefit of regular "L" energy feasts.

The most recent study on the measurable benefits of family ritual was conducted by Dr. Blake Bowden, a senior fellow in neurodevelopment disorders at Cincinnati Children's Hospital and Medical Center. The results of his survey of 527 teens aged 12 to 18 showed that those who ate a meal with an adult in their family an average of about five days a week versus three days a week tended to smoke and abuse drugs less, drink less alcohol, were more motivated in school, and were more optimistic about the future.[5] While there are many other possible explanations for these findings, including the fact that adults may not want to eat meals with children who are poorly adjusted or that troubled teens don't want to eat with their family, it is also possible that there is subtle love energy at work in the form of cardio-energetic parenting.

THE HUMAN ECG

That sitting around the family dinner table may be a form of heart energy exchange is suggested by an often neglected yet crucial medical finding: The energy generated by the heart is not contained within us. There is no shield to "L" energy, so when the heart beats, it can signal other hearts with its info-energy. Even though the doctor places her stethoscope directly on your chest and the technician attaches the electrodes of the electrocardiograph directly to your skin, the energy they are recording is not just yours. It is a spiritual admixture of the energy of all hearts coming and going, including that of the doctor and technician doing the testing.[6] Unfortunately, the invention of the stethoscope long ago removed the gentle, attentive caress of the physician's head and hand from our chest and his gentle touch from our back, but our heart still reaches out and conveys its energy into the cardiologist's and everyone else's head, heart, and soul.

Heart-to-heart info-energetic connection is not just a theoretical concept. Research shows that, by comparing electrocardiograms, one person's heartbeat can be measured in another person.[7] The impact of heart energy connection seems most measurable and noticeable when we are closest together, particularly when we physically touch. When we hold hands, we are on some level acting like two ECGs connecting, and we exchange "L" energy, creating cellular memories. Since the hands have hundreds of sweat glands that reduce skin impedance and thereby increase energy conduction, our hands serve as natural electrodes. When we hold hands, we connect heart energies, most particularly when we facilitate the polarity of that connection by holding right hand to left as when we walk with our lover rather than right to right as when we shake hands to make a business deal.[8] When a family joins hands to say a prayer or blessing prior to their evening meal, they are also joining hearts and creating an "L" energy loop.

BEYOND THE SELF

Our life experiences are influenced by a "profoundness paradox." Despite our brain's attempt at "self-fulfillment," we seem most profoundly and spiritually moved—animated or energized by a subtle life energy—when we are the least aware of our "self." At the most miraculous times in our life, we seem to overcome our xenophobia, reduce our brain's awareness of individual self, and feel completely immersed in the grandeur of just being alive. When we feel the warm love of our family, we can forget the pressures of our individual striving for success. When we have an intense sexual orgasm, are moved to tears by the birth of a new being, try to find meaning in the loss of a loved one and the reality of our own mortality in the process of our own grieving, or laugh so hard that we cry, we may experience a sudden selfless "knowing"—an energetic epiphany that we are totally connected beings and not just separate persons.[9] We may suddenly realize that we are not just particles occasionally bumping into each other but also waves of energy infinitely linked together.

Even the baby and its mother are in some ways one "L" energy system. The electrical potential generated by the heart that is detected by an electrocardiograph can be recorded from any site on the body, not just the chest. While we often think of our heart as in our chest, its energy is not "in" us—it "is" us. Modern physics, biology, and medicine speak of "volume conduction," meaning that, just as a mother whale's song travels through the ocean water to calm her calf, energy is immediately conveyed through an entire system.[10] The experience of volume conduction can take place around the family dinner table or when lovers embrace.

A well-known example of "volume conduction," or the simultaneous broadcasting of energy through a system, is noted in the concurrent recording of fetus and mother cardiac electrical fields (potentials) from the same pair of electrodes placed on the mother's abdomen.[11] The ultimate obstetrical illusion is that there is ever a time when the mother and fetus are energetically separated, either in the uterus or in later life. You have read that doctors have long considered the mother's electrocardiographic energy as a nuisance they call an "artifact" and have struggled to listen only for the fetus' heart and look for its energy on the fetus' individual electrocardiogram. Their own mechanical instruments are insistently trying to tell them, however, that the merging of mother and fetal heart energy is less "artifact" than "the fact of the art" of their systemic energy connection. Life's most basic and earliest evidence of our energetic connection, then, is the mother-fetus communal energy bath that leaves a cellular memory for the child of a safe, caring primal ocean of an infantile paradise.

TOGETHER FOREVER

As strange or science fiction–sounding as the ideas presented above may seem, these assertions are well within the explanatory power of the newest and most powerful of our Western sciences—quantum physics. In 1964, Irish physicist John Stewart Bell introduced what scientists now call Bell's theorem. Applying the logic of quantum physics and extending them in experiments consistent with its rules, Bell showed that objects, once in contact, both change if there is a subsequent change in the other, no matter how far apart they are. He showed that a photon (a quantum particle of light) always has a partner somewhere in the universe and, if the direction of one photon partner's spin is changed, the spin of its partner simultaneously changes no matter where the partner may be.[12] Bell's theorem is an expression of the principle of nonlocality you have read about.

The concept of "nonlocality" discussed in Part I means that "L" energy does not go anywhere at all in the usual way we think of "going." According to the concept of nonlocality, info-energy in the form of the "fifth force" is everywhere always. We are not just influenced by that energy but a part of it. When we pray, we don't send energy up to a High Power spiritual satellite to be relayed to or for someone else. Prayer, like love, is merging with the info-energy that we are always a part of whether our brain "knows" it or not. Energy cardiology and its many related fields of study provide the research and established theories such as dynamic system memory, speed-of-light info-energy conveyance, wave/particle duality, volume conduction, and nonlocality that help us begin to understand prayer, psychic communication, and the making of miracles. Cardiac psychology and stories from cardio-sensitives give us dramatic confirmation of the importance of a cardio-centric and energetic view of life for healing and health. Good medical advice regarding a healthy heart might include not only what and how much we should eat but how, where, and with whom.

Connecting heart to heart may be a form of praying. It is not only a matter of sending and receiving energy but of attending to the heart in order to become aware of the level on which our sharing of the infinite energy that is everywhere is primarily taking place within us. It is surrendering the self, transcending the brain's illusion of control, resonating with "L" energy, and the way the created becomes One with the Creator.

The electromagnetic energy of the heart is instantaneously registered in the electroencephalogram (EEG), an instrument that measures the bioelectric energy of the brain. This means that the brain/heart/body connection is likely to sometimes be experienced as a powerfully sudden and serendipitous event. When we focus on our heart, we connect our entire body system in a synchronized brain/heart/body energy "happening" as might take place when a frightened mother finds the sudden strength to lift a car off of her child or a person performs some other "superhuman" feat.[13] Captain Ahab expressed the intensity of this heartfelt energetic happening when his intense emotion regarding Moby Dick made him say, "If my chest were a cannon, I would shoot my heart out upon him."

I recently saw a cartoon that summarizes the essence of "L" energy connection and the difference between the ways of the brain and the heart. A couple is sitting high on a remote mountaintop looking down on a beautiful view. The man is working on his computer and says, "Cell phone, laptop, pager, satellite uplink—even way out here I feel so connected!" The woman is looking sadly alone and pensive as she peers out from the mountaintop at the beauty sprawled before her. She answers, "Strange . . . I don't think you're connected at all."

GOD'S LANGUAGE

Connecting heart to heart, like connecting with your own heart, is not something you do but more how you are. Benedictine monk Brother David Steindl-Rast clarifies the concept of connection through "just being" by observing, "As long as you know you are praying, you are not praying properly."[14] Our Western brain is so dominant and we are so used to *doing* things, or complying with advertising campaigns that tell us to "just do it," that the cardio-energetics approach of "just being" seems like "doing nothing at all." Cardio-contemplation and connecting heart to heart are both ways of living that are far from "just doing nothing." Contacting your own heart and making contact with other hearts requires intense spiritual effort.

Like physicists studying quantum events in their laboratories, cardio-sensitivity and connecting heart to heart requires invitation instead of demand, being receptive instead of prejudicial in our expectations, and being accepting and welcoming instead of seductive and controlling. If we ignore our brain and let our heart be open, our old cellular memories will leak out to help remind us how "to be," energy will pour in from other hearts to remind us why we "are," and energy from the nonlocal info-energy field in which we are immersed will guide and nurture us into loving heart-to-heart bonds.

Trappist monk Father Thomas Keating echoes the "just being" way of connection by pointing out, "Silence is the language God speaks. Everything else is a broad translation."[15] "L" or subtle energy is not as noisy as the energy the brain prefers, and its cardio-centric way of loving is not as assertive and immediately invigorating as the brain's love manuals promise, but being still, silent, open, receptive, and selfless is the only way two hearts can find each other. When we are still and "brilliantly silent," we are speaking in the language of the sacred.

WHERE TO MEET YOUR MAKER

Sara Paddison, vice president of the Institute of HeartMath, writes, "Whatever your religion or cherished beliefs, the heart is the access point in the human system for experiencing God."[16] While Western-based religions often see God, the Absolute, or the Higher Power as somewhere outside or "up there," cardio-energetics teaches that God or the Absolute manifests as a divine, nonlocal, subtle energy that is everywhere and in everything. Cardio-energetics says that the heart can serve as a magnetic pole attracting that energy.

The heart may be where God's intelligence or logic is expressed within us. Paddison writes, "In gaining heart balance, you are going back to your original state. If the real purpose of life is to 'meet your Maker' . . . re-creating . . . balancing . . . focusing your system would be the means to the end."[17] The path to paradise and the gate to heaven is through the heart, and by having a warm, open heart, we allow God's love to happen to us. It is at these times when we are our most loving and ready to receive another heart.

By being still, inviting other hearts to connect with yours, and being receptive to the subtle "L" energy that is the heart's code, you are not resting, you are awakening to your connection with everyone, everything, and every time to let your natural resonation response occur. One of my heart transplant recipients, a minister of a Unity Church, summed up the feeling of connecting heart to heart when he said, "I used this word carelessly before I got my new heart; I won't anymore. Now I know what the word ecstasy really is and I know what people mean when they say they can feel their heart bursting with joy. It's like a flower seeking the sun and connecting with a sacred kind of energy that people, places, and things give off. I can feel it in my heart, and it often brings me to tears at the strangest moments. When I look at my grandson, a sunset, or a robin, I feel overwhelmed with a warm energy in my heart, and it is ecstasy. Now when I conduct services on Sunday mornings, I don't say 'let us pray,' I say, 'Let us let prayer happen.'"

SYNCHRONIZED HEARTS

Energy cardiology researchers are now using a complex system to measure the way in which hearts can communicate with one another. CSEP, or Cardiac Synchronized Energy Patterns, is a way of detecting various types of energy associated with the heart, including electrical activity recorded by the electrocardiograph, magnetic activity recorded by the magneto-cardiograph, cardiac sounds recorded by an electronic stethoscope, and various pressure and temperature changes as recorded by specially designed quantifying instruments.[18] The sum of all of these measures constitutes a total combination of "heart energies" that carry the as yet unmeasurable "subtle 'L' energy" along with them as they course through the body.[19] Using this objective technique, energy cardiology can study synchronization between organisms that are not physically connected.

Russek and Schwartz conducted a fascinating experiment illustrating the energetic connection between hearts and between hearts and brains. They had two people sit opposite one another in the same room with their eyes closed and not communicating in any tactile, visual, or auditory way.[20] Using two of the CSEP measurement procedures, they attached separate ECGs and EEGs to both persons and recorded them simultaneously. The preliminary results of the Russek and Schwartz study indicated three possible "L" energy connections. First, it appeared that a person's own heart's energy transmits to her or his brain. Second, one person's heart seems to exchange energy with another person's brain. Finally, and most relevant to the heart-to-heart connection hypothesis, there seemed to be exchange of energy between two people's hearts. As with two tuning forks, the resonating energy from one heart interacts with the energy of our own brain, other brains, and other hearts. Russek's and Schwartz's work may help explain the apparent combining and synchronizing of energy that accounts for the "laser power" effect of group prayer discussed at the beginning of this chapter.

If the heart acts like the soul's tuning fork, it may express the soul's code with every beat. Every contraction of our heart may become the memory of another heart, and that newly created memory in someone else's heart is radiated back to us to become a new memory for our heart. A group of hearts sitting around the family dinner table together may resonate together in an infinitely complex system of memory making and

"L" energy-sending prayer. In more technical terms, each of us has our own unique CSEP signature that we constantly communicate to and receive from others.

TELESOMATIC EVENTS

Philosopher Paracelsus (1493–1541) wrote, "The vital force is not enclosed in man, but radiates around him like a luminous sphere, and it may be made to act at a distance. In these semimaterial rays the imagination of a man may produce health or morbidity."[21] Since cardio-energetics suggests that there are no barriers in time or space to separate us, that our info-energy can "act at a distance," and that there are light and dark sides to this subtle "L" energy, the consequences of connecting heart to heart may not always be pleasant. Sending "bad energy" could cause negative physical and psychological consequences "telesomatically."

Nonlocal connection is sometimes referred to as "telesomatic," a word derived from the Greek words "tele," meaning far off, and "soma," referring to the body.[22] Reports of sensing something wrong with someone far away or making a psychic connection with a person who is not present, similar to the findings regarding remote viewing in the PEAR laboratory, are common. Like the stories of the heart transplant recipients regarding their cellular memories, reports of these telesomatic occurrences that seem to illustrate our energetic and nonlocal connection have long been viewed with great suspicion. They are often dismissed as "mere coincidence" or amusing little anecdotes, but cardio-energetics provides a way to understand telesomatic connections.

An example of a telesomatic event comes from the wife of one of my patients who spoke with me in my office. Her husband was undergoing angiography and, to distract herself from her worries about her husband as she waited, she wanted to discuss my research in cardio-energetics. In the middle of a sentence, she doubled over, grabbed her chest as if in severe pain, and cried, "My God. He's had a heart attack. Joe just had heart attack." I called for a stretcher and, as we wheeled her to the cardiac unit, her husband was wheeled past her as the nurses brought him out of the exam room. Husband and wife looked at each other and, before they could speak, one of the nurses sensed the wife's fear. She said, "He's OK. He had a little trouble in there and his heart stopped for just a few seconds. We got it going again and he's going to be fine." The telesomatic connection in this case was not pleasant for the wife but illustrative of the couple's strong energetic connection with one another.

A similar story is reported by parapsychologist Loisa Rhine. She tells of a woman who suddenly "doubled over, clutched her chest as if in pain, and said, 'Something has happened to Nell; she has been in an accident.'" Two hours later the sheriff arrived to state that Nell had died on the way to the hospital following an auto accident. She was killed by a piece of the steering wheel that penetrated her chest.[23]

As remarkable as these stories of connection at a distance may seem, they are remarkably consistent from case to case in the nature of the reports. They are much more commonplace than would be expected if they were mere flukes. Moreover, they resemble nonlocal events that occur in physics laboratories in their coincidental, serendipitous appearance. Like many of the quantum physics principles, they may reveal that our classical Newtonian physics cannot explain everything. Telesomatic stories are often reported by people who seem more tuned in than most to their "hidden observer" described earlier. These stories are reported by persons who have had or now have some profound connection with the person [such as receiving a new heart] with whom they share the telesomatic experience.

When we speak about consciousness, we usually think in terms of first-person singular and how our "self" experiences the world. As individually as we experience our consciousness, it is shaped in the context of relationships. In other words, our relationships with others and other things is a crucial part of what it means to be a "me."

"Me" or "it" have been the concern, but often the issue of "us" and third-person accounts of awareness and connection with nonlocal subtle energy such as experienced by the couple above have been left out. Cardio-energetic's focus on second-person "heart-to-heart" connection suggests that there is a unique power when two hearts connect. In a review of a book summarizing a major scientific meeting to discuss consciousness and subtle energetic connections and awareness, Dr. Alexander Eliot wrote, "there is something about the nature of consciousness that requires the presence of the 'other' as another subject who can acknowledge my being. . . . Perhaps at the next . . . conference the second-person voice will also be heard."[24] The sound of the heart speaking may be heard in this "second voice."

ONE MIND AND MILLIONS OF BODIES

Here is a summary of some of the latest research supporting the power of "L" energy to connect us "heart to heart."

• Blood platelets, the tiny round disks in our blood that help clotting take place, were isolated from a healthy human volunteer and then "treated" or influenced by an energy healer, someone who claims to be able to alter the energy within living systems. In complete stillness and silence, the healer "connected" with one of the platelets' key biochemicals that help make platelets work—an enzyme called monoamine oxidase (MAO). The enzyme's activity was altered as compared with no change in the activity of "untreated" samples.[25]

• Thirty-two subjects mentally attempted to alter blood chemistry. They tried to prevent a process called hemolysis, which can cause blood cells to deteriorate. The energy connectors or healers were able to prevent this process.[26]

• In 13 experiments, the ability of 62 people to influence the physiology of 271 distant subjects was studied. A summary of the results indicated that many of these people were able or willing to tune in to their own physiology. These were the same people who also were able to alter the physiology of other persons at the "psychological distance" of 20 meters used in the experiment. Those who were able to telesomatically connect had many of the characteristics of the cardio-sensitives.[27]

• A double-blind study of 393 persons admitted to a coronary care unit examined the affect of intercessory prayer offered from great distances to half of the patients. Statistically significant fewer patients in the prayer group required intubation (mechanical ventilation) and antibiotics and were less likely to develop pneumonia or require diuretics.[28]

• Nonhuman species and even mechanical objects seem able to show the effects of the same subtle energy connections shown by humans. Researchers tested the possible influence of 80 groups of 15 chicks on a randomly moving robot carrying a lighted candle in a dark room. Baby chicks prefer light, and the experimenters were trying to determine whether the chicks' preference could influence the robot. In 71 percent of the cases, the robot spent excessive time in the vicinity of the chicks. In the absence of the chicks, the robot followed the random trajectory.[29]

• There are 54 verified accounts of animals that returned to their owners over great distances. These animals traveled to places they had never been before and therefore could not be directly influenced by prior planted sensory cues or a homing instinct.[30]

Cardio-energetics proposes that the explanation for telesomatic events relates to the subtle "L" energy mediated by the heart. Sara Paddison states, "Our research at the institute found that power to reside within the heart. It's a hidden power that operates in a higher range of frequency bands than the mind."[31] The "power" to which Paddison refers may be "L" energy, and the "mind" to which she refers may be the heartless brain, the small "m" version of the capital "M" brain/heart/body Mind of cardio-energetics.

THE "1 TO 9" RULE

Based on the research into the energy mediated by and emanating from the heart, the Institute of HeartMath proposes what they call a "1 to 9" rule of the heart's energy. Their research shows that by focusing on the heart's natural intelligence, your one energetic effort yields a ninefold return of healthy, balanced energy to you and the world.[32] They say they have found that, because the heart is so energetically powerful, it has a "multiple effect," collecting and amplifying healthy energy throughout all systems.[33]

If you have ever walked through the woods on a warm summer day, you may recall feeling the warmth of the sun drawing you toward it through the trees. Something seemed to guide and pull you along the way. You may have been working at your desk and felt a warmth tapping you on your shoulder—a signal from the sun shining through your window. This is how it feels to tune in to the energy not only of your heart but of other hearts. Fifteenth-century philosopher Marsilio Ficino suggested that everyone turn toward the mystery of his own nature the way a sunflower turns toward the sun.[34] Copying the way of the sunflower is the way of cardio-energetic heart-to-heart connection.

HAVING OUR HEART

One of the most difficult challenges in connecting heart to heart is accepting the fact that such a connection, like prayer, is not something you *do* but how you *are*. By silencing your brain and freeing yourself from its constant annoying urgings to do or think something, by being still enough in the presence of other hearts to allow your heart to be receptive and open to the energy coming to it, by allowing yourself to experience the subtle "L" energy connection in your own heart, and by being aware of the energy going out from your heart to other hearts, your heart becomes no longer just yours but ours. Cardio-contemplation helps you fully and totally have your heart, and sharing cardio-contemplation deeply and profoundly with others helps you share all of what is in and coming from all of our hearts.

The Lustful Brain and the Loving Heart

"The meeting of two personalities is like the contact of two chemical substances: If there is any reaction, both are transformed."

— *CARL JUNG*

THAT LOVING FEELING

You feel love's power when you look into your child's eyes, gaze at the wonderfully wrinkled face of a grandparent, or recall a cherished moment you shared with your family when you were growing up. As if an indication of the sudden change from using your head to deal with life to using your heart to celebrate it, you become light-headed and warm-hearted. You feel a subtle energy attracting you, and your heart may even skip a beat in its excitement that you are now connecting with life on its terms. You struggle to put what you are feeling into words, stammering or regressing to the love language your heart learned when you were a child.

Since the beginning of time, man has tried to define and understand the meaning of love—an impossible task. Love is one of the greatest examples of the power of our heart. Our brains cannot explain or define completely the amazing power of love, and yet when we are in love our hearts seem to understand it completely.

WHAT DOES "I LOVE YOU?" MEAN?

We have long been faced with the challenge of making concrete and measurable what seems to be essentially subjective and immeasurable. We know that what we think about a poem, song, book, or lover is very personal and seems related to our cultural heritage, language, imagery, interests, past life experiences, and many other factors that would seem to defy easy quantifying, yet we persist in saying things such as "I have zero interest in that book," "That view is much more gorgeous than the other view," or "He is more loveable than the other guy."[1] I have been using the letter "L" to signify both the individual's life info-energy and the connective aspects of living that might be called loving energy, and it is very difficult to represent the subtle equivalence between the energies we can more easily see and touch and the energy that seems more spiritual.

In most of our attempts to speak of love, the heart has long been a symbol we use. Based on the concepts of cardio-energetics, it may be that a key aspect of falling in love is the experience of one's own heart falling into energetic synchronization with another heart, an occurrence our brain seems to have great difficulty expressing in its form of energy. The brain is ill-equipped to translate the subtle nature and spiritual magnitude of love-energy events. It is not very good at expressing the subtle but powerful "pull" of "L" energy received from the heart from the cellular memories tapped and released by an intimate heart-to-heart connection. It does not speak the language of what the heart tells it is a "magnetic" power of attraction, attachment, or repulsion—which sometimes occurs because of its powerful positive/negative polarity. Maybe if we learn more about how the heart thinks, feels, and communicates, we will become more conversant in the language of love.

THREE HABITS OF THE HEART

You have read that the heart uses the processes of connecting, nurturing, and integrating all of our cellular memories to create who we are, what we need, and what we have to give. These same three processes are what most people refer to when they say they are in love. "I feel so connected to you," "You give me strength," and "Without you I am not complete" are sample love lines that depict the basic habits of the heart. In essence, loving someone else may be the process of projecting to another heart its own natural way of dealing with the world.

Dr. Lawrence Laskow, who proposes a system he calls "holoenergetic healing," asserts that loving energy is what connects people and makes a loving energy system. He also identifies nurturing, connecting, and integrating as the three core qualities of love.[2] Another author, Matthew Fox, identifies these same three habits of the heart as the three core concepts of spirituality, which may explain why loving can seem to feel like such a sacred occurrence representing the merging of two souls finally freed of obstacles to their energetic connection established by their selfishly defensive brains.[3]

The modern view of love is a highly romantic one. While it often speaks in terms of such things as warmth and caring, what is frequently being conveyed is a need for a lover who meets one's own selfish needs as expressed by the brain's evolutionary directive for self-advancement. If you listen with your heart, you hear less about "my heart" and more about "our hearts." The heart tends to speak in the second-person voice of "us" more than the brain's first-person "me" and third-person "you." If you want to know if you are tapping into the heart's code, try tape recording your conversations with your lover and then counting the number of "I, me, and you" words compared to "we, us, and ours."

When we say that loving is giving our heart to someone, we are describing an "L" energy donor/recipient interaction every bit as profound as a heart transplant. When loving makes us feel more fully alive and energized than at any other time in our life, it is because the power of the "L" energy synchronization between lovers activates the cellular memories of our shared infantile paradise. Perhaps we "feel young again" and regress to using the same baby talk with our lover that we use with a child, referring to him or her as "baby, sweetie, and honey," to acknowledge our sense of joining and remembering what it is like to be as energized and enchanted with life as children are.

Being in sensuous love may be a form of recovering our cellular memories of the state of paradisal infancy when we were nestled safely and lovingly in the amniotic sea inside our mother's womb. One reason we may speak of being drowned in a sea of love or of our love flowing to another person, or seem so attracted to the ocean and any body of water, may be the cellular memories activated by the sight and feeling of water.

THE MYTH OF CASUAL SEX

As you read in chapter 8, when we physically touch one another in a loving manner or join hands, we directly exchange our subtle "L" energy. Our hands act as the leads on an electrocardiograph, establishing measurable energetic connection between two hearts that is measurable in the hearts and brains of both lovers.[4] When we hug, press our chests together, and thump our hands rhythmically on the back of someone we care for, we are placing our hearts as closely together as we can so that their close proximity allows our hearts to "beat as one."[5]

From a cardio-energetic point of view, it may not be possible to engage in "casual" sex. Every mechanistic act of genital juxtaposition and mutual pelvic gymnastics may also be a vital-fluid, connective-energy exchange. What we mechanistically refer to as a climax is really a powerful end to the build-up to an energetic bond. Whenever we "make love," and whether or not we combine cells to make a new life, we are creating new cellular memories within and between two life systems. We are engaging in an energetic event that, because of the principle of nonlocality and the fact that elements once in contact are forever connected, becomes a permanent cellular memory of and for each lover. If our intent is to avoid energetic commitment, no sex is "safe" sex.

When I first presented my theories of cardio-energetic loving, one physician said, "I respect the power of the heart, but I cannot accept your radical new idea that one heart can actually physically affect another heart. That's just a throwback to vitalism and I think we long ago left that stuff behind." I responded that the idea of the heart's influence on another heart and even the impact of a transplanted heart on the feelings and behaviors of the recipient is hardly new. In the 1860s, French physician Claude Bernard circulated the blood of one dog through the heart of a second dog. After a time delay, he noted changes in the heart rate of the donor dog were accompanied by parallel changes in the recipient dog's heart rate.[6] As mentioned above, when energy cardiologists Schwartz and Russek modified this century-old approach by connecting the electrocardiographs and electroencephalographs of two persons, they too discovered that there is some vital energetic connection that takes place between humans.[7]

We can often feel the energy flowing between ourself and our lover. To be sensual is to be aware of the subtle "L" energy of the heart, and it is much more a matter of energy-field merging than just searching for erotic zones or G-spots. Because loving is more an affair of the heart than the head, when we attempt to make sensuous contact with another human being, we are literally using our basic five senses as energy conduits to and from our heart and using the mechanisms of the body to express the vitalism of the spirit. In effect, our immeasurable love code is transmitted as subtle "L" energy and carried within the measurable forms of energy we exchange, much as the meaning of the words we speak are converted to the type of energy conveyed over telephone lines. Free of the brain's defensive interference, our heart can merge with another heart in a "cardio-energetic consolidation" that we experience as consummated love.

FINDING YOUR "H" SPOT

When we become sexually aroused, our heart rate increases. Like turning up the volume on the radio, more energy is being broadcast. Because there are more and more intense contractions of our heart, more info-energy is pulsated from our heart to our lover's heart. Because sexual intimacy can be seen as energy enhancement facilitated by two hearts acting as subtle "L" energy accelerators, the heart becomes our most important erotic organ—the "H" spot from which subtle loving energy emanates. When another heart races along with and in response to our own, the contractions of both hearts intensify and transmit even more "L" energy, literally "coming together" energetically.

When we experience sexual orgasm, our heart rate more than doubles. As a result, a large amount of "L" energy is exchanged between partners because orgasm represents a cardio-energetic power surge. If body fluids are exchanged through the sex act, even more info-energy may be transmitted with the exchanged cells' memories. The sex act then becomes an info-energetic transplantation between two persons, each serving as both donor and recipient of "L" energy. Because the principle of volume conduction you read about in chapter 8 says that energy is conveyed and expressed immediately through an entire system, semen, vaginal secretions, and saliva can serve as the vital fluids physically containing and conveying a measure of each lover's heart's cellular memories.

BROKEN OR BLISSFUL HEARTS

When our love songs are not celebrating the magic of love, they are bemoaning a lost or unrequited love. Perhaps no other emotion is capable of eliciting such deeply felt highs and terrible lows. Cardio-energetics suggests that this may be so because "L" energy is the primary language of the heart and therefore is very closely connected with both the brightest and darkest energy of the brain/heart/body Mind.

Nothing in the universe is one-sided. Our life and love is a kind of systolic/diastolic dance that resonates the dark-side "L" energy, providing the necessary contrast to its light-side "L" energy. Love is not a static state of the heart but an oscillation that invigorates our loving and our life by contributing the day and night and ups and downs that make life and love possible. Because of the powerful reverberating "ups" and "downs" of "L" energy, love is not for the faint of heart. When we get ourselves involved in matters of the heart, we immerse ourselves in both the light and dark kinds of energy. If we romantically delude ourselves into believing that love is only blissfully beautiful, we are ignorantly assuming that the heart has only one side, that systole can exist without diastole, and that there can be day without night. We become love blind to the true nature and challenges of loving and set ourselves up for disappointment and relationship problems. If we mistake the necessary "diastolic" downs and stresses of love as signs that love is ending, we can become lovesick cynics who withdraw from loving. If we realize that, as with any form of energy, and just as peaceful oceans can also become destructive tidal waves, love's healing power is matched by its potential to hurt, we can enter loving bonds with a wiser and more tolerant heart. Just as the same electrical energy that lights our life can end it, the loving energy of the heart can also shake and weaken us and even be lethal. The pain of loving is the price we must pay to benefit from the healing power of love.

THE CARDIO-ENERGETICS OF HEARTBREAK

When we refer to our heart as broken, we may in part be referring to an energetic connection we experience as having ended. We may be reporting our experience of the essential complimentary sides of "L" energy, our sense of connecting with the dark cellular memories of all prior physical separations. Our loving cellular memories retain not only a joyful sense of our infantile paradise but also the pain of our fall from grace. Because of our cellular memories, which have been left within us by our heart, every time we physically or mentally end a relationship, we are recycling through the ending of every relationship we have ever experienced. We may also be experiencing the pain of an illusory separation, since all our heart wants is to help us feel connected with others.

For cardio-energetics, heartbreak is not only the disruption and/or recollection of a disruption of a prior physically activated energy connection. It is also a spiritual shock, the direct experience of the negative aspects of our lover's energy. Just as when two positive or two negative poles of a very strong magnet make contact, when we experience the wrong polarities, we feel repelled. Healthy, lasting loving is remembering that the very strength of our repulsion is evidence of the power of the loving energy available between us. The magnitude of the pull of our loving energy reveals the strength of the negative forces that are also present. The more "attracting pull" we feel from someone, the more "repelling push" that is also likely to be present. This systolic/diastolic nature of love is not one of its problems but a reflection of the challenge it poses to our soul.

When any energy connection is terminated, we say there is a disconnection. The same holds true for our heart. When the heart can no longer use its physical body to bring in the energy of the lover, it feels as if its power lines have been cut. The brain, which relies primarily on the four basic forms of energy (electromagnetic, gravity, strong and weak nuclear energy) usually processed by our five basic senses (seeing, hearing, smelling, tasting, and touching) may think that its loving energy source is gone forever. If we tune in to the heart's code, however, we will learn that our lover's energy is forever within us as a sacred cellular memory and that the energy waves of our lover are no less real than the physical particles that represented our lover. The very good news from cardio-energetics is that all endings, including death, are the brain's illusions. For the heart, what the brain sees as an ending is only a starting point of info-energetic transition and transformation.

HOW TO MEND A BROKEN HEART

Cardio-contemplation and the cardio-coherence that accompanies it is one way to mend a broken or energy-disconnected heart. By using the techniques presented in chapters 7 and 8, we can hear our heart telling us that our lover may be gone physically from our daily life but will always be in our heart and in our soul. Cellular imprints left within us are not erased. By tapping into the heart's energy and wisdom, we can be energetically "with" our lover no matter where she or he may be.

The word "bereaved" means "to have taken away." The word "grieve" refers to a feeling of weight or heaviness.[8] Our heart feels "heavy" when a physical loving bond is disrupted because some of the energy of our loved one that so lightens our heart is diminished. Our heart is made lighter again by tuning in to our heart to recover the cellular memories that forever contain the energy of our lover even when he or she is no longer physically with us.

Energy healer Julie Motz writes, "It is our emotions, which, I believe, are waves of energy moving through our bodies, that tell us what we fear, what we desire, who we are, and to whom we are connected."[9] Once we understand cardio-energetics' concept of loving as an info-energetic spiritual event rather than a romantic brain occurrence, our heart is free to fulfill the promise we often make to one another when we feel the most loving—that we will love and be loved forever.

THE IMPORTANCE OF BEING A BI-SENSUAL

The word "sensual" as used by cardio-energetics refers to the various ways we become aware of the subtle "L" energy of love. Our heart acts like a Geiger counter, sensing various aspects and intensities of loving energy. To love wisely and permanently, we must be "bi-sensual" and alert to and tolerant of the two natures of love as a strong attracter and also sometimes a strong repeller.

In my clinical work with families with very troubled children, I have noticed an info-energetic paradox. The child who seems to cause the most disruption in the family system is also often the child who seems to elicit the most loving energy from the parents even when there is also a very dark side to the loving. Describing her love of her rebellious teenage daughter, a mother said, "I love her so much it hurts, and she hurts me so much I love her. If I didn't love her as much as I do, I'd hate her. She causes me so much more heartache than my other daughter, yet my connection with her seems the strongest. It would break my heart if I could not be with her but sometimes she breaks my heart when she is with me. I have to take the good with the bad. That's what real love is." This mother was describing not only the nature of both sides of the heart's loving energy but the fact that the intensity of a profound loving connection is often accompanied by an equally challenging and intense agitation and suffering.

Those we connect with intimately and with whom we share intense "L" energy will always bring us both great peace and great pain, and we will always do the same to them. When it comes to loving energy, delight and disgust are not far from one another. If we deny that fact, it is a sign that our romantic brain is dominating our wiser, loving heart and that the brain is desperately clinging to its evolutionary imperative of self-advancement.

SEXLESS IN SEATTLE

I recently spoke to a large group of heart patients and their spouses in Seattle, Washington. Some were awaiting a new heart and I took the opportunity to interview them for this book. All of them were experiencing various levels of cardiovascular disease. I was able to interview eight men and seven women heart attack survivors and their spouses. As I always do, I heard many explanations for their heart disease, including rich diet, obesity, high blood pressure, genetic predisposition, lack of exercise, smoking, and stress. I had been introduced to my audience with all of my former professional positions, and when my interviewees found out that I was former director of professional education at the Kinsey Institute for Research in Sex, Gender, and Reproduction at Indiana University, had studied at the Masters and Johnson Institute, and had founded and directed a sexual dysfunction clinic in Michigan, they disclosed with varying levels of discomfort a concern they said none of their doctors had discussed in any detail with them. All of the patients and their spouses with whom I spoke said that, for more than a year prior to their heart attack, they had not been sexually active.

Current research on the sexual lives of heart patients shows that more than half of heart attack victims have one thing in common: They did not have any sexual activity of any kind for the entire year preceding their heart attack.[10] If it was discovered that over half of the five hundred thousand people who have a heart attack each year never ate carrots, there would probably be a rush to the vegetable market and Bugs Bunny would be the American Heart Association's poster child. However, while lack of sex and deprivation of the immense "L" energy that accompanies it seems to be at least a contributor to vulnerability to heart disease, little has been made of this finding.

Another study also showed the impact of erotic deprivation of the heart. Twelve hundred men and five hundred women were confidentially interviewed about their sexual activity in the hours, days, and year preceding their heart attack. From these interviews, it was learned that lack of sexual activity was one characteristic shared by those who had a heart attack. This study was published in the *Journal of the American Medical Association,* one of the most prestigious medical journals in the world, yet this finding has been largely ignored by most physicians.[11] In another example of the heartlessness of medicine, those physicians who did read and respond to the journal article said only that the data from the study showed that having sex *after* a heart attack did not seem too likely to be fatal.

Cardio-energetics suggests that lack of intimate physical contact may deprive the heart of a form of much needed regular "L" energy boost and the intense proximity of the energetic presence of another heart that helps it stay in "synch." Sudden cardiac death is the ultimate lack of life rhythm, and sensual contact may be important to providing energetic nurturing and rhythmic synchronization to the heart from another heart, just as a low-fat diet, regular exercise, and less stressful life helps protect it.

Despite all of the progress we have made in identifying the risk factors for cardiovascular disease, such as obesity, sedentary lifestyle, high blood pressure, and stress, more than 50 percent of heart attack victims have none of these risk factors, and most people who have one or more of these risk factors will never have a heart attack.[12] Currently, only about 50 percent of the time can mechanistically oriented physicians account for why we get sick and get well, yet we seem to live as hostages of a health terrorism that warns us away from the simple pleasures of living so we can have a longer but often less joyful life as the "worried well."[13]

Despite the evidence you have read about in this book, modern medicine clings to the image of the body as a machine serviced by the heart as a biomechanical pump. By doing so, it neglects many of cardio-energetics', energy cardiology's, and cardiac psychology's important findings about the heart as a loving, energetic organ. The remainder of this chapter is about one of life's potentially greatest and most healthy pleasures—loving, sensual connection—and how connecting heart to heart may be the ultimate health maintenance program.

STEMMING THE FLOOD

Psychologist John Gottman has done extensive research on intimate relationships, and some of his work may reveal the role of "L" energy in these relationships and its implications for physical and mental health.[14] His work illustrates the role of the heart in marital conflict. He reports that a psychophysiological response called "flooding" occurs in partners in relationships who are critical of each other, "stonewalling," and refusing to engage emotionally. Flooding is primarily the rapid increase in heart rate.[15] Depending on body size, a man's heart beat at rest tends to be about 72 beats per minute and a woman's heart beats at about 82 beats per minute.

Flooding, according to Gottman, is when the heart rate increases about 10 beats per minute. Some people, usually those whose temperament may cause them to have a more highly reactive heart, experience such immediate and severe flooding in response to emotional conflict that their heart accelerates 30 beats per minute in the space of a single heartbeat.

In what author Daniel Goleman calls a "limbic tango," partners cycle through a spousal conflict usually initiated by the woman who tends to be the emotion manager of most relationships. Since she is usually the partner who is more relational and "heart" focused and vigilant for relationship problems, she complains about a problem she feels in her heart but her spouse does not sense in his.[16] The man, who usually has his heart less into the relationship, tries to use his brain to try to figure out the "substance of the problem" and how it might be immediately fixed. His protective and selfish brain personalizes the complaint as its own failure. Since the problem was detected by the woman's heart and the man is trying to solve it with his head, many relationship problems may be due to speaking in two different codes. The man's brain feels its heart starting to flood and tells him to withdraw. It says, "Go golfing, watch a ball game, cut the grass, but do anything to just get me away from this hassle for awhile."

When a man withdraws, or intellectualizes a complaint, the woman goes from emotional disappointment to intellectual disgust and becomes critical. Failing to connect "heart to heart," she now uses her brain more than her heart and tries to find her partner's weak mental point in order to make her emotional point. She exaggerates, sulks, or initiates a subtle emotional vendetta intended to teach her love-blind partner a lesson "the hard way." Because Gottman's research shows that men tend to be more "hot-hearted" and cardio-vascularly reactive than women during conflicts, the man's heart begins to flood.

When a man's heart floods, his brain detects a vague sense of dread caused by a physiological reaction to a sense of helplessness in the face of his partner's disappointment and disgust. Wanting to stem the flood, the man "stonewalls" or tries to sever the intensified energetic connection with his partner, which is now a dark-side connection. He tries to block or deflect the energy, which his heart senses is coming at it, by being abrupt, curt, and unresponsive. When a man stonewalls, the negative energy his partner is sending bounces right back to her off his emotional wall. As a result of this toxic energy rebound back to *her* heart, now *she* begins to flood.

When a man's heart floods, he stonewalls and tries to block off or send the disruptive energy away in an attempt to maintain his own cardiac coherence. When a woman's heart floods, she tends to send the disruptive energy inside, somaticizing her cardiac incoherence, which weakens her immune system. As a result, she experiences various infections, allergies, headaches, and, in a genitalia-manifested metaphor of her rejection of her partner and the toxic nature of her relationship with him, may even experience recurrent vaginitis. There is no more direct evidence of the impact of the thinking, feeling, loving, and angry heart than an exhausting spousal limbic tango.[17]

SEXUAL VIBRATIONS

You have read that, because of volume conduction, the electrical potential generated by the heart, as identified by the electrocardiograph, can be recorded from any site on the body.[18] Not only does each beat of the heart generate patterns of energy that have the potential to influence the function of every cell, but these patterns of energy also serve as a synchronizing and integrating force. Because the heart's energy arrives at every one of our 75 trillion cells virtually at the same time, love happens all at once all over our body. Because the blood is such a good conductor of sound, our heart's sounds travel through the blood to everywhere within us. Because the heart's energy is everywhere all of the time, the entire body system becomes an erogenous zone.

I first noticed the significance of the energetic vibrations surging through the body when I worked with paraplegics who came to my clinic attempting to recover their sexual lives. Because of a break in the neural conduction of sexual impulses from the genitals to their brain, most paraplegics reported nearly complete numbness in their genitalia. They assumed that, because of the loss of pelvic sensations, they would never again experience orgasm. Cardio-energetics, however, offered a creative nongenital, energetic way to help these patients return to a pleasing sexual intimacy.

Spinal-damaged patients coming to my clinic at Sinai Hospital of Detroit were first given a complete physical and neurological examination to determine or confirm the exact level of neurological damage. They then took part in a seminar on the basics of human sexual response and were helped to examine their own attitudes toward sexuality, intimacy, loving, and their own damaged body. Using the H*E*A*R*T* questionnaire and the CSI, they were also helped to assess and understand the nature of their "cardio-match" with their partner. They were then asked to return to their hotel with their partner to do a "sensual energy scan."

The sensual energy scan consisted of a partner of the paraplegic going over every inch of the body of the paraplegic partner. Using a brush to gently stroke the skin, a straw to focus the breath on a specific area, and cold and hot liquids to warm and cool the lips of the scanning partner, he or she searched the body of the partner for areas that led to a feeling of sensual arousal. These areas usually turned out to be "pulse points" where the partner could actually see and feel the heart beating. In almost every case in which partners were willing to take the time and have the patience, the paraplegics were helped to return to orgasms. Most reported that their orgasms were even more intense and fulfilling than their prior genitalia-focused orgasms. In keeping with the "let it happen" approach of cardio-connection discussed throughout this book, orgasms seemed to happen most easily, often, and most intensely for those couples most "in love" (as described in this chapter) and most willing to be patient, take their time, and be available to the energetic event.

Cardio-energetics sees sexual intimacy as energy connection. Since energy is everywhere, that connection can take place anywhere. Patients reported "neck-gasms," "ear-gasms," and even "inner-arm orgasms." One couple in which the man was unable to move or feel beneath his waist developed a form of sexual interaction that involved the man rubbing the inner surface of his forearm, where his pulse could be observed, firmly and rhythmically against the clitoris of his partner. The result was mutual orgasm.

One paraplegic man summarized the "sensual scanning technique" as follows: "When I broke my neck, I thought that was that. I thought I would never have sex again and I couldn't think of any way I could possibly have an orgasm since I could not feel my penis. When you showed us the energy scanning thing, we finally found that I really responded to my neck being licked with my partner's cold tongue. I would never know when it would happen, but all of a sudden, and when we seem to not even be trying, it seems to happen. Now, she keeps ice tea next to the bed and we have a great time. I'd say I'm orgasmic about 50 percent of the time, but who's counting? I know I'm a much better lover now than before I broke my neck."

Just as we all might learn more about a more connected, caring, balanced life from the characteristics of those heart transplant recipients who seem more cardio-sensitive, we might also enhance our own sexual intimacy by being less genitalia dependent and capitalizing on the cardio-energetics principles of volume conduction and dynamic systemic energy available throughout our body.

WEARING OUR HEART ON OUR FACE

You read in chapter 6 about the face of an angry heart and the thin smile, bulging cheeks, wide eyes, and jutting chin of the hot and agitated heart. Love energy can also show on our face in the form of at least eighteen different smiles that signal "come here and connect with me." Anthropologist Helen Fisher has identified the look of a loving heart as expressed on the face. She calls one of these facial expressions a "copulatory gaze."[19] When we look into our lover's eyes for several moments to establish an ocular energetic connection, then lower our eyelids and look down toward our genitalia to direct the energy to that area, we are acknowledging that our lover's energy has been received into our pupils, and our eyes point the way to another place for a physically sensual energetic connection.

Any positive effect of sending and receiving energy eye to eye is negated, however, by the "look of disgust." No matter what our brain is making us say, when our heart distorts our face by curling our lips firmly to one side and wrinkling our nose, in what Charles Darwin suggested is a primordial attempt to close the nostrils against a noxious odor or to spit out a poisonous food, we are saying "get away."[20]

The energy of the heart molds our body and face. It creates a mask that, over time, becomes etched with the tracings of the energy we send. Leftover wrinkles from the too-frequent look of disgust show us that the heart has had trouble connecting, just as the smile marks next to the eyes indicate that a loving heart has been energizing this body.

THE POWER OF PROPINQUITY

Another principle from the "cardio-energetics of sensuous love" is the influence of propinquity, or close physical proximity on loving connection. As would be predicted by biophysiology, energy systems near to one another often show a more profound energy connection. Nearness, not absence, makes the heart grow fonder. The more often we are exposed to someone, the more we are soaked in their energy and the more we become attracted to and bonded with them. Psychologists call this the "repeated exposure effect," a law of propinquity that teaches that quantity of time together is at least if not more important than the quality of time we spend with one another.[21]

The myth of "quality time" may be a major stressor for our loving relationships. What we need is not to try to make the most of a little time spent with those we love but to spend much more of the time we have loving. No matter how busy we become, the fact is that long, restful, quiet periods of heart-to-heart contact are the essential energy connections that tend to keep love growing and alive.

Cardio-energetics suggests many other lessons of love. Here are some examples of findings from cardio-energetics regarding healthy loving that challenge the brain's selfish romanticism.

• *The brain says "opposites attract." The heart knows that similarities strengthen attraction.* While it is true that opposites attract, research shows that they do not connect for long. The more similar a person is to us, particularly in their energetic temperament (inhibited or uninhibited) and heart reactivity (hot or cold), the more likely it is that a loving energy connection will grow and develop.[22]

• *The brain says to "assert and represent ourselves" in our relationships. The heart knows to listen, receive, and be open to our lover's energy.* Cardio-energetics teaches that humble ingratiation—working hard to agree with, praise, and flatter our partner—is crucial to maintaining an energetic relationship. When it comes to the matter of "L" energy exchange, "fair fighting" does not cause the brain-to-brain confrontation to be less destructive.[23]

• *The brain says the lover's friends and family matter less than who our lover is. The heart knows that we love an entire energy system, not just one individual.* Cardio-energetics warns that our parents and those who were around us as we developed have left a permanent loving energy imprint within our heart, and that learning to recognize, respect, tolerate, and share that imprint is crucial to mature, lasting loving and to our total health.[24]

• *The brain believes in the "just world hypothesis" of beauty, that attractive people deserve their attractiveness, but the heart knows that beauty evolves as loving energy "creates" our lover in our own eyes.* The brain thinks that attractive people are better people because they were rewarded for their cleverness and goodness by their good looks.[25] Cardio-energetics teaches that the more time we are with our partner, the more we will began to physically look like them and be molded by their heart's energy. For cardio-energetics, beauty is not "in" the eyes of the beholder but created "by" the eyes of the beholder by the energy he or she sends to the partner.

The idea of "romantic love" is a relatively new one that emerged well into the seventeenth century at the same time the brain rose to power over the heart.[26] Cardio-energetic love is heart-centered and based on the idea that the heart gets the brain to decide to love rather than being led by its lower, limbic romantic impulses. Cardio-energetic love involves the decision to attempt to connect deeply and lastingly with the heart energy of the partner and not to "fall into love" just because the brain sees a person who will meet its every need.

A LOVING TRINITY

Psychologist Robert Sternberg has proposed a triangular theory of love that provides a summary of the sensuous nature of "L" energy.[27] He says that the three key components of loving are passion, commitment, and intimacy. Passion refers to those drives that lead to feelings of romance, physical attraction, and sexual consummation. This is primarily a neuro-chemical bodily reflex, and without the brain to reflect on it and the heart to give it meaning, it alone is not fulfilling and is not likely to maintain a relationship, particularly at times of stress and challenge to that relationship.

The second of Sternberg's components of love, commitment, is the rational decision to stay with a lover in the short and long term. This is primarily the work of the brain seeking support in its struggles through life. Without the thrill from the body's connection with another body or the intimacy of the heart's energetic connection, commitment alone leads to what Sternberg calls an "empty," and cardio-energetics calls an "energy-less," love.

The third component of loving, according to Sternberg, is intimacy, which Sternberg defines as feelings in a relationship of closeness, bonding, and intimate connection. These feelings are similar to the three loving habits of the heart identified at the beginning of this chapter—connecting, nurturing, and integrating. Where passion is the work of the body and commitment is the job of the brain, intimacy is an affair of the heart.

Without the heart to coordinate our loving, we have only what Sternberg calls infatuated, empty, and unrealistic or romantic love. When we put our heart into our loving by being more cardio-sensitive, we love "Mind to Mind," as two trinities of brain/heart/body energetically connected. When such a profound connection occurs, our heart is made happy and content as we find meaning together in the chaos of living.

OVERCOMING THE BRAIN'S LOVE BLINDNESS

When we are still enough to establish the cardio-coherence that makes us peaceful enough to love and be loved, and allow ourselves to suspend the brain's defensive vigilance and arrogant prejudices, then we can become more aware of what our heart is trying to tell us about another heart, and compassionate enough to be receptive to the subtle energy coming from that heart. That is when our brain can overcome its innate love blindness. Suddenly, and often without warning and far beyond its powers of reason, the brain realizes that there is a much higher power than the power it seeks in its daily struggle for dominance. At such times, it surrenders its control, allows its heart to join freely and fearlessly with another heart, and, speaking for the heart, says, "I love you."

CHAPTER TEN

A Hassled Brain and a Happy Heart

"When you're not trying to make the heart into something you think is proper, it showers you with its magic, and even in the midst of pain it can offer moments of rapture."

— *THOMAS MOORE*

THE SWINGING PHILOSOPHER

"Stop it, you're killing me," said my nurse Judy. Laughing so hard she could barely stand up and bending over as if in pain, she had to lean on my bed for support. Tears streamed down her face as she pleaded, "No more. Please. I can't take it. Please stop." Her laughter was so loud that other nurses and patients hurried to see what was causing the raucous laughter coming from the hospital room of a man dying of cancer.

I had been in the hospital for several weeks. Chemotherapy and a bone marrow transplant had left me so weak I had to be lifted from my bed by a crane-like device called a Hoyer that swung me in the air suspended by a belt. The machine had jammed and the nurse struggled with the controls as I hung helplessly suspended over the scale used to weigh me every morning. I was being rocked back and forth wildly and nothing Judy tried seemed to help her regain control of the machine.

As I spun around, something about my helplessness and humiliation made me begin to laugh. The absurdity of my situation seemed to touch my heart and to make me reflect on the meaning of my illness. Between each laugh, I delivered philosophical punch lines to Judy as she worked to free me. I told her how bizarre it seemed that brilliant minds could transplant organs person to person but had difficulty moving one man, who now weighed little more than one hundred pounds, from his bed to a scale that showed every morning the gradual disappearance of his body. I told her how often we seem to be servants of the very machines our brains construct to serve us, how these mechanistic slaves seem to play such exacerbating tricks on their masters, and how we are controlled by the very technology we have developed in order to give us more control. I told her how our brain's creations seem to turn on us and muddle our life by creating the chaos that can be the curriculum for learning the lessons of more balanced living. I told her about the turmoil and upheaval in my life caused by my cancer and the irony that I could be killed by one of medicine's machines running amuck with a mysterious energy all its own just when my life was being saved by the best mechanistic biomedicine had to offer. Still trying desperately to free me, my nurse replied without looking up, "What are you, the swinging philosopher?"

I could not control my arms or legs, but I could feel my heart racing as the machine swung me in circles it seemed to select on its own. I could feel energy from my heart shaking my entire body with its every beat, and I thought how my heart seemed to be the only part of me that kept tapping out a steady rhythm even as the malignant cells in my body had totally lost their synchronization. I thought how its animated rhythms, stable or unstable, healthy or pathological, so precisely measured the difference between my life and my death. As these thoughts raced through my mind, my entire situation struck me as a tragic farce and Judy and I started to laugh even harder.

As she gave up trying to control the machine and sat frustrated and helpless on my bed, Judy sighed, "OK Harold the Hoyer, you win." Her naming of the machine only made us laugh harder, and with that laughter my swinging seemed less chaotic and began to fall into a natural rhythm simulating the beating of my heart. The energy of my nurse's and my own heart seemed to merge and the machine ceased its wild movements. Something about the "L" energy bond between Judy and me reflected in our shared laughter seemed to take control of the machine. Like the subjects in the PEAR program whose loving bond altered the behavior of machines and whose joyful shared being rather than hard individual effort resulted in the most effective energy connection with the machines, my nurse and I had finally seemed to become the energetic "operators" of the machine only when we stopped trying to control it.

STRUMMING THE STRINGS OF THE HEART

Judy said later that the absurdity of a man dying of cancer, and so frail and helpless that he could barely lift his arms, preaching from the sling of an out-of-control machine had "struck a cord" in her heart that led to her uncontrollable laughter. After several minutes and after it seemed to sense that it had taught me enough for one day, the machine lowered me gently back onto my bed.

My informative ride on the machine and the laughter it induced was as emotionally and physically intense as those times when my awareness of the threat of death had resulted in tearful sobbing. Deep in my heart, I could feel the warmth and joy of the energy of Judy's and my shared good humor, and as I write these words, I smile as my heart still remembers. Something about that event also struck a chord in my heart, and I remembered one of my favorite quotes about humor by Reinhold Niebuhr: "Humor is a prelude to faith and laughter is the beginning of prayer."[1]

JOCULAR EPIPHANIES

Science has no satisfactory explanation for why humans can laugh. While laughter has positive health benefits, most animals get along fine without it. Cardio-energetics suggests that laughter is, as happened with my nurse and me, the music played when a familiar chord—a cellular memory—is strummed on the strings of our heart. It occurs when we experience a "jocular epiphany" or cardio-coherence of the kind that seems to happen whenever the brain's illusion of its ultimate control over our destiny is exposed and when its arrogance is juxtaposed with the reality that we all get "the" and not "our" way.

Researchers at the PEAR program found that those persons who made a game of trying to energetically connect with and influence the machines did better than those who tried harder and harder to control it. Those who laughed and played "with" the machines and named them did better than those who tried to focus on and manipulate them. As you have read, since the PEAR laboratory was established in 1979, their millions of trials have shown the subtle but real proactive role of consciousness ("L" or life/love energy) in the behavior of random physical systems. The Princeton group found that the most effective way of connecting with devices via "L" energy is "to speak of the devices in frankly anthropomorphic terms, and to associate successful performance with the establishment of some form of bond or resonance with the device, or with some self-sacrificial immersion in the machine's operation."[2] This seems to be what happened when Judy and I gave up trying, started laughing, and joined energetically and lovingly together in our laughter, and when Judy named the machine. As my nurse indicated by saying our laughter was "killing her" as she lost all sense of self-control, humor, much like the loving and sensual connection you read about in chapter 9, is a form of "selfless resonance" of a heart-to-heart subtle energy connection.

GETTING A BRAIN BYPASS

While we occasionally giggle when we are alone, our biggest and hardiest laughter usually occurs when we are with others. Whenever two or more hearts are gathered to share a very intense, intimate, stressful, helpless situation, they seem to gang up on their owners' brains to make them calm down. They perform a "brain bypass" and allow our souls to comfort and revel with one another as we are allowed a peek at the always present chaos of the world and the laughable ridiculousness of our brain's illusion that it is in charge and can impose its form of order on the universe.

One of my patients described a jocular joining of "L" energy by saying, "It seems to be at the worst of times when people are touched in their hearts and seem to have to make a joke. I think it's because we are being mooned by the cosmos and Mother Nature has dropped her pants to show us how silly we are when we think we are the boss." When people are interviewed following a tragedy such as a severe storm or flooding, they very often joke. While this may be a form of psychological defense against their vulnerability, it is also a heartfelt expression of the sense that none of us is immune from the randomness of life. Several years ago, the suburbs of Chicago experienced the worst flooding in a hundred years. Thousands of people were left homeless. When interviewed for television, most of the flood victims joked and laughed about their misfortune.[3]

TWO FEELINGS FOR THE PRICE OF ONE

Comedian Lily Tomlin said, "When I'm happy I feel like crying, but when I'm sad I don't feel like laughing. I think it's better to be happy. Then you get two feelings for the price of one."[4] When the brain feels sorry for itself it makes us cry, but when our heart realizes that all life is a form of suffering that all of us share, it makes us laugh. When we cry so hard we laugh, we are usually feeling alone and helpless in the situation that brought on our sadness. When we laugh so hard we cry, it indicates that something about our situation has touched our heart and we can feel completely and profoundly connected in our mutual participation in the natural chaos of life. It seems as if the heart is our primary sensor of humor and that we need both our tears of sadness and tears of joy. It is our tears of laughter that are a form of the heart crying with the joy of a profoundly realized sense of "L" energy connection with another heart.

Kurt Vonnegut wrote, "Laughter and tears are both responses to frustration and exhaustion . . . I myself prefer to laugh, since there is less cleaning up to do afterward."[5] Not all of our laughter comes from the heart or leads to tears. As you will read below, the brain has its own sense of humor that tends to be more controlling, cynical, and sarcastic, but when our heart laughs, our eyes often flood with tears from the recognition of the divine wonderfulness of the futility of our attempt to approach life's challenges exclusively on a rational basis.

HEAVY AND LIGHT TEARS

A few months ago, I lectured at a children's hospital on the topic "Healthy Tears of a Healing Heart." A very sick little girl came up to talk to me and said, "I know how to tell what kind of tears I have. Tears of sadness make me feel 'heavy' and tears of laughter make my feel 'light.' " This child's heartfelt wisdom reveals the knowledge that laughter tears connect us with others energetically to lighten our burden, while tears of sadness often express our sense of loneliness. Both the tears of sadness and the tears that flow when we laugh very hard contain proteins that are not present in tears from cutting onions or irritated eyes.[6] The presence of these proteins indicates that tears can cleanse us of stress chemicals. Laughter's tears cleanse the body of the same harmful toxins as tears of sorrow, but there is one major difference. Laughter helps us transcend our suffering by sharing with others our connection with the natural randomness of life. Laughter tends to turn us outward while crying from sadness usually turns us inward. People often cry for us, but it may be equally important to our healing that they learn to laugh more often with us.

Anyone who has been around a person who is laughing very hard has felt the energy from that laughter as pent-up "L" energy is sprayed everywhere. Research shows that laughter is one of the best ways to discharge constricted emotional energy.[7] When we say we are "laughing our head off," we may really be saying that, at least for one merry moment, we are free of our brain's control to interact with our world purely from the heart.

When I am asked how to tell if someone has learned to "tap the energy and wisdom of the heart," I answer, "Look for someone who has been in a loving relationship for a very long time and who can laugh very easily, often, and hard with their lover. They may be the true gurus of cardio-energetics."

ANOTHER FINE MESS

Laughter is the heart's public address system. It is where announcements of our ability to be less arrogantly "me" and more humbly "us" are broadcast. We laugh at Laurel and Hardy's Sisyphus-like piano struggle because we are all pushing our own version of a piano up hundreds of stairs only to have it come rolling back down again. We are not laughing at but with them because we all have experienced our own version of their frustration.

Laughter is the outward manifestation of increased heart rate and oxygen intake accompanied by some of the most healthy physiological changes that can happen to our body. Psychologist William Fry Jr.'s research shows that twenty seconds of guffawing gives the heart the same beneficial workout as three minutes of hard rowing.[8] While the increased heart beat that accompanies anger leads to toxic changes in the cardiovascular system, the rhythm of a joyful "hearty" laughter produces more healthy hearts for everyone within range of its influence.

We cannot have our "heart broken" unless we have extended it and known not only deep pain but also intense pleasure. We cry hardest for those losses that the energetic heart treasures most in our life, and those who cry the most have often lived the most intensely.

Just when I was being saved from cancer, I was almost killed by a hospital machine that slung me through the air. I began to feel angry, sad, and sorry for myself until I realized that what I was experiencing could and did happen to other patients. Perhaps that machine, by flying me through the air, forced me to take myself more lightly and, when I joined with the nurse in laughter, it "knew" to let me down tenderly from my spiritually instructive flying lesson. Our heart seems to have its own way to instinctively know how to humble the brain enough to make it pause and lighten up and see the ultimate uselessness of its compulsive attempts at constant control. The magical light-heartedness of healthy laughter is reflected in

Peter Pan's words: "When the first baby laughed for the first time, the laugh broke into a thousand pieces and they all went skipping about, and that was the beginning of fairies."[9]

THE CHAOTIC HEART

Cardio-energetics suggests that, while the brain is made to help us negotiate our way through the chaos of our life, the heart is made to help us accept and find meaning within this voyage. It is the constantly oscillating, pulsating organ that seems able to find patterns and rhythms amidst the incessant disarray of the cosmos. Writing about the new science of chaos, author James Gleick points out that, just beneath the apparent order of the universe, there is chaos and at the same time, within that chaos, there is an order we are still far from understanding.[10] Cardio-energetics suggests that our heart is sensitive to the dynamic hidden order beneath the chaos and, when it finds it, it often makes us laugh until we cry at our recognition of our brain's foolish pride in its illusion of mastery of destiny. Through its hard, tear-inducing laughter, the heart tells us that, for at least a few moments, our "self" as perceived by the brain has escaped the stress of life and temporarily "died" laughing and gone to quantum heaven.

Author John Updike writes, "Human was the music, natural was the static." He was referring to the wonderful and awesome chaotic energy of life that flows within, around, and from us. The science that studies chaos is concerned with the irregular side of nature, the puzzles of life's tragedies, miracles, and monstrosities, and the nature of the loaded dice God plays with in His making of the universe. Like the heart itself, chaology looks for the hidden rhythms amidst the apparent disharmony of life. It looks for the infinite patterns amidst the local or immediate disarray and, like a person with a good sense of humor, it is always ready to "get the joke" and find a fascinating enchanted message in what seems like just another fine mess we have gotten ourselves into.

The heart itself is a chaotic organ. Dozens of disorganized "irregular rhythms" of the heart are described by cardiologists who, like other bioscientists, often take comfort in naming what they really don't fully understand. They refer to ectopic beats; parasystole, high-grad block and escape rhythms; simple and complex Wenckebach rhythms, and on and on. When I was intubated and helpless in the intensive care unit, I remember watching the machine that measured my heart rhythm and hearing the doctors point and name each variation as if identifying a cartoon character hidden in a maze of lines. I have a prolapsed mitral valve and experience several types of cardiac arrhythmia, so my electrocardiogram was a cardio-kaleido-scope for my doctors. In a sense, I naturally have a chaotic heart rhythm that my heart has found for me to allow me to live. New research derived from chaos theory suggests that cardiologists might consider the heart as a dynamical chaotic energy system rather than just an electro-mechanical pump, and that doctors are inadvertently using limited, superficial classifications of the heart's rhythms based on a brief and limited sample of its behavior that may mask the heart's true nature.[11] Doctors have the parts of the heart down pretty well, but they still too often fail to see the heart and health in general as a whole, interactive, remembering, dynamic energy system.

When we laugh and say, "Oh yeah, I get it," we are announcing that we have recovered a cellular memory of our common suffering amidst the chaos. Our sense of humor is our heart's sense of connection, and by developing that sense, we heal our own and others' hearts.

COSMIC SENSE AND EERIE ORDER

When doctors looked at my heart tracings when I was a patient in the intensive care unit, one of them said, "Boy. Look at that rhythm. That's eerie." What cardiologists call arrhythmias are really images of what scientist Douglas Hofstatter describes as "an eerier type of order."[12] Just as the "eerie order" of life is what seems to pop into our awareness when we are moved to our strongest laughter, "eerie order" and not a mathematical average may be the ultimate code of a uniquely adaptive and healthy heart. Looking at the heart as a dynamic energy system operating by principles being learned from the study of chaos, rather than as a mechanical pump that sometimes loses its stroke, allows us to learn the true nature of the organ that helps us flow with the natural instability of life.

In simple terms, the study of chaos is the search to find the miraculous patterns in what formerly seemed to be only erratic and unpredictable events. It is the science of clouds, rainbows, dripping faucets, and floods, and at its very best, it is uncovering the punch line for the subtle jokes nature plays on us when it shows us nonsense in order to tease us into finding the deeper cosmic sense of life. Applied to cardio-energetics, chaos theory challenges doctors to develop their sense of "humor" and to look for and go more willingly into the mysterious eerie order just beneath the chaos of heart and other "dys-rhythmic" states we call "dis-ease."

A CARDIAC CAN OF WORMS

When a doctor listens to our heart, she hears the swooshing and pounding of fluids and the soft opening and closing of valves. She listens for the sounds of a pump but may be insensitive to the energy of the organ or the fact that she is sending energy into the heart to which she is listening. If she used a computer to model any one aspect of the heart's behavior, she would require the most powerful of our newest supercomputers. A model of the whole energy system of the heart would be beyond the range of any known computer.[13] A few minutes' tracing of electrical energy on a piece of paper is but the crudest of estimates of one tiny aspect of the heart's behavior. With every swoosh and click, there is always a vibration of energy that contains the information of our soul, the chaos of our life, and the meaning of our living.

So complex is the heart's energy that, when it becomes seriously disturbed, it can cause the heart muscle—as if it were crying or laughing too hard for too long—to fibrillate. Ventricular fibrillation causes hundreds of thousands of sudden deaths each year. It is a form of stable chaos that kills and that can only be corrected by a jolt of electric energy that creates a different chaos and suggests a new order to which the heart can return. A cardio-energetic definition of physical death is losing and not being able to recover the cellular memories of the natural beat and rhythm of life. While the cause of fibrillation is often traced to blockage of the arteries, many times the cause of fibrillation is unknown. A person with a seemingly healthy heart is just as (if not more) likely to have a heart attack as someone who has some of the major risk factors such as obesity and high blood pressure.[14] Saving the life of a person whose heart is attacking him is substituting a new form of more stable chaos for the lethal chaos of fibrillation and a way of helping energetically enlighten a confused heart.

Cardiologists refer to fibrillation as a condition in which the heart acts "like a can of worms" writhing in an uncoordinated mass. In fact, the problem is not with the "stuff" of the heart but with the energy of the heart as its energy waves "break up," much as strong electromagnetic energy can interfere with the reception of a broadcasted signal. When fibrillation occurs, the individual parts of the heart are usually working perfectly. The fibrillation that can lead to death is a disruption of the heart's rhythmic energetic whole, a sign of a complex info-energy system gone awry due to a lethal form of cellular amnesia.

"Chaotic heart," or fibrillation, is not just a malfunction in a pump's apparatus. Its onset remains mysterious to cardiologists. Cardio-energetics suggests that, if cardiologists can learn to look for and understand the subtle "chaotic" energies and patterns of the heart instead of just labeling and trying to biochemically control them, and if they can learn that all hearts are energetically connected to other hearts and everything, energy cardiology can provide ways to a more energetically enlightened medicine.[15]

FROM THE "AHA" OF THE HEAD TO THE "AHA HA-HA" OF THE HEART

When my nurse Judy said laughingly, "Stop it. You're killing me," it was a message of surrender from her brain as it failed to figure out what to do and a joyful "aha ha-ha" of cardio-connection established by her heart. Within, and perhaps because of, the chaos of my experience, a cellular memory from my nurse's system was released and expressed in her hardy, or "hearty," laughter.

A few years ago, I talked with Judy about our shared struggle that special morning. She told me that, when she was a little girl, her grandfather had spent years assisted with a Hoyer like the one that entrapped me. One day, as she watched her mother swinging her grandfather in the same type of apparatus used with me, she giggled about how strange it looked to her. Her mother became angry and slapped her on the arm. "I don't think I ever thought about that slap until that morning," she said. "For the first time, I could feel the energy my mother must have felt in her helplessness with her father and me laughing about it. It all came back to me and I think that's why I laughed so hard I cried. I think I even felt that little sting on the same arm my mom slapped. Something about the whole mess seemed to flash that memory right to my heart and suddenly it all made a very weird kind of sense and made me laugh so hard I cried."

When the brain struggles to figure out why things have gone wrong and cannot make an "aha" to solve a problem, it makes us impatient with our "self" and makes us cry at its individual helplessness and martyrdom. The heart can find a natural connective rhythm at the chaotic moments of our life and, when it does, it experiences an "aha ha-ha" similar to Judy's empathetic memory of her mother's helplessness.

CREATIVE CATASTROPHIZING

Psychologist Jon Kabat-Zinn, in his book *Full Catastrophe Living,* refers to Zorba the Greek as "dancing in the gale of the full catastrophe."[16] Our heart is made to provide the beat for that dance and to help us find something powerfully spiritual and enlightening even at our darkest moments. The brain's self-survival posture defines any catastrophe as disaster, but the heart seems somehow to understand catastrophe as what Dr. Kabat-Zinn calls awareness of the "poignant enormity" of the full experience of the energy that constitutes life.

Psychoanalyst Mart Grotjahn notes that, "To have a sense of humor is to have an understanding of human suffering and misery. Humor bespeaks a sad acceptance of our weakness and frustration. But laughter also means freedom."[17] Cardio-energetics teaches that by letting our heart "break open" with full immersion in and receptiveness to the catastrophes of life, and laughing freely and openly with others, we can regain an energetic balance. Author Allen Klein, who calls himself a "joyologist," writes, "Once we find some comedy in our chaos, we are not long caught up in it." The heart's sense of humor allows our brain not to be "caught up" and carried away by chaos even as we are, as I was in that swinging machine, forever whirling about as a part of and contributing our own energy to that chaos.

LAUGHTER IN THE CAVES

Sir Boss, Mark Twain's hero in *A Connecticut Yankee in King Arthur's Court,* complains about the old and tired jokes being shared around a sixteenth-century campfire. He says he had heard them all before when he was in the nineteenth century. No one knows for sure how long one of our most profoundly important human senses, our sense of humor, has been around, but anthropologists studying what they call EEA—environment of evolutionary adaptedness (how well things cope with their changing surroundings)—suggest that, had Sir Boss gone all the way back to the Stone Age, he would have moaned or at least grunted about a primitive form of the same old jokes bantered back and forth in some form between our ancient cousins.[18] From the teaching jokes of Zen Buddhism to the simple lessons of the Laurel and Hardy movies, the wisdom of the heart is revealed in the laughter it elicits from us when something outside touches our heart and reminds us of our ageless and common joys and sorrows.

When something touches our "funny bone" and we "get" the cosmic joke on our brain's arrogant illusion of power, we are bent over in humble acknowledgment of our place in the universe. Anyone who has been profoundly disappointed when their most carefully arranged objectives crumple because of some unexplainable and random cruel twist of fate knows that, when the brain plans, God laughs.

FRACTAL FUNNINESS

The brain follows what author Riane Eisler describes as the "dominator" model as it tries to control, master, subdue, and conquer nature.[19] The heart follows what Eisler calls the "partnership" model, marked by respect, cooperation, openness, and harmony with instead of control over nature. Despite our brain's best intentions and efforts on its body's behalf, things will inevitably go what it considers wrong and mess up its attempts to get its way. The heart knows we are all partners, sharing, experiencing, and trying to learn and live with "the way."

Scientists studying chaos refer to "fractals," jagged, tangled, twisted shapes representing organizing principles within the chaos that characterize all of nature. A cosmic clowning affects us all, and the rough sharp edges of chaos can wound us. Even when we are hurt by life's turmoil, the heart helps us find a kind of "fractal funniness" in the chaos of life.

ON BEING A GOOD SPORT

No matter how much our brain prides itself on establishing a perfectly ordered and controlled life, and no matter how many beepers, cellular phones, answering machines, and day-planners it uses, we all fall victim to the ever-present effects of what physician Larry Dossey calls "the trickster."[20] Within the chaos of life, there seems to be some self-correcting force of nature drawing us back from our reliance on our brain's rationality to the natural turbulent irrationality of life with which the heart deals much more easily.

As someone who lives in Hawaii, I have long known about the "trickster effect." The demigod Maui was called "the Trickster," and he was constantly playing tricks on his brothers. Polynesia is populated with thousands of gods and sacred ancestors who are known to play tricks on the islanders every day. The menehune, a legendary race of tiny people, still fool Hawaiians with their unpredictable and remarkable feats performed in the dead of night, and ancient ancestors (aumakua) constantly trip us up just to slow us down. In my travels around the world, I have found that every indigenous culture has its own unique version of one or more "tricksters" that play major roles in their mythology.

Like the tricksters in other cultures, demigod Maui was, like all of us, part buffoon and part philosopher, partly human and partly divine. If we are to be more cardio-sensitive and learn to benefit from the divine energy of our heart as well as the human rationality of our brain, we must be willing to invite the trickster to come to play with us. We must be willing to be more gracefully forgiving of his (in most cultural myths, most tricksters are male) often cruel jokes, and open our heart to the lessons even his meanest hoaxes can teach us.

The trickster effect is experienced when our expectations are not met, when we spill gravy on our tie just before an important meeting, or our shoelace breaks when we're late and trying to run out the door. These little tricks are like the heart's gentle love taps on our brain's shoulder meant to remind us to fully experience life rather than just leading or being led by it. They are honks on the trickster's clown horn meant to get our attention and to slow us down when we are racing too fast to allow our heart to be a part of our living.

LIFE'S NOT-SO-LITTLE HASSLES

Little things stress us a lot.[21] Recent research shows that the heart reacts intensely to the small, unexpected "hassles" of daily life. Unless we pay attention the pestering and gentle teasing of the trickster that teaches us to slow down, be still, be quiet, and listen to our heart, he will play even bigger tricks that are more disruptive to our life in order to get our attention. Sometimes he will frustrate us so that our heart throws a fibrillation fit or chaotic tantrum. A review of sudden cardiac death revealed that lethal arrhythmias are most commonly precipitated not by major stressors but by the small, unexpected hassles that occurred within one hour before the episode of arrhythmia.[22]

Research shows that we can all expect approximately thirty of these little "heart hassles" each day of our life, what psychologists define as "irritating, frustrating, distressing" mini-crises.[23] These little nuisances seem to be the puff of air from chaology's metaphoric butterfly's wings flapping. If we do not sit down and listen to our heart's warning to take it easier, these little "heart hassles" become the chaotic hurricane that blows us away. The problem is less the nature of the emotions provoked by these events than the prank they play on us with their abrupt, surprising upset of our brain's best and most carefully laid plans.[24] When the trickster hides our keys or squirts ketchup on our white sweater, our heart jumps more severely and rapidly than it does in reaction to the major crises of our life.[25]

We cannot deal with the trickster by using our brain to try to outwit him. The more our brain plans, the more sneaky the trickster becomes. The more we try to outsmart and outrush the trickster, the more we are his helpless foils and the victims of his even more disruptive tricks. We can only deal with the trickster in two ways. First, we must go along with his pranks and share a "hearty" laugh when the joke is on us and our ineptitude, frailties, and lack of competence is exposed for all to see. Second, when we experience the surprise setbacks that make us pause from our hectic life pace, we have to become even more alert for what psychologists call "life's uplifts," the simple little pleasures of life such as a smiling child, a lovely flower, a powerful storm, or a gorgeous sunset.[26]

Psychologist Richard Lazarus writes, "a person's morale, social functioning, and health don't hinge on hassles alone, but on a balance between the good things that happen to people that make them feel good and the bad."[27] A heart with a good sense of humor easily laughs at the bad and gently celebrates the good, and the result is a healthy energy balance between the dark and light side of our subtle "L" energy. The wise heart knows that the trickster most often appears at those times when the brain thinks everything is going just the way it planned. The trickster's job is to be the jester of chaos, to remind us that nothing goes perfectly for too long, and to trick us into enjoying good times while they last.

If we are not open to the trickster effect, he will keep coming back until we learn what he has to teach us about humility. Author Richard Smoley writes, "As long as we lie to ourselves, the Trickster will be with us. He'll show up just when we least want him, to embarrass us on a first date, to prove us fools in front of the learned company we're trying to impress, to make us miss a power breakfast with that all-important business contact. Yes, he'll leave at our bidding, but he always comes back with a vengeance. The only way to get rid of him is to listen to his message—and to admit the truth about ourselves in all its beauty and ugliness."[28]

We need the trickster's little jokes on us to remind us to pay more attention to the gift of being alive. He teaches us about who we are and what we can and can never be, even if his lessons are often clumsy and disturbing to our plans and image of who our brain thinks we are. Our brain would like to keep the trickster out of our life, but our heart knows well how to play, learn, and laugh with the trickster. Dr. Larry Dossey writes, "We can never banish the Trickster. To do so would be to amputate a vital part of ourself, including our need to create, to frolic, to love, to be—in a word, human."[29]

HOW THE HEART'S HUMOR HEALS

Serious research into our sense of humor began in the late 1980s. The healing effects of humor identified by psychologists relate to the psychology of the heart. By understanding how humor works, we may be better able to understand the code that reveals how our heart thinks, feels, and behaves. Here are some things psychologists have learned about humor that are also habits of the heart.

• The heart is an organ of connection and seeks interrelationship. Psychologists now know that humor can be one of the best ways to diffuse interpersonal conflicts and to experience and express intimate connection.[30]

• The heart constantly is trying to teach us to pay attention to life's "uplifts" and that we need the energy of other hearts that comes from forming new bonds. Humor has been shown to be one of the most effective ways of teaching, so when we laugh with someone, we are teaching and learning with them about the ups and downs of daily life.[31]

• The heart seeks lasting connections, abhors disconnection, and cannot laugh when it is losing a connection. Research shows that lack of humor and shared laughter is one of the earliest and most predictive signs of a failing intimate relationship.[32]

• The heart is inclusive in its oscillating nature and teaches us to be aware of both sides of any life experience. Persons with a sense of humor can see several sides of an issue and are able to "break out of a perceptual set" and think and feel creatively. This ability to tune in to the heart's sense of balanced humor allows us to see problems coming from any side. As author Jeremiah Abrams writes, "The one-sided get blind-sided."[33]

• Through its energy, the heart draws other hearts to it and is drawn to other hearts. Unlike the brain's sardonic humor that can drive people away, healthy humor, the kind that leads to strengthened immunity, healing, and cardiovascular health, is "attracting humor" that narrows social distances.[34]

• The heart enjoys making other hearts "feel good." Healthy humor makes everyone feel better, but the brain's humor is often intended to disparage others to make itself look good.[35] The brain's humor is represented in author and magazine editor C. L. Edson's observation, "We love a joke that hands us a pat on the back while it kicks the other fellow down the stairs."

• Unlike the brain, the heart knows that it alone cannot be "the mind" but that together with the brain and body it forms a Mind of which it is a key part. By its nature, the heart is a partner seeking to "be a part of" rather than "in charge of." By contrast, the dominating brain's humor is often a "control device" it uses to assume superiority over other brains.[36]

• The heart loves and uses humor to express love. The brain's humor is often used to express its dislike of another person.[37]

• The partnership-oriented heart gets along well with the trickster and loves surprises, incongruity, and anything that annoys the arrogant brain. The brain's humor is defensive and, envying the Trickster's power, the brain often heckles him and tries to be like him, much as a rude heckler mocks a comedian and tries to steal the limelight away from the performer.[38]

• When the heart is in healthy energetic balance, its rhythm is steady and the energy it sends attracts others and conveys its healthy state to their hearts. Researchers now know that easy, honest, connecting laughter is a key sign of health.[39]

• Humor is one of the best ways of avoiding aggression, releasing tension, reducing anxiety, and enhancing immune function, all of which are healthy states for and of the heart.[40, 41] One of the best preventers of heart disease is humor.[42]

• When the brain is quieted, the heart is free to laugh. During laughter, there is a decrease in the flow of blood to the prefrontal and temporoparietal cortical areas of the brain, suggesting that the positive emotional state induced by humor puts the brain momentarily at rest.[43]

All of the above positive effects of humor require heartfelt compassionate laughter, not mocking, disparaging laughter.[44] Those moments we are laughing the hardest are likely to be those when we are the most directly tuned in to our heart's code. At these times, we are suspending the brain's often oppressive pressuring control and egoistic sense of self and connecting with the world on a heart level. Zen scholar R. H. Blythe writes, "When we laugh, we are free of all the oppression of our personality."[45]

DO BE SILLY

The word "silly" derives from the Greek "selig" meaning "blessed." There is something sacred in being able to be silly, living in tolerant peace with the Trickster, and being aware of the heart's wisdom as revealed by its humor. Germany's great sixteenth-century mystic Jakob Böhme wrote that those who seek the path of the heart are often seen as fools and pointed out that "the way to the love of God is folly to the world, but is wisdom to the children of God. Hence, whenever the world perceiveth this holy fire of love in God's children, it concludeth immediately that they are turned fools, and are beside themselves."[46] Cardio-energetics teaches that it is healthy to be childish if childishness means re-enchantment with living and the ability to "get beside our cerebral self" to join hearts joyfully with others.

The heart teaches us that we do not laugh because we are free of suffering but because we know and accept that life is suffering. Philosopher Friedrich Nietzsche pointed out that "the most acutely suffering animal on earth invented laughter." The more you find yourself laughing at others, the more likely it is that you are dealing with the brain's code. The more you find yourself laughing with others, the more likely it is that you have tuned in to the heart's code and are receiving one of the most neglected presents our bodily system has to offer—a joyful, happy heart. Norman Cousins, who healed himself from a life-threatening illness in part with laughter, wrote, "Of all the gifts bestowed by nature on human beings, hardy laughter must be close to the top."[47]

You have read about how to contact your own and other hearts, about the heart's way of loving, and the power of a happy heart. The last chapter of this book puts all of these characteristics of the heart's code together to suggest how the heart may be our own individual inner healer and the healer of all systems.

CHAPTER ELEVEN

Healing from the Heart

"Who hath put wisdom in the inward parts? or who hath given understanding to the heart?"

—*BOOK OF JOB* (38:36)

A COCK FOR HYGEIA

Just before his death, Socrates recalled a debt he felt he owed to the Greek god of medicine that had cared for him throughout his life. Referring to the Greek tradition of compensating the god Asclepius for his care, he said, "I owe a cock to Asclepius." He was following the Greek custom of honoring the Asclepian repair-approach to medicine, the ancient version of the modern biomechanical medicine that saved my life. Western medicine continues to evolve as the most powerful, effective system for dealing with trauma and disease ever devised but often fails when it comes to Asclepius' daughter Hygeia's more heart-oriented approach to well-being. Hygeian medicine recognizes that the body has its own natural wisdom, an intuitive integrative capacity that, with very little thought on our part and even when we are sleeping, is at work every moment of our life. It acknowledges the subtle info-energetic intelligence field that is our body and the natural oscillation between health and sickness as essential parts of the same life continuum. Asclepian medicine does things to us to fix us, but Hygeian medicine helps healing happen within us by allowing the natural "L" energy from our heart to flow freely.

This chapter is about the preliminary attempt to apply what is known so far about the energy of the heart and cellular memories to a cardio-energetic model for healing. Healing from the heart begins with asking and answering ten questions, and the way the Asclepian brain and Hygeian heart answers these questions illustrates a different focus to healing than typically proposed by Western cerebral-centric biomedicine.

1. What is healing?

The Brain: Healing is the biomechanical influencing of the body's systems by direct attempts to fix, correct, and restore a mechanical system to its version of "normal" functioning. Modern Asclepian medicine is the most effective body repair system in history.

The Heart: Healing is making whole, reconnecting, recovering molecular memories that promote healing, and being alert to risks to our well-being from being out of balance with the energy of all systems around us. Psychiatrist David Benor has made a detailed study of healing initiatives, and his definition of healing fits the cardio-energetic definition. He sees healing as the intentional influence of one or more persons upon a living system without using known physical means of intervention."[1] For cardio-energetic healing, "influence" means focusing on the wisdom and energy coming in subtle fashion from the heart and not just brain-invented manipulations and techniques. Healing with the heart is not "trying to heal" but allowing the heart's natural healing energy and all the memories of healings that have ever occurred to resonate within you, and being still and "thoughtless" enough to allow one's own heart to fall into a shared coherence with other hearts in a form of compassionate prayer beyond words.

2. Why heal?

The Brain: We heal to be able to keep going, do more, have more, live longer, and get the most out of our individual life.

The Heart: We heal in order to be whole with the systems around us and to be able to care for, heal, and protect those systems, including people, plants, animals, and places.

3. Who needs healing?

The Brain: Sick or "broken" biosystems need mending because they have fallen into a state of disrepair. Anyone who is not "healthy" and "normal" according to bioscience is in need of its intervention.

The Heart: Everyone and everything everywhere needs healing all the time, because healing is the process of keeping healthy energy connection flowing within all systems. Systems, not individuals, get sick. Health and sickness are not opposite ends of a continuum. All of us are sick and healthy at the same time all the time because we are chaotic energetic systems in the process of self-correction. Stability does not mean never changing. The systemic stability of cardio-energetics is indicated by a system's constant energetic readjustments.

In 1900, French physiologist Charles Richet said that "instability is the necessary condition for the stability of the organism." In other words, chaos is sickness to an Asclepian but a form of dynamic health to a Hygeian. Amidst the infinite patterns of snowflakes, there is no one right way to be a "healthy" or "right" snowflake. The ocean is not "sick" when it is in turmoil. We should not waste the magic of healing connection by employing it only when we think we are sick. There is a mysterious reciprocity at work in the relationship between illness and health, and the best model of healthy balance is not someone standing firmly on the ground but someone walking high on a tight-rope, balance bar in hand and constantly readjusting and adapting.

4. How do we heal?

The Brain: The credo of Asclepian or brain-oriented healing is "don't just sit there, do something." There is no better system for making quick diagnoses and taking quick immediate action than modern biomedicine, and most of us have experienced its lifesaving power. It is a system designed to locate failure in a specific biomechanical part and then correct and stabilize the problem by chemical or mechanical means.

The Heart: The credo of Hygeian or heart-oriented healing is "don't just do something, sit there." If you take a lot of over-the-counter medications, your cold will probably go away in about fourteen days. If you do nothing at all but take it easy, it will probably go away in about two weeks, and in the process you may realize how too much stress lowered your immunity and that you should be spending more time in your daily life doing what a bad cold often makes you do—staying home, cozying up under a warm blanket, having some chicken soup, and reading a good book. A cold can be the body's expression of the spirit's cry to "go home." Healing is enhanced when we remember that we seem to have an internal drive toward health and that most problems correct themselves if we allow our body's natural healing wisdom to do its job. Hygeian heart healing is becoming aware of where and how in our lives we have become disconnected or have lost touch with our primary stabilizer—the heart. Heart healing requires that, like the operators in a Princeton laboratory, we let, rather than try to make, an energetic re-connection happen.

Physician Larry Dossey refers to the value of what he calls "the great wait."[2] While there are times when urgent lifesaving action is necessary, such times are rare compared to those when "just being" is the healing thing to do. Through stillness and gentle, repetitive ritual more than intense action and procedures, we can recover the cellular memories left by those who have gone before us. These memories teach us how to be whole again and how to connect with the energy we share with all systems. Like a tightrope walker, if we try too hard, worry too much, and think too hard, we may become insensitive to the very signals that help us readjust and maintain our state of dynamic, often shaky, but adaptive, life-maintaining balance.

5. Where do we heal?

The Brain: We remove ourselves from nature and go within the most modern, technically advanced, airtight building we can find that is staffed with the most brilliant, sophisticated, well-known, objective, highest-paid healers. We take off our clothes, replace them with a ritualistic robe that allows others easy access to our body (particularly from behind), climb into a high bed that restricts any quick escape, surrender various body fluids, allow ourselves to be submitted to study by student priests who are often exhausted from the requirement of their constant participation in an ongoing hazing ceremony, and turn our body over to the Asclepian priests and maidens for repair. A few floral cuttings and traces of nature may be brought to the temple by visitors, but the idea is to have as little of the natural world and as few loving family members around as possible so as to not disrupt the sanctity, codes, procedures, policies, hierarchy, and bureaucracy of Asclepius' temple. The more and newer the machines, the better our chances to heal.

The Heart: We heal by finding a very energy-friendly place that allows us to connect more intensely with the natural aspects of our living and by being immersed in the energy emanating from the plants, animals, and loving people around us and of which we are an integral part. An ocean or a forest are good places to heal because they resonate directly with our healing center, our heart.

6. By whom are we healed?

The Brain: We are taken from our family and healed by a parade of

smart strangers who look at written tracings that are symbolic approxima-
tions of our body's functioning and who then prescribe the action to be
taken and what should be done "to us" by them or their medicinal approx-
imations of natural substances. If we are "compliant," we may heal. If not,
we may be viewed by the priests of the temple as having "failed to respond
to treatment."

The Heart: We are not healed "by" but "with." We are healed with the
presence of healing hearts all around us joining with our heart and not just
doing things "to it." Research shows that the need for the most common
surgical procedure performed in the United States, Cesarean section, can
be reduced more than 50 percent when a mother has the continuous presence of a supportive woman (called a "doula") during labor and delivery.[3]
Cardio-energetics suggests that we check the heart and not just the diplo-
mas of our physician and pick one that our heart tells us "has a good
heart" and gives off "good healing energy."

7. When do we know we are healed?

The Brain: We know we are healed when numbers from machines tell
us we are "back within the normal range," our doctor tells us we are
healed, or an insurance plan has informed us that our allotted healing time
has run out. We are healed when we have managed to delay death or are
able to return to the same frenzied, hectic life that caused us to require
healing in the first place.

The Heart: Whether or not we are cured, we are healed when we feel
whole, when others say they feel more connected with us, and when something in our heart makes us feel re-enchanted and energetically recon-
nected with the world again. We are healed when we have learned to
celebrate life rather than just struggle to prolong it and when we have
learned how to be more aware of the oscillating subtle instability that is
just beneath what we may experience as "stable health."

8. How does healing happen?

The Brain: Once we find the part of the mechanical system that is
broken and repair it, healing has happened because we have been returned
to "normal function." There is nothing "vitalistic," energetic, or spiritual
about getting better, only the reestablishment of biomechanical function.

The Heart: Healing happens when we feel a loving energy flowing
freely within us again and when the subtle "L" energy of life, our ancestors, the trees, the birds, the flowers, the animals, and the life system tell us
through our cellular memories that we have opened our heart sufficiently

to let the energy flow again. Healing happens when the field of energetic intelligence within the body system exercises its intuitive powers to restore a more adaptive balancing between ourselves and our world.

9. What happens after we heal?

The Brain: After we are healed, we go back about our daily life business. We may be more vigilant for another breakdown in a body system and alter some of our behaviors to lessen the chance of relapse or recurrence, but healing usually allows us to resume more than change our prior life. At least temporarily, until the brain resumes its urgent pressures and forgets our prior suffering, we may become a member of the group of the worried well and practice "preventive" medicine.

The Heart: There is no "after" healing because we are constantly aware of being whole, connected, and sending and receiving energy from the systems around us. Sickness is as much a part of life as health, so we learn when we suffer the pain of sickness to attend more to a healing style of living. We can also learn from others when they suffer that, by helping them heal, we are energized in our own healing. Instead of self-oriented "preventive" medicine, we practice enhancement healing with all systems.

10. What makes a healer?

The Brain: A healer is someone who has learned all about how the body systems work and for several years has sacrificed much of his or her own mental and physical health in order to pass the tests required to be declared legally allowed to try to heal others and work in the healing temples. The healer is objective, emotionally distant, mechanistic, skeptical, and unbelieving of anything that cannot be seen or touched.

The Heart: All of us are healers, but some are more healing than most because they have been transformed by serious illness and, as a result, are more cardio-sensitive than those who have not yet had their turn at confronting their own mortality. The cardio-sensitives know that self-care begins with caring for others and with the awareness that none of us is ever truly emotionally distant or totally objective. The two criteria of a more cardio-sensitive healer are having learned through a crisis and, in part because of that crisis, having developed a profound compassion for the energy of and from one's own heart and the hearts of others.

OF A MIND TO HEAL

Mind/body healing has seen a significant increase in acceptance, supportive research, and both professional and public awareness. Cardio-energetics proposes, however, that biomedicine and many forms of so-called mind/body medicines often see the "mind" as somewhere in the brain and as in charge of the body, not as a coupling of brain and body as coordinated by the heart and its rhythmic info-energy. For cardio-energetics, healing is less a process of mind over matter than of using our heart to unite the rational power of the brain and the spontaneous healing powers of the body so that the triune Mind's healing intuition can work its daily miracles.

You have read that our brain is our primary health maintenance center. Research from fields such as psychoneuroimmunology shows that how our brain thinks translates directly to how our body and all of its systems operate.[4] There is no doubt that thinking more rationally about life, dealing less reactively with stress, and using visualization, imagery, and the relaxation response to help focus and direct the biomechanical body systems can be extremely beneficial in health and healing. Without the heart, however, the brain is like a partially sighted surgeon. It can put us at risk of further disconnection by its narrow view of protecting its own body's health at the expense of the overall health of the system in which it lives and worrying more about not being sick than celebrating being alive to share life with others.

There is abundant evidence to show that a moderate, low-calorie, low-fat, high-fiber diet, regular exercise, and stress-reduction techniques can help keep the body well. While many of us have responded by working out regularly or eating more low-fat foods, too many of us have turned obsessive about fitness and health. Trying to avoid dying rather than enjoy living, we use strict eating and exercises regimens that take all the pleasure out of eating and all the fun out of physical fitness. We might make our attempts at more healthy living more effective if we stopped just trying to avoid a heart attack and started putting more heart—more shared joy and less guilt—into those things we do that we hope will protect our health. It is senseless to almost kill ourselves in the effort to live longer.

CHURCHILL'S BLACK DOG

Winston Churchill helped save the world. His courage and leadership in the face of Nazi tyranny are still idolized by those who remember how his valor and inspiration helped defeat Hitler. His wit and particularly his subtle humor are well known. Less known is the fact that, throughout his life, Churchill was plagued by severe depression and what he called his "heavy heart," followed by his "black dog" of chronic depression.[5] This great man, whose character energized the free world, was in part motivated and given strength as much by the "dark" energy of his life as his lighter, more joyful energy. Churchill's life offers a model for healing somewhat different from that typically used by mind/body healing advocates because it redefines a "positive attitude" as one that includes full awareness and acceptance of the dark side of "L" energy and that the only negative emotion is a "stuck" emotion that dominates and suppresses the emergence of other emotions.

Two of the best-known contributors and heroes in the field of mind/body medicine are Norman Cousins and Dr. Bernie Siegel. Norman Cousins was a brave and creative man who described his self-assertiveness, enlightened cooperation with his physician, and his use of laughter and a positive attitude to carry him through several serious illnesses.[6] Dr. Siegel has written and spoken courageously about the healing power of love well before such ideas were discussed at medical meetings.[7] While the popular press interpreted the lessons from both of these men to mean that an upbeat, Pollyannaish attitude heals, both men emphasized in their own ways the importance of full understanding of the dark side of one's life.

Churchill's life presents two key components to be added to the powerful healing influences identified by mind/body writers such as Cousins and Siegel. His story illustrates how cellular memories of his depression-prone ancestors were a source of Churchill's resilience in the face of overwhelming odds. Such cellular memories also provide impetus and endurance in the form of a "stress hardiness" that helps even the suffering to be great healers themselves. Full awareness of the influence and origins of one's cellular memories and willingness to use their energy no matter its nature provides the necessary instability that creates the adaptive stability of great Minds.

The brain abhors the leftover sadness within our cellular memories and our individual heartfelt depressive reactions because they are distractions from its primary mission of seeking pleasure for its body. The heart, however, is nurtured not only by gladness but by facing rather than avoiding or denying what psychologist Carl Jung called the "shadow" of our personality and all prior personalities.

ANCIENT MOOD MAKERS

Author Anthony Storr states that it was the persistence of Churchill's recurrent fits of depression that seemed to follow him everywhere that caused Churchill to name his recurrent emotional state his "black dog."[8] He referred to it as always being with him and said that, as painful as his realization of this dark energy was, he felt this awareness of his inner shadow was a key component of his ability to sense, understand, and deal with the dark energies that swirled from hearts such as Hitler's and the other murderers of World War II.

Churchill's "black dog" was not only his. The cellular memories of his ancestors seemed to echo within him. Many of his ancestors were accompanied through their own lives by the same "black dog" that walked at Churchill's side. Historian A. L. Rowse described Churchill's dark-side legacy of depression as derived to some extent from his ancestors, primarily the first duke of Marlborough. He quotes the duke as saying, "I am extremely out of heart."[9] As his black dog bit at his heels, the duke was motivated to reach out for healing and love. He wrote to his lover, "My dearest soul, pity me and love me."[10]

Cardio-energetic healing requires being clearly and directly aware of the black dog that walks with all of us. While positive affirmations are a key part of mind/body healing, brain/heart/body cardio-energetic healing also requires affirming the negative energy of our life and opening our heart to not only the love but the hurt that comes with the inheritance of the cellular memories made by our own experiences and by all hearts that came before ours.

LESSONS FROM CHIRON

According to Greek mythology, the centaur Chiron taught the art of healing. He was wounded by a poisoned arrow and carried that poison forever in his body. He was both healer and in need of healing, and awareness of that need made him a better healer of others. Cardio-energetics says that we all have some poison within our cellular memories and that we are all both healers and in need of healing. Such poison can serve as a stimulant to make us more sensitive, tolerant, understanding, and willing to help with the pain of others. It can throw us "off balance" just enough that we learn more about how to better keep our balance.

Almost every great leader, gifted artist, or brilliant scientist has had his or her own "black dog," a form of their own Chironic poisoning that motivated them toward their personal, "abnormal" uniqueness, and that contributed to their extraordinary accomplishments.[11] William Black, Lord Byron, Alfred Lord Tennyson, John Berry, Anne Sexton, Vincent van Gogh, Robert Schumann, Franz Kafka, and Isaac Newton all suffered throughout their lives with an indolent depression. The greatest levels of sensitivity, alertness to the body's own intuitive healing processes, creativity, and well-being seem to carry with them the necessary alternating current of the negative dark subtle "L" energy. Without close knowledge and awareness of the lingering cellular memories in the form of the shadow of our personality, we cannot be healed or offer healing to others.

Much of our dark energy is left as cellular memory imprints from our parents and ancestors. Viewing depression as a singular mood state experienced by one person neglects the fact that much of the dynamic info-energy discussed throughout this book exists as a collective cellular memory and not just the result of our individual life experiences. Cardio-energetic healing views a positive attitude as an obstinate resistance to the temptation to seek only the wonderful aspects of living and the tenacious willingness to get down and dirty with the more base and even mean-spirited quality of our spiritual energy. Some of our most powerful healers have not been those with angelic serene faces and calm voices. They have often appeared battle-weary from their courageous continuing skirmishes with life's challenges and from having picked themselves up again and again after being knocked down by a cruel joke of the trickster. They often appear drawn, hardened, and sad, their faces twisted and wrinkled with the battle scars from having fully engaged all the chaos that life has to offer.

DOES DEPRESSION HAVE TO BE SO DEPRESSING?

One reason depression has been increasing over the last decades may be that we have become so fixated on our pursuit of happiness that we become angry and impatient with any unhappiness at all. We seem to have lost much of what poet John Keats represents in his poem "Ode to Melancholy" and refers to less metaphorically in his personal correspondences as our "negative capability," a personal attribute he defines as "being capable of being in uncertainties, mysteries, doubts, without any irritable reaching after fact and reason."[12] Without our negative capability, we can feel deprived instead of challenged when what we see as our natural birthright to constant delight is not forthcoming. It seems to be our brain that feels "entitled" while our heart is more appreciative. In our heart, we seem to know that sadness is as essential to life as joy and have learned that we benefit from a good cry as much as a good laugh. Our heart seems more able than our brain to enjoy a little "down time" from the intensity of elation and to be reenergized, to feel more alive, by experiencing a full range of emotion.

Another reason statistics show a rise in rates of depression across all age groups may be that our brain is getting better at facing reality. While a little creative denial is essential to healing, so is some fact-facing no matter the grave nature of those facts. One common characteristic of depressed people is, unlike those who are less often sad, they seem to be too good at facing reality. They seem more keenly aware of violence, unfairness, and the cruel randomness of life that the less depressed manage to more effectively deny most of the time. If depression-prone people keep facing reality and living only in the shadows of their brain's defensive way of living, they become seriously and chronically depressed.

When we say someone is "unbalanced," we are being cardio-energetically accurate because they are leaning too far to only one side of the emotional spectrum. As proposed by the opponent process theory you read about in chapter 6, we are—like our heart—oscillating beings. Healing and well-being requires that we deny the brain's version of reality just enough to enjoy our life without constant fear, while at the same time accepting the necessity of life's essential down times as spiritual nudges toward establishing a better and more adaptive fulcrum point in our life balancing act.

ABOVE ALL, BALANCE

Cardio-energetic healing, then, is first and foremost energetic balance, or perhaps more accurately, constant rebalancing. Too much happiness can cause the heart's energy to be disrupted and even cause death.[13] In a study of 170 cases of sudden death over a six-year period, 6 percent of these deaths were immediately preceded by the experience of sudden happiness.[14] To heal and be a healer, we have to enhance our spiritual "resistance" to the forces of life that push against us by dancing in, rather than fighting against, or allowing ourselves to be swept away by, the inherent chaos of life.

Too little unhappiness can diminish our mental, physical, and spiritual stamina. Cardio-energetic healing is pragmatic hedonism. It is not just feeling good, but it *is* profoundly feeling. A Zen saying is, "After ecstasy, the laundry." In our eagerness to return to paradise, we must remember to brush our teeth, water the plants, and feed the cat. In our modern emphasis on the value of self-happiness and fear of unhappiness, we are becoming spiritually soft. Cardio-energetic healing requires a focus on the heart to recover more of the energy of our cellular memories, both glad and sad, old and new, so that we develop a healing hardiness. The healing heart is one that tries to connect more than perfect and make everything in our lives wonderful. It helps us sometimes to "just be" rather than always trying to "be happy." As George Orwell pointed out, "Men can only be happy when they do not assume that the object of life is happiness."[15]

SENSUOUS HEALING

The word "sensuous" means "perceived by or affecting the senses" and "readily affected through the senses."[16] Another component of cardio-energetic healing is to develop our sense, our cardio-intuitiveness, for our innate healing propensity. Immunologist Dr. J. Edwin Blalock of the University of Alabama, Birmingham, describes the immune system as a sensory organ that "senses" cells and substances that are not recognized by other body systems.[17] Our immune system does not simply react to invaders, it can also sense and remember them. There is no more direct proof of cellular memory than the conduct of the cells of our immune system as they seek, find, dispose of, and remember until their death any substance that enters or is generated from within the body itself that does not belong there.

Cardio-energetics shows that our heart, because it is a thinking, feeling, endocrine organ, acts in conjunction with our immune system and serves as its surveillance system. As you read in Part I, the heart's cells are full of neurohormones that communicate back and forth with our immune system, the heart regulates its own rhythm, and it contains its own nervous system. It is "sensuous" because it can sense and react to the outside world and then tell us when someone, someplace, or something "feels good for us" or may not be good for us. When we say, "Something in my heart tells me this is no good," or "I sense this is not good for my system," we are speaking for and from our heart.

Dr. Robert Ader coined the term "psychoneuroimmunology" to refer to the study of the interaction between the brain, the immune system, and our reactions and interpretations of the outside world. Along with his colleague Nicholas Cohen of the University of Rochester, Dr. Ader showed that the immune system not only can sense what is not good for us but can also remember and learn. Ader and Cohen's research proved that immune cells "remember" and can be "conditioned" to respond to a neutral stimulus. They administered an immune-suppressing drug and a placebo (a dummy pill) together and, as a result, the immune system finally responded to the neutral system alone without the presence of the drug. If the immune system learns, and the immune system is also in our heart, our heart can learn too. Learning is a form of remembering, so the cellular memories of our immune system are crucial to our health and healing. The process of inoculation is a biochemical tutoring of the immune system and a way to create vigilant cellular memories within its cells for a future invader.

SENSE-ABLE CELLS

Cardio-energetics says that we have "sense-able" cells. The fact that human cells can sense and learn has been known for more than seventy years. The learning and remembering abilities of immune system cells were first reported in 1926 by Drs. Metal'nikov and Chrine of the Pasteur Institute in Paris.[18] Because the healing Mind (brain/heart/body) senses, learns, and remembers, and because cardio-energetics asserts that the heart is at the center of the Mind and sender of the info-energy being pumped to and stored in our cells, healing from the heart means going beyond mind-over-body to seeing and tuning in to the heart as the core of the holistic healing energy system.

The healing system mediated by the heart is a new field that combines several areas of study and their findings: what we know about the functioning of the heart (cardiology) and the healing brain (neuropsychology); what we know so far about the immune system and its interactions with all systems (psychoneuroimmunology); what know about the endocrine and nervous system within the heart (neurocardiology); what we have learned about the brain's and body's interactions with the world as they affect the heart (cardiac psychology); the new ideas about the dynamic energetic system of the heart (energy cardiology); and the concepts about learning to "read and listen" to the heart's energy and wisdom (cardio-energetics). While no journal would fit it in, this new field that studies the role of the heart in healing might be called "psycho-neuro-energeti-cardio-neuro-immunology." Taking the time to slowly pronounce each of the eighteen syllables of this made-up word and to get the brain to even try to say it would at least cause most of us to slow down enough to be able to pay more attention to our heart.

HEALING RHYTHMS AND TENDER TEMPOS

There is no more obvious evidence of connection between our heart and energy outside the body than our heart's response to musical rhythms. As far back as 1929, researchers tried to measure the effect on the cardiovascular system when a person listened to a gramophone.[19] More recently, it was discovered that the human heart rate could be varied over a certain range by synchronizing the sinus rhythm—the normal heart rhythm—with an external auditory stimulus such as a steady clicking sound.[20] Our heart is the metronome of our body's biorhythm, and health happens when we are in rhythm within ourselves, synchronized with other living systems, and moving to our preset beat rather than trying to respond to the driving beat of the stressful outside world.

Professor David Aldridge at the University of Witten Herdecke in Germany suggests that disease is a type of musical dyslexia and the inability to "keep our rhythm" while living with and being bombarded by the varied rhythms of the world around us.[21] Healing, then, becomes the ability of our heart to improvise and develop its own new rhythms to the chaotic rhythms that continually emerge in our daily life. For example, type A behavior (hurried and hostile living) may be seen as the heart's musical inability to play its own natural, steady, gentle song because we allow it to be aggravated and thrown off beat by our environmentally reactive brain, or to react to other type A brains and their agitated hearts.

Cardio-energetic healing views all disease as "arrhythmia." When our heart is sick, it beats irregularly, and when our cells lose their natural rhythm of division we develop cancer. The Greek word "chronos" refers to clock time, but "kairos" time is a natural rhythm of life emanating from our own heart and its energy translated throughout our body system. Cardio-energetic healing requires tuning in and living by our heart's own good "kairos" time, and not always allowing "chronos" or clock time to dictate our life.[22]

Most of my heart transplant recipient patients report changes in their musical preferences after receiving their new heart. In effect, they have had a new human tissue pacemaker placed in their chest. Even though doctors may regulate the new heart's beating with medication, that heart's cells still have their memory of their original rhythm, which may manifest itself in changes in musical taste as often as it does changes in tastes for food.

A cardio-energetic healing technique I have used with my own cancer and heart patients is to have them select music they feel represents their heart and, if necessary, select music for listening that helps quiet their heart. I ask them if the music they have selected shows the type of heart they want to have or the heart they now have. I also ask them to select music that represents the heart of parents and family members. My type A patients almost always select fast, loud, high volume music as representative of their heart, but report that this is not the type of heart energy they think is good for them. My cancer patients tend to select slower, quieter music, perhaps in an attempt to help their cells get their rhythm back.

I sometimes play samples of restful works such as the first movement of Beethoven's Symphony no. 6 or Smetana's *The Moldau*. More often, I ask my patients to select the works they think represent healing and health. I ask them to spend a few minutes every day at work listening with earphones to a slower, quieter music. They almost always select music that resonates at about 70 to 80 beats per minute, a rhythm characteristic of a coherent heart. Most patients report that this simple and brief exercise helps them get back to at least a little more peaceful state.

THE FOURTH CHAKRA

Cardio-energetic healing derives some of its approaches from many of the ancient forms of medicine. Chinese medicine, one of the oldest, longest tested, and most powerful and trusted medical systems in the world, views the body as an eco-energetic system. It speaks of vibrational subtle energy that must be integrated into the cellular matrix by passing through a specialized step-down system of "transformer" stations that yogic tradition calls "chakras."[23] These are the relay stations used by the heart in its communicating of info-energy to the body's cells.

According to the Chinese system, energy storage and conveyance centers contribute and distribute a type of subtle nutritional energy throughout the body. There are seven of these energy transforming centers: the coccygeal, sacral, solar plexus, heart, throat, third eye, and head chakras. Each center is closely associated with its own physiological endocrine system, and neuro-emotional system. Of concern to cardio-energetics is the fourth chakra, the heart.

Chinese medicine sees the fourth chakra as one of the most important centers for the conveyance and storage of subtle "L" energy. Unlike Western medicine, which sees the brain as the core of the body system, Chinese medicine sees the fourth energy zone, the heart, as the center of all the energy centers. It is seen as our primary energy connection station, mediating between the lower physical ("earthly") and higher energy centers. It is seen as the transitional point where our physical essence connects with heaven, or the cosmos.

Alternative medicine researcher Dr. Richard Gerber writes, "One of the most important links between the heart chakra and a physical organ is seen in the association of the heart chakra with the thymus, a primary mediator of the development of immune cells called T lymphocytes.[24] Cardio-energetics sees the heart as an immune organ, and psychoneuroimmunologists trying to clarify the connection between human emotions and illness would be well advised to follow the Chinese medicine lead and look not only at biochemical connections but also the energy connection between the heart, thymus gland, and our immunity. Chinese medicine has long asserted that there is a subtle energy flow through the heart and on to the thymus gland and thus to and throughout the body's immune system. These ancient healers knew that what we feel in our heart is conveyed to our immune system.

THE MIND IS ALL BODY

Another source of support for the concepts of cardio-energetics is the recent documentation of the existence of a miraculous neurochemical information system within our body. Dr. Candace Pert, the neurobiologist and former chief of brain chemistry at the National Institute of Mental Health, whose work I referred to earlier in this book, describes the body's communication system as containing two key elements—the chemical substances known as neuropeptides and the receptors into which these neuropeptides fit.[25] Neuropeptides are produced by nerve cells in the brain and are made up of amino acids. They serve as neurotransmitters or the communicating connectors of the entire nervous system. Pert's groundbreaking work gives credence to the idea that there is a complex, body-wide systemic memory including our cellular system.[26]

Cells throughout the body, including cells in the immune system, the stomach, and the heart, have receptors made just for these neuropeptides. Dr. Pert writes, "the more we know about neuropeptides, the harder it is to think in the traditional terms of a mind and a body. It makes more and more sense to speak of a single integrated entity, a "body-mind."[27] Because it is the energy of the heart that helps to propel the neuropeptides throughout the body, cardio-energetics suggests that it makes sense to speak of the heart not just as another organ influenced by the neuropeptides but as the energy core of a healing Mind composed of a brain/heart/ body dynamic system.

Dr. Pert writes, "In the beginning of my work, I matter-of-factly presumed that emotions were in the head or the brain. Now I would say they are really in the body as well. They are expressed in the body and are part of the body. I can no longer make a strong distinction between the brain and the body."[28] When I spoke with Dr. Pert about my theories of cellular memories and related the stories of my heart transplant patients, she was not surprised. She pointed out that, since the cells in the heart are loaded with molecules that necessarily contain at least some form of memory, these memories could well come along with the heart to join with the new body and brain.

Dr. Pert speculates, "I think it is important to realize that information is stored in the brain, and it is conceivable to me that this information could transform itself into some other realm."[29] Cardio-energetics says that this "realm" is the subtle "L" energy, which may be mediated by the heart. Assumptions such as that the brain thinks independently of the body and heart, our heart is merely a powerful but dumb pump, and that our cells cannot remember are not in keeping with either the newest scientific knowledge from cellular biology or the oldest wisdom of ancient traditional medicines.

Since energy and the information it carries cannot be destroyed, where does the information (energy) go after the destruction of the molecules or neuropeptides (mass) that contained it are destroyed? Cardio-energetics says that it does not go anywhere; it just is and it is forever. It walks with us as a black dog and a playful, happy puppy left in our care by those who lived before us. It remains all around us, permeating everything and everyone and enveloping us with a scintillating energy like an omnipresent quantum heaven. Ultimately, cardio-energetic healing is enhanced when healing is not viewed as a way of avoiding death but of becoming re-enchanted with all aspects of the subtle "L" energy of the heart, the energy of all systems, and all feelings both good and bad. The "Mind," as I have proposed it, is an interactive, energetic, dynamic, remembering system functioning as a single whole, coordinated by the power of the heart and maintaining the connection between the brain and the body. Dr. Pert and her colleagues have suggested, with her discoveries, a neurohormonal correlate for this interactive system.[30]

Dr. Herbert Weiner, in his book *Psychobiology,* anticipated the role of cellular memories in healing more than twenty years ago when he first proposed the idea that disease is a breakdown of communication with and between cells, leading to an abnormal regulation of bodily functions and behavior.[31] Cardio-energetic healing is based on this old but increasingly research-supported idea that "dis-ease" is a perturbation of the info-energetic system composed of the brain, the heart, and the 75 trillion cells in the body.

LOVE HEALS THE HEALER

Cardio-energetics says that our capacity for and willingness to give love is at least if not more important than how much we are loved. It is not so much "feeling loved" as "loving others" that is the way of the healing heart. As you learned in chapter 9, the brain is romantic. It is sentimental, easily influenced by the neurohormones of our reactive physical senses, and the source of the popular psychology notion that we must first love ourselves before we can love someone else. Most research on loving has focused on people's rational or brain-oriented view of love, but pioneering research from the field of psychoneuroimmunology shows that the cardio-energetic view of "giving love to others first" is the way to a physically and emotionally healthy self.

Dr. David McClelland at Boston University defines love as a body/mind state that occurs on all levels of the human system, including the immune system and the heart.[32] His research involved tapping into the hearts instead of the heads of his subjects by asking them to tell stories and fantasize about past or future life experiences as a means of uncovering the code of the heart instead of the mental malarkey of the brain. Author Henry Dreher writes that McClelland's goal "was to measure the seemingly immeasurable; the heart within the mind [brain/body] of his subjects."[33] (brackets mine)

McClelland's work showed that a love for power negated the power of love. He studied men with what he called "inhibited power syndrome," a high need for control accompanied by the brain's inevitable disappointment with the reality that none of us has all that much control over anyone or anything. By their early fifties, these frustrated lovers of power were two and one half times more likely to develop heart disease or what cardio-energetics calls "a chaotic incoherence of the heart."[34]

McClelland also showed that the immune systems of the lovers of power were weaker than those who knew the power of love.[35] To show the healing power of a coherent and caring heart on the immune system, Mc-Clelland showed college students a documentary about the life of a person who is the perfect example of a cardio-energetic healer who knew well the code of the heart, the late Mother Theresa. Another group of students was shown a film about Nazi triumphs during World War II. The students who watched Mother Theresa experienced a profound increase in their immuno-efficiency as compared to those who watched the war film.[36] Watching a person with a coherent, open heart, what McClelland called "affiliative trust," seemed to make the students' hearts more coherent, open, and more able to tap into their own heart's affiliative trust code, and these changes were accompanied by a lasting enhancement of their immunity.[37]

THE DULCINEA EFFECT

In the novel *Don Quixote,* the poet-knight Cervantes meets a street prostitute. He sees this woman not as a whore but as someone with great beauty, kindness, and virtue, and his perception of her transforms her. He gives her a new name, Dulcinea, and his loving energy changes her and helps her begin to see herself as a more loving, caring person. When the knight is dying, he calls his lover to his bed to solidify the cellular memory of his loving image and to remind her that, even in his physical absence, she will now always be Dulcinea. This "Dulcinea Effect" represents the transformative power of love, the exact opposite of the systemic disruption caused by a love of power. It is an example of the registering of one heart's code in another heart, a transplantation of cardio-energy that influences both donor and recipient.

WITNESSING THE DEVELOPMENT OF THE SOUL

Cardio-energetics proposes that, ultimately, healing is a matter of the heart, not the head. It is a choice to tune in to another realm beyond that with which the brain is more comfortable, the realm of subtle "L" energy dancing between all systems. It is realizing what my mother told me when I was a little boy: When my grandfather died and we were all crying, I asked her if everyone had to get old. Her answer left a cellular memory in my heart that is being recovered and sent with this book. She said, "The body gets old, but never your mind. Even if the brain seems to fail and the body gets weak, the heart stays strong and its energy is forever. In the central place of every heart, there is a recording and sending chamber; so long as you see to it that your heart keeps sending loving signals to other hearts even when you are sad, your heart will get loving signals back. If what you sent was beautiful, cheerful, hopeful, and caring, that is what your heart will eventually receive, and no matter what happens to your brain or your body, who you are and have been to others will make you forever young at heart."

Dr. Pert writes, "The nature of the hypothetical 'other realm' is currently in the religious or mystical dimension, where Western science is clearly forbidden to tread."[38] Our increasingly urgent need to be healed and to heal our world requires that modern bioscience transcend its fear and tread cautiously but courageously into the other realm where the many as yet mysterious secrets of the heart's code are still hidden.

From the first miracle of the beginning of life to the final miracle of transcendence beyond life, you have your own spiritual recording chamber vibrating in the center of your being. Every beat of your heart shapes the memories that will forever be your legacy, the infinite echoes of your soul that will resonate long after your body and brain have ceased to serve your soul's needs. If you close this book, sit back, become very quiet, ignore your brain's urging to get up and get going, and take plenty of time to sense the subtle code tapping in your heart and the other hearts around you, you will have the wondrous privilege of being a participant observer of the forging of your soul.

Glossary

ANF: Atrial Naturetic Factor, referring to a peptide or substance secreted from the atrium (upper-chamber area) of the heart, that conveys information immediately from the heart to various organs of the body including the endocrine organs (adrenal glands, pancreas, etc.) and the brain.

Asclepian Medicine: Based on the mythic Greek physician-hero Asclepius, this form of medicine emphasizes repair of the body's breakdown through external manipulations, control, and treatment.

ATP: Adenosine triphosphate, a tiny molecule made from the food and sunlight we take in every day. There are at least 2 million ATP molecules vibrating every one ten-thousandth of a second in each of our 75 trillion cells to serve as a powerful info-energetic source.

Bell's Theorem: Physicist John Stewart Bell's mathematical theorem that when one member of a quantum pair (such as two electrons spinning in space or two persons falling in love) is interfered with in any way, its partner is also altered at exactly the same time. Bell's theorem is evidence of the nonlocal nature of "info-energy" called "action at a distance" (two objects influencing others irrespective of time and space). It is also evidence of the "sticky" nature of "L" energy, which means that all connections exist on some level forever, everywhere, and for all time. Despite many attempts by scientists to disprove this challenge to our brain's mechanistic view of the world, Bell's theorem still stands as a fundamental quantum physics principle.

Bioenergetics: The branch of biology that deals with the energy generated within and from living systems.

Chaology: The mathematical science that seeks patterns and mysterious forms of order amidst the apparent meaningless disorder, or chaos, of the world.

Cardiac Coherence: A state of cardiovascular and neurophysiological balance indicated by smooth, steady cardiac tracings as measured by electrocardiographs conducted by the HeartMath Institute.

Cardiac Conduction System: Cardiology's name for the complex bundle of fibers relaying info-energy within and from the heart.

Cardiac Psychology: The field of health psychology that identifies psychosocial risk factors for the development of cardiovascular illness and proposes lifestyle changes to help prevent and heal heart disease.

Cardio-contemplation: A technique to draw the brain's attention toward its heart. It involves being quiet, still, and allowing (not trying to make) the resonance response occur. It is a derivation of the "Freeze Frame Technique" developed by researchers at the Institute of HeartMath in California in which stressful situations or scenes are "frozen" to be considered from a more heart-focused, calmer perspective. Cardio-contemplation, however, is less "consideration" than full awareness of experiences in the center of the body.

Cardio-energetics: The field that combines findings from cardiology, cardiac psychology, energy cardiology, neurocardiology, psychoneuroimmunology, and the basic principles of quantum physics with the idea that energy and information are interchangeable and that this info-energy is primarily conveyed and communicated by the heart.

Cardio-sensitive: A sensitivity to the heart's code, that is, the subtle "L" energy. Based on interviews with seventy-three heart transplant recipients and sixty-seven recipients of other organs, as well as interviews of transplant patients by other researchers, there appear to be seventeen characteristics of cardio-sensitive people—those who are able to recover some form of the cellular memories of their donor. These persons may serve as models for any person wishing to learn to better read the heart's code.

Cell: From the Latin "cellula" meaning small room, one of the 75 trillion building blocks of the body that constitute about two thirds of the body's weight. Every cell is highly energized, uses a form of memory to conduct its work, and is directly and immediately influenced by the heart's "L" energy.

Cellular Memory: The theory that each of the 75 trillion cells in the body have various levels of stored information left there by the heart's conduction of "L" energy, which can be retrieved by focusing less on the brain and more on the heart. The impact of cellular memory is illustrated by the recall of heart transplant recipients of various forms of their donor's memories. Since information is a form of energy and, like matter, energy can not be destroyed, cellular memories are infinite.

Chakra: From the Sanskrit meaning "wheel," chakras, according to Indian yogic teachings, are the body's energy centers, resembling whirling vortices of subtle ("L") energy. There are seven chakras, the fourth being the central or "heart" chakra. These energy centers relate to the levels of flowing Qui (pronounced "chee"), referred to in the two-thousand-year-old system of Chinese medicine.

CSEP: Standing for "Cardiac Synchronized Energy Patterns," these are recordings of the heart's info-energy, including its electrical potential as measured by the electrocardiograph, its magnetic energy as measured by the magnetocardiograph, acoustical energy as measured by ultrasound techniques and the electronic stethoscope, and various other pressure- and temperature-detecting instruments.

Cytoplasm: A gelatinous protoplasmic fluid in the cells of the body in which several cellular parts (organelles) are located.

Dynamic Energy System: The central concept of a new interdisciplinary science proposed by psychologists Schwartz and Russek that integrates the more relational, subjective, vitalistic, and holistic medicinal approaches, which often originated in ancient cultures, with the more substantive, objective, mechanistic, reductionist, modern biomedical approaches. A "dynamic energy system" is one that is connected energetically with all other systems, "remembers" that interaction, and is primarily coordinated and integrated by the info-energy of the cardiovascular system as conveyed by the heart.

Dynamic System Memory: As proposed by Schwartz and Russek, the theory that, just as two tuning forks' vibrations become a characteristic part of each other's vibratory patterns, all systems interact in an info-energetically systemic manner to constantly create one another's memories of their interaction.

DNA: The body's basic genetic remembering and coding system made up of thin strings of deoxyribonucleic acid and including adenine, guanine, cytosine, and thymine.

Energy Cardiology: Schwartz and Russek's newly proposed field that combines alternative and conventional medicines in an interdisciplinary approach that applies the concept of systemic info-energy to the cardiovascular system and, because of the heart's centrality and immense energetic power, emphasizes the role of the heart as the coordinator and communicator of many forms of energy including "L" energy.

Environmental Determinism: The theory that a person does not act on the world but is essentially reactive to and a product of environmental and behavioral circumstances.

Flashbulb Memories: Enduring and detailed recollections of particularly significant, often negative, events.

Freeze Frame Technique: This HeartMath Institute–researched process involves mental recognition of a specific stressful feeling, making a mental effort to shift focus to sensations coming from the area of the heart instead of the head, recalling a very positive event of the past, and mentally asking the heart for its insights on what might be a better way of dealing with the stressful situation that could induce a state more like that of the past positive event.

Frustration/Aggression Hypothesis: The psychological theory that people automatically react with aggression when encountering a barrier to a goal. Some psychologists offer a new version of this hypothesis in which they suggest that the aggression is not elicited by feelings of frustration but by the intervening feeling of anger.

Heart's Code: The subtle info-energetic ("L" energy) signals from the heart that contain encoded memories of each person's cells and heart, and of all people's cells and hearts.

Hidden Observer: The hypnotized person's "self," or consciousness, that is not subject to the hypnotist's command. Under hypnosis, a hypnotized subject follows the instructions of the hypnotist but still retains a subconscious alertness because he or she has a vigilant sensitivity despite his or her altered state of awareness. Cardio-sensitives seem to demonstrate a high degree of "vigilant sensitivity," as if their hearts recognize truth when the brain is tricked or distracted.

Hygeian Medicine: Based on the Greek goddess Hygeia, daughter of the Greek mythic physician-hero Asclepius, this form of medicine focuses on the natural rhythm of health and illness, the body's instinctual drive to heal, and its innate cellular memory of the state of well-being.

Iconic Memory: "Afterimages" of physical stimuli, such as the tracings of light from a candle moved through a dark room.

"L" Energy: The info-energy of the heart's code, it is the "fifth force" that is related to—but transcends in its nonlocal nature—the known four energy forces of gravity, electromagnetism, strong nuclear energy, and weak nuclear energy. Like everything in the cosmos, it has a "light" (positive) and "dark" (negative) side. Cardio-energetic "stability" is a continually creative "instability" that balances both sides of "L" energy.

Meme: A small mental representation of cultural information, such as a commercial jingle, car design, clothing fashion, dance step, or simple phrase. The "science" of memetics studies the ways in which memes can act as "brain viruses" and "infect" our consciousness by becoming annoying, dominating, distracting memories.

Microtubules: Hollow tubes in every cell in the body latticed with kernel-like hexagons that contain and convey intracellular information. It is possible that, on the most basic level, cellular memories are stored in microtubules.

Modal Memory Theory: Psychologists identify three types, or "systems," of memory: sensory, short-term, and long-term memory. Cellular memory can manifest itself as any and all of these types of memory but can transcend them by storing more subtle "L" energy tracings of events and experiences as "senses from the heart."

Na'au: Hawaiian word for the "gut" of the soul where the heart/mind unity is located. The na'au constantly sends out "mana," or "info-energy," and is where all the wisdom of ancient ancestors (cellular memories) are stored. This is one of many centuries-old examples of traditional peoples' knowledge of the heart's code and cellular memories. (Ancient Hawaiians said "Ho'opa'ana'au," pronounced "hoh-oh-pa-ah-na-ow" and meaning to learn by and within the heart forever).

Neurocardiology: The field that studies the heart as a neurohormonal organ.

Nonlocality: The quantum physics principle that distance and barriers of time and space are illusions of the materialistic, substantiality-oriented brain and that there are no limits of distance, time, or barriers in the transmission of "L" energy, as illustrated by prayer, remote viewing, and other so-called psychic phenomenon.

Neurotransmitter: A chemical emitted from nerve fibers that carries messages that make body systems remember, within a fraction of a second, how to behave.

Neuropeptides: Neurotransmitters made up of amino acids (the building blocks for the proteins that are crucial for all life processes) that are active not only in the brain but, like microcosmic keys fitting into tiny keyholes in the cells of the body, act like "bits of brain" that float throughout the body and help unlock a cell's memory.

Organelles: Specialized parts of cells, each with its own function and unique way of communicating its information within the cell.

Oscillation: The alternation of energy patterns as shown in the heart's rhythm. Cardio-energetics suggests that the heart's oscillation is a model for our "oscillating self-structure" (alteration patterns of info-energy resonating in the body system). It is composed of male/objective/substantiality and female/subjective/relationality. Two persons "oscillating together" in a loving bond can exert the most influential and distinct "L" energy because they unite in a balanced energy system.

Parapraxes: "Slips of the tongue" or faulty acts that some psychologists suggest reveal feelings emerging from the unconscious, and that cardio-energetics suggests are "slips of the heart": the recovery of cellular memories.

Psychoneuroimmunology: The field that studies the interaction between the mind, body, and social systems and how this interaction influences health and healing.

PEAR: The Princeton Engineering Anomalies Research program at Princeton University in New Jersey. For twenty years, this highly scientific center has identified subtle energy ("L" energy) connections between people and machines and between people and remote places. These connections seem most profound when the "percipients" (participants who are indeed able to achieve these "L" energy connections) show many of the same characteristics of heart transplant "cardio-sensitives."

Psychic-spurt Phenomenon: As shown in the PEAR program, "L" energy connection (tapping the heart's code) seems to be sudden, then diminishes, and then resumes its initial profound but very subtle influence. The U-shaped curve of their experience is similar to the cardio-sensitivity connection between heart transplant recipients and their donors. Resumption of the "L" energy connection seems to depend on the ability to be "loving"—quietly selfless and connected enough to allow the heart to fall into info-energetic resonance with the natural rhythms of the outside world.

Pu'uwai: Hawaiian word for the heart (pronounced "poo-oo-vī"), literally "lump of water," and referring to the ancient Polynesian concept of the heart as the primary matter (lump) representation of the source of basic life-sustaining energy (water). This is a two-thousand-year-old precursor of the basic quantum physics premise of wave/particle duality that is characteristic of "L" energy.

Reciprocal Determinism: The theory that individuals can be self-directive and exercise some control over their thoughts, feelings, and actions through conscious decision.

Rejection Phenomenon: When tissue is transplanted from one body to another, the immune system of the recipient xenophobically identifies the new tissue as a "stranger" and attacks it. Rejection is a threat to the success of transplantation, and researchers are now looking at better ways to reduce biological rejection and also how to make two systems more "info-energetically" friendly to one another.

Relationality: Often seen as the "feminine connectiveness" orientation to life, the concept that all persons, places, and things share a common, subtle info-energetic field of intelligence beyond their "substance" nature.

Resonance Response: The body has several automatic responses such as the fear, sexual, and relaxation responses. The resonation response is the heart's innate capacity to fall into synch with the natural rhythms of life and to help calm its brain and body by its synchronization with other hearts and the subtle energy of the natural world.

Sinoatrial (SA) Node: The heart's rhythmic center. It is a tiny patch of tissue in the heart's back wall near the top of its right atrium (collecting chamber) that is the center of the "cardiac conduction system." It functions as the heart's own internal pacemaker and is central to the complex "nervous system" of the heart.

Substantiality: Often associated with the "masculine separateness" orientation to life, the concept that all persons, places, and things are substances made of a mass of stuck-together particles.

Systems Theory: The concept that all people, places, things, and forces in the universe are integrated into a hierarchy of mutually influential matter and energy.

TABP: Type A Behavior Pattern. Originally, type A referred to a hurried, rushed personality; now, called type A Behavior Pattern, it refers to a set of behaviors primarily consisting of impatience, hostility, and cynicism. Type A Behavior Pattern is associated with the development of heart disease.

Temperament: A set of individual characteristics that remain relatively stable in the face of intense emotional reactions. Evidence shows that every heart may have its own "cardio-temperament" (an "overreactive" or "underreactive" heart) that is influenced by its "cellular memories," which were implanted primarily by one's mother but also by other hearts.

Volume Conduction: Based on a concept from physics and biology, the fact that the electrical potential generated by the heart and as measured by an electrocardiograph can be recorded from any site on the body. Cardio-energetics asserts that the reason volume conduction exists is because the entire body is a moment-to-moment expression of the info-energy of its heart. Since the heart is not shielded, it sends its "L" energy outward at the speed of light to connect with other energy systems.

Quantum Heaven: A phrase used by energy cardiologists Schwartz and Russek to refer to a field of nonlocal intelligence or enveloping infinite info-energy that "is" everything.

Wave/Particle Duality: The quantum physics principle that everything in the cosmos, and the cosmos itself, is both "stuff" and "process," both "matter" and "energy." All particles are waves and vice versa; whether the particle or wave nature of something is observed is determined by what is being looked for and when.

Xenophobia: The brain's evolutionary fear and even hatred of strangers and any "thing" perceived as other than the self. A major factor in organ transplant rejection.

Endnotes

INTRODUCTION: THE SPIRIT'S ENERGY AND THE SOUL'S HEART

1. A forum regarding the emergence of a field or fields to begin to explore the complex new issues related to what I am calling the heart's code—the relationship between information, energy, and mind/body medicine—published in *Advances: The Journal of Mind-Body Health* Vol. 13 (1997): pp. 3–46.

2. There is currently a debate regarding the challenges involved in working toward one integrated model of medicine and whether or not there should be just one model or perhaps many models that we should learn to understand better so we can, as University of Maryland anthropologist Dr. Claire Monod Cassidy suggests, free ourselves from reliance on any one paradigm and become better able to "surf" the entire web of knowledge from all sources of healing. See *Advances* Vol. 13 (1997): pp. 6–30.

3. Dr. Larry Dossey examines the persistent need of healers to attribute many of the miracles they see to the effects of a "subtle" invisible energy or force that passes between healer and patient in his article "The Forces of Healing: Reflections on Energy, Consciousness, and the Beef Stroganoff Principle." *Alternative Therapies* Vol. 3 (1997): pp. 8–16. Dossey suggests that, just as it was important in the development of medicine to understand and accept the existence of new forces such as infection, it may also be important to accept as yet immeasurable nonlocal "forces" or subtle energy to understand some forms of healing. What I call "subtle" or "L" energy throughout this book may be a metaphor for a complex princi-

ple of life we cannot yet understand or explain but can experience or choose to "see" as another "force" of life.

4. The "Yan Xin Qiqong" phenomenon, the Chinese concept of healing "subtle" energy, has been practiced and treasured in China for over seven thousand years. The first book written in English about this process is titled *Secrets and Benefits of Internal Qiqong Cultivation*. This book is a collection of Dr. Yan Xin's lectures edited by H. Lin, R. Cohen, M. Cohen, and B. Campton (Malvern, Pennsylvania: Amber Leaf Press, 1997).

5. C. Sylvia and B. Novak, *A Change of Heart* (New York: Little, Brown, 1997).

6. E. Laszlo, *The Interconnected Universe: Conceptual Foundations of Transdisciplinary Unified Theory* (Singapore: World Scientific Publishing, 1995).

7. B. Siegel, "Emotions, Energy, and Healing," *Advances* Vol. 13 (1997): pp. 4–5.

8. The field of energy cardiology was named and developed by Gary E. Schwartz, Ph.D., and Linda G. Russek, Ph.D. They first proposed their theories about an interdisciplinary approach to study how the concept of energy and information conveyed within that energy applies to the cardiovascular system in "Energy Cardiology: A Dynamical Energy Systems Approach for Integrating Conventional and Alternative Medicine," *Advances* Vol. 12 (1996): pp. 4–24.

9. Their most recent publication combines several theories of health and healing from around the world into a set of "world medicine hypotheses" that serve as a starting point for the development of a comprehensive theory of mind/body medicine that can incorporate the strengths of many models. See G. E. Schwartz and L. G. Russek, "The Challenge of One Medicine: Theories of Health and Eight 'World Hypotheses,'" *Advances* Vol. 13 (1997): pp. 7–23.

10. J. G. Miller, *Living Systems* (New York: McGraw-Hill, 1978).

11. D. J. Chamoers, *The Conscious Mind: In Search of a Fundamental Theory* (New York: Oxford University Press, 1996).

12. S. Mead, *The Lively Experiment: The Shaping of Christianity in America* (New York: Harper and Row, 1963), p. 129.

Chapter 1: BREAKING THE LETHAL COVENANT

1. W. B. Mendelssohn, M. Maczaj, and J. Holt, "Bupirone Administration to Sleep Apnea Patients," *Journal of Clinical Psychopharmacology* Vol. 23 (1991): pp. 71–72.

2. T. Moore, *Care of the Soul* (New York: HarperPerennial, 1992), p. 278.

3. M. Csikszentmihalyi, *The Evolving Self* (New York: HarperCollins, 1993).

4. *Ibid.,* p. 36.

5. The issue of healthy balance between the necessary unhappiness that comes with the privilege of living and the happiness derived from the more splendid moments of daily life is creatively presented in Dr. Larry Dossey's "In Praise of Unhappiness," *Alternative Therapies* Vol. 2 (1996): pp. 7–10. He reviews the work of psychologist Mihaly Csikszentmihalyi, Alan Watts, and others who have observed the brain's natural evolution-based negativity. This quote is on p. 7.

6. A. Watts. "Odyssey of Aldous Huxley," *Original Live Recordings on Comparative Philosophy* (San Anselmo, California: The Electronic University, 1995).

7. P. MacLean, "On the Evolution of Three Mentalities," in *New Dimensions in Psychiatry: A World View, Vol. II,* eds. S. Arieti and G. Chrznowki (New York: Wiley, 1977).

8. H. Beinfield and E. Korngold, "Chinese Traditional Medicine: An Introductory Overview," *Alternative Therapies* Vol. 1 (1995): pp. 44–52.

9. *Ibid.,* p. 45.

10. N. Sivin, *Traditional Medicine in Contemporary China* (Ann Arbor, Michigan: University of Michigan Press, 1987), pp. 47–53.

11. W. Brugh Joy, *Joy's Way* (Los Angeles: Jeremy P. Tarcher, 1978).

12. For a full discussion of the oceanic Polynesian model of well-being, see my *The Pleasure Prescription: To Love, To Work, To Play—Life in the Balance* (Alameda, California: Hunter House Publishers, 1996).

13. See M. Friedman, N. Gleischmann, and V. A. Price, "Diagnosis of Type A Behavior Pattern," in *Heart and Mind,* eds. R. Allan and S. Scheidt (Washington, D.C.: American Psychological Association, 1996), pp. 179–196.

14. L. H. Powell, "The Hook: A Metaphor for Gaining Control of Emotional Reactivity," in *Heart and Mind,* eds. R. Allan and S. Scheidt (Washington, D.C.: American Psychological Association, 1996), pp. 313–328.

15. A. Bandura, *Social Foundations of Thought and Action: A Social-Cognitive Theory* (Englewood Cliffs, New Jersey: Prentice-Hall, 1986).

16. B. F. Skinner, *Beyond Freedom and Dignity* (New York: Bantam Books, 1971), p. 211.

17. H. Tennen and G. Affleck, "Blaming Others for Threatening Events," *Psychological Bulletin* Vol. 108 (1990): pp. 209–232.

18. F. Kafka, *The Trial* (New York: Schocken Books, 1974), pp. 213–215. This reference and a discussion of the comparison between the often less spiritually and intellectually demanding writings of "self-help books" and the more substantial, challenging work are presented in a wonderfully insightful book by Wendy Kaminer, *I'm Dysfunctional–You're Dysfunctional* (New York: Addison-Wesley, 1992).

19. E. M. Ozer and A. Bandura, "Mechanisms Governing Empowerment Effects: A Self-Efficacy Analysis," *Journal of Personality and Social Psychology* Vol. 58 (1990): pp. 472–486.

20. A. Bandura, *Social Foundations of Thought and Action.*

21. L. Berkowitz, "Frustration-Aggression Hypothesis: Examination and Reformation," *Psychological Bulletin* Vol. 106 (1989): pp. 59–73.

22. For a discussion of the limits of the usual risk factors, such as smoking and obesity, in predicting who will develop heart disease, see S. L. Syme, "Social Support and Risk Reduction," *Mobius* Vol. 4 (1984): pp. 44–54.

23. R. Mulcahy, L. Daley, I. Graham, and N. Hickey, "Level of Education, Coronary Risk Factors, and Cardiovascular Disease," *Irish Medical Journal* Vol. 77 (1984): pp. 316–318.

Chapter 2: UNRAVELING THE MYSTERY OF THE FIFTH FORCE

1. For an exploration of the "energy-information" relationship, see B. Rubik, "The Unifying Concept of Information in Energy Medicine," *Alternative Therapies in Health and Medicine* Vol. 1 (1995): pp. 34–39.

2. For an easy-to-understand review of energy, force, and fields as applied to biological systems, see J. G. Miller, *Living Systems* (New York: McGraw-Hill, 1978).

3. S. B. Nuland, *The Wisdom of the Body* (New York: Alfred A. Knopf, 1997), p. 123–124.

4. *Ibid.,* p. 123.

5. J. Hillman, *The Soul's Code* (New York: Random House, 1996).

6. E. B. Tylor, *Primitive Culture, Vol. I* (London, 1871), p. 387.

7. *Webster's Third New International Dictionary* (Springfield, Massachusetts: Merriam-Webster, 1993) p. 2176.

8. J. Motz, "Everyone an Energy Healer: The TREAT V Conference in Santa Fe." *Advances* Vol. 9 (1993): pp. 95–98.

9. R. C. Byrd, "Positive Therapeutic Effects of Intercessory Prayer in a Coronary Care Unit Population," *Southern Medical Journal* Vol. 81 (1988): pp. 826–829.

10. J. Motz, "Everyone an Energy Healer," p. 98.

11. R. G. Jahn and B. J. Dunne, "Science of the Subjective," *Technical Notes* (New Jersey: Princeton University, March 1997).

12. R. G. Jahn, "Information, Consciousness, and Health," *Alternative Therapies* Vol. 2 (1996): p. 34.

13. R. G. Jahn and B. J. Dunne, *Margins of Reality: The Role of Consciousness in the Physical World* (New York: Harcourt Brace Jovanovich, 1987).

14. A. L. Lettiere, "Toward a Philosophy of Science in Women's Health Research," *Journal of Scientific Exploration* Vol. 10 (1996): p. 539.

15. E. H. Hess, *The Tell-Tale Eye* (New York: Van Nostrand Reinhold, 1975).

16. J. J. Woodmansee, "The Pupil Response as a Measure of Social Attitudes," in *Attitude Measurement,* ed. G. F. Summers (Chicago: Rand-McNally, 1970).

17. M. Ullman and L. Krasner, *Dream Telepathy* (New York: Macmillan, 1973).

18. K. M. Hearne, "A Nationwide Mass Dream-Telepathy Experiment," *Journal of the Society for Psychical Research* Vol. 55 (1989): pp. 271–274.

19. R. Gerber, *Vibrational Medicine* (Sante Fe, New Mexico: Bear Company, 1988), p. 44.

20. J. Biggs and F. Peat, "David Bohm's Looking-Glass Map," in *Looking-Glass Universe: The Emerging Science of Wholeness,* eds. J. Biggs and F. Peat (New York: Simon and Schuster), 1984.

21. T. Moss, "Puzzles and Promises," *Osteopathic Physician* Vol. 4 (February 1976): pp. 30–37.

22. T. Moss, *The Body Electric* (Los Angeles: Jeremy P. Tarcher, 1979), p. 219.

23. B. Grad, "Some Biological Effects of Laying On of Hands and Their Implications," in *Dimensions in Holistic Healing: New Frontiers in the Treatment*

of the Whole Person, eds. B. Otton and R. Knight (Chicago: Nelson Hall, 1979), pp. 199–212.

24. For an excellent discussion of "vital subtle energy" and a summary of its characteristics, many of which I include in my list of the characteristics of "L" energy, see J. White, *The Meeting of Science and Spirit* (New York: Paragon House, 1990), pp. 70–75.

25. J. Clarke, "SQUIDS," *Scientific American* (August 1994): pp. 46–53.

26. Researcher Lawrence Beynam examined the nature of what I am calling "L" energy and he called "X" energy. Results of his work and a description of some possible primary characteristics of "L" energy presented here are based on his work and the work and theories of other scientists as summarized in J. White, *The Meeting of Science and Spirit,* pp. 73–74.

27. J. Eisenbud, *Parapsychology and the Unconscious* (Berkeley, California: North Atlantic Books, 1984), p. 100.

28. H. Motoyama, *Theories of the Chakras* (Wheaton, Illinois: Theosophical Publishing House, 1981).

29. S. Karagulla, *Breakthrough to Creativity* (Marina Del Rey, California: De Vorss, 1967), p. 39.

30. M. Ficino, *Commentary on Plato's Symposium on Love,* translated by Jane Sears (Dallas: Spring Publications, 1985).

31. J. Motz, "What Energy 'Knows,' " *Advances* Vol. 12 (1996): p. 33.

Chapter 3: THE CHANGING PORTRAIT OF THE HEART

1. L. Watson, *Lifetide: The Biology of Consciousness* (New York: Simon and Schuster, 1980).

2. Plato, *The Collected Deluges,* eds. E. Hamilton and H. Cairns, Bollinger Series Number LXXI (New York: Pantheon Books, 1961).

3. J. C. Pearce, *Evolution's End: Claiming the Potential of Our Intelligence* (New York: Harper San Francisco, 1992), p. 104–105.

4. The field of energy cardiology owes its theoretical and research origins to the creativity of Dr. Linda G. Russek and Dr. Gary E. Schwartz. For a pioneering description of energy cardiology and the measurement of the energy of the heart, see Linda G. Russek and Gary E. Schwartz, "Energy Cardiology: A Dynamical Energy Systems Approach for Integrating Conventional and Alternative Medicine," *Advances* Vol. 12 (1996): pp. 4–24.

5. J. S. Wilentz, *The Senses of Man* (New York: Thomas Crowell, 1968), p. 10.

6. For an excellent description of the physical power of the heart, see C. Hocrine, *Nutrition Plan for High Blood Pressure* (San Francisco: Jove Publications, 1977).

7. *Ibid.*

8. D. Ackerman, *The Natural History of the Senses* (New York: Random House, 1990): pp. 178–179.

9. M. Wentzel, "Voices of Their Ancestors," *Sheraton's Hawai'i* (Summer 1997), p. 70.

10. J. Bernard and L. Sontag, "Fetal Reactions to Sound," *Journal of Genetic Psychology* Vol. 70 (1947): pp. 209–210.

11. J. C. Pearce, *Evolution's End,* p. 106.

12. *Ibid.,* p. 103.

13. *Ibid.,* pp. 103–104.

14. J. Lacey and B. Lacey, "Conversations Between Heart and Brain," *Bulletin of the National Institute of Mental Health,* Rockville, Maryland (March 1987).

15. C. B. Clayman, ed., *The American Medical Association Encyclopedia of Medicine* (New York: Random House, 1989): pp. 142–143.

16. M. Cantin and J. Genest, "The Heart as an Endocrine Gland," *Scientific American* Vol. 254 (1986): p. 76.

17. J. Kabat-Zinn, *Full Catastrophe Living* (New York: Delta, 1990), p. 47.

18. J. Fisher, "Is There a Need for Cardiac Psychology? The View of a Practicing Cardiologist," in *Heart and Mind: The Practice of Cardiac Psychology,* eds. R. Allan and S. Scheidt (Washington, D.C.: American Psychological Association, 1996). The first text in this field is by R. Allan and S. Scheidt, *Heart and Mind* (Washington, D.C.: American Psychological Association, 1996).

19. M. B. Straus, *Familiar Medical Quotations* (Boston: Little, Brown, 1968), p. 38.

20. W. Harvey, *Anatomical Studies on the Motion of the Heart and Blood,* translated by C. D. Leake (Springfield, Illinois: Charles C. Thomas, 1928). (Originally published in 1628.)

21. W. Osler, *Lectures on Angina Pectoris and Allied States* (New York: Appleton-Century-Crofts, 1897), p. 154.

22. Osler, W., "The Lumelian Lectures in Angina Pectoris," *Lancet* (1910): p. 839.

23. M. Friedman and R. H. Rosenman, "Association of Specific Overt Behavior Pattern with Blood and Cardiovascular Findings: Blood Cholesterol Level, Blood Clotting Time, Incidence of Arcus Senilis, and Clinical Coronary Artery Disease," *Journal of the American Medical Association* Vol. 169 (1959): pp. 1286–1296.

24. G. Burell et al., "Modification of Type A Behavior Patterns in Post-Myocardial Infarction Patients: A Route to Cardiac Rehabilitation," *International Journal of Behavioral Medicine* Vol. 1 (1994): pp. 32–54.

25. R. Allan, "Introduction: The Emergence of Cardiac Psychology," in *Heart and Mind,* eds. R. Allan and S. Scheidt.

26. D. M. Ornish et al., "Can Lifestyle Change Reverse Coronary Heart Disease? The Lifestyle Heart Trial," *Lancet* Vol. 336 (1990), pp. 129–133.

27. L. G. Russek and G. E. Schwartz, *Energy Cardiology,* p. 4.

28. P. A. Ragan, W. Wang, and S. R. Eisenberg, "Magnetically Induced Currents in the Canine Heart: A Finite Element Study," *IEEE Transactions on Biomedical Engineering* Vol. 42, (1995): pp. 110–115.

29. R. O. Becker and G. Selden, *The Body Electric* (New York: Morrow, 1985). See also R. O. Becker, *Cross Currents* (Los Angeles: Jeremy P. Tarcher, 1990).

30. J. G. Miller, *Living Systems* (New York: McGraw-Hill, 1978).

31. S. Paddison, *The Hidden Power of the Heart* (Boulder Creek, California: Planetary Publications, 1992).

32. J. Malmivuo and R. Plonsey, *Bioelectromagnetics* (New York: Oxford University Press, 1995).

33. W. A. Tiller, R. McCraty, and M. Atkinson, "Cardiac Coherence: A New, Noninvasive Measure of Autonomic Nervous System Disorder," *Alternative Therapies* Vol. 2 (1996): pp. 52–65.

34. R. McCraty, M. Atkinson, W. A. Tiller, "New Electrophysiological Correlates Associated with Intentional Heart Focus," *Subtle Energies* Vol. 4 (1995): pp. 251–268.

35. W. Brugh Joy, *Joy's Way* (Los Angeles: Jeremy P. Tarcher, 1978).

36. The clearest description of how systems combine to create memories is in G. E. Schwartz and L. G. Russek, "Do All Dynamic Systems Have Memory? Implications of the Systemic Memory Hypothesis for Science and Society," in *Brain and Values: Behavioral Neurodynamics V,* eds. K. H. Y. Pribram and J. S. King (Hillsdale, New Jersey: Lawrence Erlbaum Associates. 1996).

Chapter 4: RECEIVING THE MOST PRECIOUS GIFT

1. S. B. Nuland, *The Wisdom of the Body* (New York: Alfred A. Knopf, 1997), pp. 220–222.

2. *Ibid.,* pp. 245–246.

3. *Ibid.,* p. 246.

4. An experienced research physicist and director of the Institute for Advanced Studies at Austin, Texas, H. E. Puthoff supports further research and theoretical development of the field of energy cardiology. See his "Technological Problems, Bold Possibilities," *Advances* Vol. 12 (1996): pp. 35–36.

5. W. F. Kuhn, B. Myers, A. F. Brennan, et al., "Psychopathology in Heart Transplant Candidates," *Journal of Heart Transplant* Vol. 7 (1988): pp. 223–226.

6. W. James, *Psychology: Briefer Course* (New York: Holt, 1890).

7. B. Bunzel et al., "Does Changing the Heart Mean Changing Personality? A Retrospective Inquiry on 47 Heart Transplant Patients," *Quality of Life Research* Vol. 1 (1992): pp. 251–256.

8. L. A. Kraft, "Psychiatric Complications of Cardiac Transplantation," *Seminars in Psychiatry* Vol. 3 (1971): pp. 89–97.

9. J. B. Rauch and K. K. Kneen, "Accepting the Gift of Life: Heart Transplant Recipients' Post-Operative Adaptive Tasks," *Social Work Health Care* Vol. 14 (1989): pp. 47–59.

10. R. I. Frieson and S. B. Lippman, "Heart Transplant Patients Rejected on Psychiatric Indications," *Psychosomatics* Vol. 28 (1987): pp. 347–355.

11. B. Bunzel, "Does Changing the Heart Mean Changing the Personality?" pp. 251–256.

12. T. P. Hackett and N. Cassem, "Development of a Qualitative Rating Scale to Assess Denial," *Journal of Psychosomatic Research* Vol. 18 (1974): pp. 93–100.

13. F. M. Mai, "Graft and Donor Denial in Heart Transplant Recipients," *American Journal of Psychiatry* Vol. 143 (1986): pp. 1159–1161.

14. N. Haan, *Coping and Defending—Processes of Self-Environment Organization* (New York: Academic Press, 1977).

15. B. D. Colen, "Organ Concert," *Time* (Fall 1996): pp. 71–74.

16. *Ibid.,* p. 71.

17. P. Castelnuovo-Tedesco, "Cardiac Surgeons Look at Transplantation—Interviews with Drs. Cleveland, Cooley, DeBakey, Hallman, and Rochelle," *Seminars in Psychiatry* Vol. 3 (1971): pp. 5–16.

18. *Ibid.,* p. 6.

19. E. R. Hilgard, *Divided Consciousness: Multiple Controls in Human Thought and Action* (New York: Wiley, 1977).

20. C. Gilligan, *In a Different Voice: Psychological Theory and Women's Development* (Cambridge, Massachusetts: Harvard University Press, 1982).

21. C. Gilligan and J. Attanucci, "Two Moral Orientations," in *Mapping the Moral Domain: A Contribution of Women's Thinking to Psychological Theory and Education,* eds. C. Gilligan, J. V. Ward, and J. M. Taylor (Cambridge, Massachusetts: Harvard University Press, 1988).

22. J. Piaget, *The Origins of Intelligence in Children* (New York: International Universities Press, 1952).

23. H. Gardner, *Frames of Intelligence: The Theory of Multiple Intelligences,* 2nd ed. (New York: Basic Books, 1993).

24. S. J. Lynn and J. W. Rhue, "The Fantasy-Prone Person: Hypnosis, Imagination and Creativity," *Journal of Personality and Social Psychology* Vol. 51 (1986): pp. 404–408.

Chapter 5: CELLULAR MEMORIES ARE MADE OF THIS

1. I have referred to the writings of Dr. S. B. Nuland throughout this book. He presents a brilliant description of the energy of the body from a mechanistic point of view. See his *The Wisdom of the Body* (New York: Alfred A. Knopf, 1997), p. 122.

2. S. Ohno and M. Ohno, "The All-Pervasive Principle of Repetitious Recurrence Governs Not Only During Sequence Sontrionic but Also Human Endeavor in Musical Composition," *Immunogenetics* Vol. 24 (1986): pp. 71–78.

3. S. Ohno and M. Jabara, "Repeats of Base Oligomers (N = 3n + − 1 or 2) as Immortal Coding Sequences of the Primeval World: Construction of Coding Sequences Is Based upon the Principle of Musical Composition," *Chemical Scripta* 26B (1986): pp. 43–49.

4. For an entertaining description of the workings within the human and other bodies, see J. Treffil, *Sharks Have No Bones* (New York: Simon and Schuster, 1992).

5. S. R. Hameroff and R. Penrose, "Orchestrated Reduction of Quantum Coherence in Brain Microtubules: A Model for Consciousness," in *Toward a Science of Consciousness: The First Tuscon Discussions and Debates,* eds. S. R. Hameroff, A. Kaszaniak, and A. C. Scott (Cambridge, Massachusetts: MIT Press, 1996).

6. B. Horrigan, "Stuart Hameroff: Consciousness and Microtubules in a Quantum World," *Alternative Therapies* Vol. 3 (1997): p. 72.

7. *Ibid.,* p. 70.

8. For a discussion of our accelerating switch from a sense of the eternal to the computer-based sense of time measured in one-billionth of a second, see J. Rifkin, *Time Wars* (New York: Henry Holt, 1987).

9. R. Heinberg, *Memories and Visions of Paradise* (Los Angeles: Jeremy P. Tarcher, 1989), p. 195.

10. As quoted in T. Moore, *The Re-Enchantment of Everyday Life* (New York: HarperCollins, 1996): p. 229.

11. R. Cooke, "Cell Transplants Can Alter Behavior," *The Detroit News,* March 10, 1997, p. E 1.

12. B. D. Colen, "Organ Concert," *Time* (Fall 1996), pp. 70–74.

13. R. Cooke, "Cell Transplants," p. E 1.

14. G. E. Schwartz and L. G. Russek, "Do All Dynamic System Have Memory? Implications of the Systemic Memory Hypothesis for Science and Society," in *Brain and Values: Behavioral Neurodynamics V,* eds. K. H. Pribram and J. S. King (Hillsdale, New Jersey: Lawrence Erlbaum Associates, 1996).

15. A. Tomatis, "Chant, the Healing Power of Voice and Air," in *Music, Physician for Times to Come,* ed. D. Campbell (Wheaton, Illinois: Quest Publishers, 1991).

16. R. Axel, "The Molecular Logic of Smell," *Scientific American* Vol. 273 (1995): pp. 154–159.

17. J. Martin and M. T. Jessell, "The Sensory System," in *Essentials of Neural Science and Behavior,* eds. E. R. Kandel, J. H. Schwartz, and T. M. Jessell (Norwalk, Connecticut: Appleton and Lange, 1995).

18. R. C. Atkinson and R. M. Shiffrin, "Human Memory: A Proposed System and Its Control Processes," in *The Psychology of Learning and Motivation: Advances in Research and Theory, Vol. 2,* ed. K. W. Spence, (New York: Academic Press, 1968), pp. 89–195.

19. R. A. Baron, *Psychology,* 2nd ed. (Boston: Allyn and Bacon, 1992), p. 211.

20. R. C. Atkinson and R. M. Shiffrin, "Human Memory" pp. 16–37.

21. E. Poppel, "Oscillations as Possible Basis for Time Perception," in *The Study of Time: Proceedings of the First Conference on the International Society for the Study of Time,* Oberwolfach, West Germany, eds. J. T. Fraser et al. (New York: Springer-Verlag, 1969).

22. This numerical limit was described in a classic paper by psychologist George Miller, "The Magical Number Seven, Plus or Minus Two: Some Limits on Our Capacity for Processing Information," *Psychological Review* Vol. 101 (1986): pp. 343–352.

23. R. A. Brown and J. Kulik, "Flashbulb Memories," *Cognition* Vol. 5 (1977): pp. 73–99.

24. F. Heuer and D. Reisberg, "Vivid Memories of Emotional Events: The Accuracy of Remembered Minutiae," *Memory and Cognition* Vol. 18 (1990): pp. 496–506.

25. H. L. Roediger and K. B. McDermott, "Creating False Memories: Remembering Words Not Presented in Lists," *Journal of Experimental Psychology: Learning, Memory, and Cognition* Vol. 21 (1995): pp. 803–814.

26. G. R. Marek, *Toscanini* (London: Vision Press, 1975).

27. L. G. Russek and G. E. Schwartz, "Energy Cardiology: A Dynamical Energy Systems Approach for Integrating Conventional and Alternative Medicine," *Advances* Vol. 12 (1996): pp. 4–24.

28. C. Siebert, "Carol Palumbo Waits for Her Heart," *New York Times Magazine,* April 13, 1997, p. 81.

29. *Ibid.*

30. J. L. Swerdlow, "Quiet Miracles of the Mind," *National Geographic* Vol. 187 (1995): pp. 2–41.

31. For example, see R. McCraty, M. Atkinson, and W. A. Tiller, "New Electrophysiological Correlates Associated with Intentional Heart Focus," *Subtle Energies* Vol. 4 (1995): pp. 251–268.

32. R. Sheldrake, *The Presence of the Past* (New York: Random House, 1981).

33. L. Dossey, "What's Love Got to Do With It?" *Advances* Vol. 2 (1996): pp. 8–15.

Chapter 6: THE TEMPERAMENTAL HEART

1. Domino transplantation is still rare. A similar occurrence to the one I have reported here is described by a London, England, newspaper reporter, Daniel Jeffreys. He reported that a heart and a heart-lung transplant patient ran a race against each other in the transplant olympics and that the heart-lung recipient lost to the man who now had his heart. The two men who had shared the same heart discussed their new food cravings; the heart recipient reported that he had the same food cravings as his donor had. See "Have These Transplant Patients Inherited the Donor's Character?" *London Daily Mail,* June 4, 1996, p. 51.

2. R. A. Baron, *Psychology,* 2nd ed. (Needham Heights, Massachusetts, 1992): p. 307.

3. A. Thomas, S. Chess, H. G. Birch, "The Origins of Personality," *Scientific American* Vol. 223 (1970): pp. 102–109.

4. *Ibid.,* p. 104.

5. A. Thomas and S. Chess, *Temperament and Development* (New York: Brunner/Mazel, 1977).

6. D. D. Jackson, "Reunion of Identical Twins, Raised Apart, Reveals Some Astonishing Similarities," *Smithsonian* (October 1980): pp. 48–56.

7. For elaboration of the issues and implications of nonlocal consciousness connection as manifested between identical twins, see L. Dossey, "Lessons from Twins: Of Nature, Nurture, and Consciousness," *Alternative Therapies* Vol. 3 (1997): pp. 8–15.

8. For a discussion of the myths regarding twins in virtually every culture, see H. Teich, "Sun and Moon," *Parabola* Vol. 19 (1994): pp. 55–58.

9. C. Holden, "Identical Twins Reared Apart," *Science* Vol. 207 (1980): pp. 1323–1328.

10. L. G. Russek and G. E. Schwartz, "Energy Cardiology: A Dynamical Energy System Approach for Integrating Conventional and Alternative Medicine," *Advances* Vol. 12 (1996): p. 9.

11. J. Motz, "What Energy 'Knows,' " *Advances* Vol. 12 (1996): p. 34.

12. *Ibid.*

13. J. Kagan, *Galen's Prophecy* (New York: HarperCollins, 1994).

14. K. A. Matthews et al., "Are Cardiovascular Responses to Behavioral Stressors a Stable Individual Difference Variable in Childhood?" *Psychophysiology* Vol. 24 (1987): pp. 464–473. See also J. R. Turner, "Individual Difference in Heart Rate Response During Behavioral Challenge," *Psychophysiology* Vol. 26 (1989): pp. 497–505.

15. J. Kagan, *Galen's Prophecy,* p. 50.

16. R. S. Eliot and D. Breo, *Is It Worth Dying For?* (Toronto and New York: Bantam, 1984).

17. M. Friedman, N. Fleisschmann, and V. A. Price, "Diagnosis of Type A Behavior Pattern," in *Heart and Mind,* eds. R. Allan and S. Scheidt (Washington, D.C.: American Psychological Association 1996), pp 179–195.

18. R. Williams and V. Williams, *Anger Kills* (New York: HarperPerennial, 1993).

19. R. Williams, *The Trusting Heart: Great News About Type A Behavior* (New York: Times Books, 1989).

20. M. Friedman et al., "Diagnosis of Type A Behavior Pattern."

21. J. J. Lynch, *The Broken Heart: The Medical Consequences of a Broken Heart* (New York: Basic Books, 1979).

22. S. R. Bard, "Healing the Heart: An Interview with Dean Ornish, M.D.," *Noetic Sciences Review* Vol. 20 (1991): pp. 5–13.

23. B. Rubik, "Energy Medicine and the Unifying Concept of Information," *Alternative Therapies* Vol. 1 (1995): p. 35.

24. L. G. Russek and G. E. Schwartz, "Narrative Descriptions of Parental Love and Caring Predict Health Status in Midlife: A 35-Year Follow-Up of the Harvard Mastery of Stress Study," *Alternative Therapies* Vol. 2 (1996): pp. 55–62.

25. M. Csikszentmihalyi, *The Evolving Self* (New York: HarperCollins, 1993).

26. D. Jameson and L. Hurvic, "Essay Concerning Color Constancy," *Annual Review of Psychology* Vol. 40 (1989): pp. 55–73.

27. R. L. Solomon, "The Opponent Process in Acquired Motivation," in *The Physiological Mechanisms of Motivation,* ed. D. W. Pfaff (New York: Springer-Verlag, 1982).

28. W. Tiller, R. McCraty, and M. Atkinson, "Cardiac Coherence: A New, Noninvasive Measure of Autonomic Nervous System Order," *Alternative Therapies* Vol. 2 (1996): pp. 52–65.

Chapter 7: MAKING CONTACT WITH YOUR HEART

1. R. G. Jahn, "Information, Consciousness, and Health," *Alternative Therapies* Vol. 2 (1996): pp. 32–38.

2. This concept is described in J. T. Fraser, *Time: The Familiar Stranger* (Redmond, Washington: Tempus Books of Microsoft Press, 1987).

3. R. Gerber, *Vibrational Medicine* (Santa Fe, New Mexico: Bear and Company, 1988).

4. D. H. Hockenbury and S. E. Hockenbury, *Psychology* (New York: Worth Publishers, 1997).

5. For a current review of meditation, see M. Schlitz and N. Lewis, "Meditation East and West," *Noetic Sciences Review* Vol. 42 (1997): pp. 34–38. For a source that lists 1,253 references regarding meditation, see *The Physical and Psychological Effects of Meditation,* eds. M. Murphy and S. Donovan (Sausalito, California: Institute of Noetic Sciences, 1997).

6. A. M. West, "Traditional and Psychological Perspectives on Meditation," in *The Psychology of Meditation,* ed. M. A. West (New York: Oxford University Press, 1987).

7. C. T. Tart, *Living the Mindful Life: A Handbook for Living in the Present Moment* (Boston: Shambhala, 1994).

8. A. Deikman, "Deautomatization and the Mystic Experience," *Psychiatry* Vol. 29 (1966): pp. 329–343.

9. P. A. Norris, "Clinical Psychoneuroimmunology," in *Biofeedback: Principles and Practice for Clinicians,* ed. K. J. V. Basmahjian (Baltimore: Williams and Wilkins, 1988).

10. H. Benson, *Beyond the Relaxation Response* (New York: Times Books, 1984).

11. S. Holst, *Prose for Dancing* (Barrytown, New York: Station Hill Press, 1983).

12. S. Rechtschaffen, *Timeshifting* (New York: Doubleday, 1996).

13. M. Csikszentmihalyi, *Flow: The Psychology of Optimal Experience* (New York: Harper and Row, 1990).

14. As quoted in S. Rechtschaffen, "Shifting Time: How to Pace Your Life to Natural Rhythms," *Noetic Sciences Review* Vol. 42 (1997): p. 19.

15. A. D. Watkins, "Intention and Electromagnetic Activity of the Heart," *Advances* Vol. 12 (1996): pp. 35–36.

16. A. D. Watkins, "Letter to the Editor," *Advances* Vol. 13 (1997): p. 3.

17. Author Daniel Goleman suggests that awareness of one's own emotional state is a key factor in "emotional intelligence" in his book *Emotional Intelligence* (New York: Bantam Books, 1995), p. 46.

18. W. A. Tiller, R. McCraty, and M. Atkinson, "Cardiac Coherence: A New, Noninvasive Measure of Autonomic Nervous System Disorder," *Alternative Therapies* Vol. 2 (1996): pp. 52–65.

19. D. L. Childre, *Freeze Frame: Fast Action Stress Relief* (Boulder Creek, California: Planetary Publications, 1994), p. 132.

20. G. Rein and R. McCraty. "Long-Term Effects of Compassion on Salivary IgA," *Psychosomatic Medicine* Vol. 56 (1994): pp. 171–172.

21. D. L. Childre, *Freeze Frame,* p. 132.

22. S. Rechtschaffen, "Shifting Time: How to Pace Your Life to Natural Rhythms." *Noetic Sciences Review* Vol. 42 (1997): p. 18.

23. Dr. Robert Gerzon differentiates between what he calls "toxic, natural, and scared" anxiety and suggests that, instead of trying to reduce anxiety, which is essentially a brain-oriented function, that we try to transform it into an awareness of the vital power of life. See his *Finding Serenity in the Age of Anxiety* (New York: Macmillan, 1997).

24. R. McCraty et al., "The Effects of Emotions on Short-Term Heart Rate Variability Using Power Spectrum Analysis," *American Journal of Cardiology* Vol. 76 (1995): pp. 1089–1093.

25. G. Rein, R. M. McCraty, and M. Atkinson, "Effects of Positive and Negative Emotions on Salivary IgA," *Journal of Advanced Medicine* Vol. 8 (1995): pp. 87–105.

26. J. Achterberg, *Imagery in Healing* (Boston: Shambhala, 1985).

27. R. McCraty, *Stress Medicine* (In press, 1997).

28. L. Dossey, *Prayer Is Good Medicine* (New York: HarperCollins, 1996), p. 83.

Chapter 8: MAKING CONTACT WITH OTHER HEARTS

1. J. Polkinghorne, "Can a Scientist Pray?" *Explorations in Science and Theology* (London: The Royal Society for the Encouragement of Arts, Manufactures, and Commerce, 1993), pp. 17–22.

2. W. T. C. Boyce, C. Schaefer, and C. Uitti, "Permanence and Change: Psychosocial Factors in the Outcome of Adolescent Pregnancy," *Social Science and Medicine* Vol. 21 (1985): p. 1281.

3. A. Antonovsky, *Unraveling the Mystery of Health: How People Manage Stress and Stay Well* (San Francisco: Jossey-Bass, 1987).

4. E. W. Jensen, "The Families' Routine Inventory," *Social Science and Medicine* Vol. 7 (1983): pp. 210–211.

5. "Eating with Teens Linked to How Well They Adjust," *Maui News,* August 17, 1997, p. A6.

6. L. G. Russek and G. E. Schwartz, "Energy Cardiology: A Dynamical Energy Systems Approach for Integrating Conventional and Alternative Medicine," *Advances* Vol. 12. (1996): pp. 4–24.

7. R. McCraty and A. Watkins, *Autonomic Assessment Report Interpretation Guide* (Boulder Creek, California: Institute of HeartMath, 1996).

8. L. G. Russek and G. E. Schwartz, "Energy, Information, and the Essence of Integrated Medicine," *Advances* Vol. 13 (1997): pp. 74–77.

9. I described the psychological implications of the quantum physics "wave-particle" duality theory in my *Making Miracles* (New York: Avon Books, 1991), pp. 100–101.

10. J. Malmivuo and R. Plonsey, *Bioelectromagnetics* (New York: Oxford University Press, 1995).

11. R. T. Wakai, M. Wang, and C. B. Martin, "Spatio-Temporal Properties of

the Fetal Magnetocardiogram," *American Journal of Obstetrics and Gynecology* (March 1994): pp. 770–776.

12. The concept of nonlocality is explained clearly by physician Larry Dossey in his *Healing Words: The Power of Prayer and the Practice of Medicine* (San Francisco: Harper San Francisco, 1993).

13. E. E. Green et al., "Anomalous Electrostatic Phenomena in Exceptional Subjects," *Subtle Energies* Vol. 12 (1996): pp. 69–94.

14. K. Woodward et al., "Talking to God," *Newsweek,* January 6, 1992, pp. 38–44.

15. *Ibid.,* p. 44.

16. S. Paddison, *The Hidden Power of the Heart* (Boulder Creek, California: Planetary Publications, 1992), p. 9.

17. Ibid., p. 250.

18. L. G. Russek and G. E. Schwartz, "Energy, Information," pp. 15–21.

19. Similar measurement approaches have been used for years by psychophysiologists. They often refer to their techniques as "Event-Related Potentials." See M. G. H. Coles, G. Gratton, and M. Fabini, "Event-Related Brain Potentials," in *Principles of Psychophysiology: Physical, Social, and Inferential Elements,* eds. J. T. Cacioppo and L. G. Tassinary (New York: Cambridge University Press, 1990).

20. L. G. Russek and G. E. Schwartz, "Interpersonal Heart-Brain Registration and the Perception of Parental Love: A 42-Year Follow-Up of the Harvard Mastery of Stress Study," *Subtle Energies* Vol. 5 (1994) pp. 195–208.

21. F. Hartmann, *Paracelsus: Life and Prophecies* (Blauvelt, New York: Teiner Books, 1973), p. 133.

22. B. E. Schwartz, "Possible Telesomatic Reactions," *Journal of the Medical Society of New Jersey* Vol. 64 (1973): pp. 600–603.

23. L. E. Rhine, "Psychological Processing in ESP Experiments, Part I: Waking Experiences," *Journal of Parapsychology* Vol. 29 (1962): pp. 88–111.

24. A. Eliot, "The Hermit's Message," *Noetics Sciences Review* Vol. 42 (1997): pp. 29–33. See also S. Hameroff, A. Kaszniak, and A. Scott, *Toward a Science of Consciousness: The First Tucson Discussions and Debates* (Cambridge, Massachusetts: MIT Press, 1996).

25. G. Rhine, "A Psychokinetic Effect on Neurotransmitter Metabolism: Alterations in the Degradative Enzyme Monoamine Oxidase," in *Research in Parapsychology,* eds. D. H. Weiner and D. Radin (Metuchen, New Jersey: Scarecrow Press, 1985), pp. 77–80.

26. W. Braud, "Distant Mental Influence on Rate of Hemolysis of Human Red Blood Cells," *Journal of the American Society for Psychical Research* Vol. 84 (1990): pp. 1–24.

27. W. Braud and W. Schlitz, "Methodology for the Objective Study of Transpersonal Imagery," *Journal of Scientific Exploration* Vol. 3 (1989): pp. 43–63.

28. R. Byrd, "Positive Therapeutic Effects of Intercessory Prayer in a Coronary Care Unit Population," *Southern Medical Journal* Vol. 81 (1988): pp. 826–829.

29. R. Peoch, "Psychokinetic Action of Young Chicks on the Path of an Illuminated Source," *Journal of Scientific Exploration* Vol. 9 (1995): pp. 223–229.

30. J. B. Rhine and S. R. Feather. "The Study of Cases of 'Psi-Training' in Animals," *Journal of Parapsychology* Vol. 1 (1962): pp. 1–21.

31. S. Paddison, *The Hidden Power of the Heart,* p. 7.

32. *Ibid.,* p. 97.

33. *Ibid.,* p. 97.

34. As quoted in T. Moore, *The Re-Enchantment of Everyday Life* (New York: HarperCollins, 1996), p. 3.

Chapter 9: THE LUSTFUL BRAIN AND THE LOVING HEART

1. Dr. Robert G. Jahn raises this issue of "object-subjective" information and its measurement in his "Information, Consciousness, and Health," *Alternative Therapies* Vol. 2 (1996): pp. 32–38.

2. L. Laskow, *Healing with Love: The Art of Holoenergetic Healing* (New York: HarperCollins, 1992).

3. M. Fox, *A Spirituality Named Compassion* (San Francisco: Harper and Row, 1979).

4. L. G. Russek and G. E. Schwartz, "Interpersonal Heart-Brain Registration and the Perception of Parental Love: A 42-Year Follow-Up of the Harvard Mastery of Stress Study," *Subtle Energies* Vol. 5 (1996): pp. 36–45.

5. P. A. Ragan, W. Wang, and S. R. Eisenberg, "Magnetically Induced Currents in the Canine Heart: A Finite Element Study," *IEEE Transactions on Biomedical Engineering* Vol. 42 (1995): pp. 110–115. See also G. Stroink, "Principles of Cardiomagneticism," in *Advances in Biomagnetism,* eds. S. J. Williamson et al. (New York: Plenum Press, 1989): pp. 47–57.

6. C. Bernard, *An Introduction to the Study of Experimental Medicine* (New York: Macmillan, 1927).

7. L. G. Russek and G. E. Schwartz, "Interpersonal Heart-Brain registration."

8. *Webster's Third New International Dictionary* (Springfield, Massachusetts: Merriam Webster, 1993).

9. J. Motz, "What Energy 'Knows,' " *Advances* Vol. 12 (1996): pp. 33–35.

10. R. F. DeBusk, "Sexual Activity Triggering Myocardial Infarction: One Less Thing to Worry About," *Journal of the American Medical Association* Vol. 275 (1996): pp. 1447–1448.

11. J. E. Muller, M. A. Mittleman, M. Maclure, et al., "Triggering Myocardial Infarction by Sexual Activity: Low Absolute Risk and Prevention by Regular Physical Exertion?" *Journal of the American Medical Association* Vol. 275 (1996): pp. 1405–1409. See also D. Sobel and R. Ornstein, "Sexual Activity and Heart Attack: Not to Worry," *Mind/Body Health Newsletter* Vol. 5 (1996): pp. 2–3.

12. For a summary of data supporting this finding and other research that calls into question the justification for our modern health terrorism, see R. Ornstein and D. Sobel, *Healthy Pleasures* (Reading, Massachusetts: Addison-Wesley, 1993).

13. My book *The Pleasure Prescription: To Love, To Work, To Play—Life in the*

Balance discusses this issue in detail. (Alameda, California: Hunter House Publishers, 1996.)

14. J. Gottman, *Why Marriages Succeed or Fail . . . and How You Can Make Yours Last* (New York: Simon and Schuster, 1994).

15. J. Gottman, *What Predicts Divorce: The Relationship Between Marital Processes and Marital Outcomes* (Hillsdale, New Jersey: Lawrence Erlbaum Associates, 1993).

16. D. Goleman, *Emotional Intelligence* (New York: Bantam Books, 1995).

17. J. Gottman, *What Predicts Divorce.*

18. J. Malmivuo and R. Plonsey, *Bioelectromagnetics* (New York: Oxford University Press, 1995).

19. H. E. Fisher, *Anatomy of Love: The Natural History of Monogamy, Adultery, and Divorce* (New York: W. W. Norton, 1992).

20. As described in Goleman, *Emotional Intelligence,* p. 7.

21. R. F. Bornstein, "Exposure and Affect: Overview and Meta-Analysis of Research," *Psychological Bulletin* Vol. 106 (1986): pp. 265–289.

22. G. R. Goethals, "Fabrication and Ignoring Social Reality: Self-Serving Estimates of Consensus," in *Relative Deprivation and Social Comparison: The Ontario Symposium on Social Cognition IV,* eds. J. Olson et al. (Hillsdale, New Jersey: Lawrence Erlbaum Associates, 1986).

23. R. C. Liden and T. R. Mitchel, "Ingratiatory Behaviors in Organizational Settings," *Academy of Management Review* vol. 13 (1988): pp. 572–587.

24. L. G. Russek and G. E. Schwartz, "Perceptions of Parental Caring Predict Health Status in Midlife: A 35-Year Follow-Up Study of the Harvard Stress Study," *Psychosomatic Medicine* Vol. 59 (1997): pp. 144–149.

25. K. L. Dion and K. K. Dion, "Belief in a Just World and Physical Attractiveness Stereotyping," *Journal of Personality and Social Psychology* Vol. 52 (1987): pp. 775–780.

26. L. Stone, *The Family, Sex, and Marriage in England: 1500–1800* (New York: Harper and Row, 1977).

27. R. J. Sternberg and M. Barnes, eds., *The Psychology of Love* (New Haven, Connecticut: Yale University Press, 1988).

Chapter 10: A HASSLED BRAIN AND A HAPPY HEART

1. R. Niebuhr, *Discerning the Signs of the Times,* as quoted in L. Dossey, "Now You Are Fit to Live: Humor and Health," *Alternative Therapies* Vol. 2 (1996): p. 11.

2. B. J. Dunne and R. G. Jahn, *Consciousness and Anomalous Physical Phenomenon Technical Notes* (Princeton, New Jersey: Princeton University Press, 1995), p. 10.

3. In a study of coping styles, 40 percent of subjects under severe stress used humor to deal with their problems. R. R. McCrae, "Situational Determinants of Coping Responses: Loss, Threat, and Challenge," *Journal of Personality and Social Psychology* Vol. 46 (1984): pp. 919–928.

4. As quoted in A. Klein, *The Healing Power of Humor* (Los Angeles: Jeremy P. Tarcher, 1988), p. xvii.

5. *Ibid.,* p. 19.

6. W. Fry Jr., and M. Langsath, *Crying: The Mystery of Tears* (New York: Harper and Row, 1985).

7. N. F. Dixon, "Humor: A Cognitive Alternative to Stress?" in *Stress and Anxiety* vol. 7, eds. I. G. Sarason and C. D. Spielberger (Washington, D.C.: Hemisphere, 1980).

8. W. Fry Jr. and W. Allen, *Make 'Em Laugh: Life Studies of Comedy Writers* (Palo Alto, California: Science and Behavior Books, 1975).

9. J. M. Barrie, *Peter Pan,* Act I, 1928.

10. J. Gleick, *Chaos: Making a New Science* (New York: Penguin Books, 1988).

11. *Ibid.,* pp. 281–283.

12. *Ibid.,* back cover.

13. *Ibid.,* p. 282.

14. *Ibid.,* p. 283.

15. A. L. Goldberger, V. Bhargava, and B. J. West, "Nonlinear Dynamics of the Heartbeat," *Physica* Vol. 17D (1985): pp. 207–214.

16. J. Kabat-Zinn, *Full Catastrophe Living* (New York: Delta, 1990), p. 5.

17. M. Grotjahn, *Beyond Laughter: Humor and the Subconscious* (New York: McGraw-Hill, 1957).

18. As quoted in R. M. Nesse and G. C. Williams, *Why We Get Sick: The New Science of Darwinian Medicine* (New York: Random House, 1994), p. 142.

19. R. Eisler, *The Chalice and the Blade* (San Francisco: Harper and Row, 1987).

20. L. Dossey, "The Trickster: Medicine's Forgotten Character," *Alternative Therapies* Vol. 2 (1996): pp. 6–14.

21. R. S. Lazarus and S. Delongis, "Psychological Stress and Coping in Aging," *American Psychologist* Vol. 38 (1983): pp. 245–253.

22. The influence on the heart of small hassles is reported by L. H. Powell, "The Hook: A Metaphor for Gaining Control of Emotional Reactivity," in *Heart and Mind: The Practice of Cardiac Psychology,* eds. R. Allan and S. Scheidt (Washington, D.C.: American Psychological Association, 1999), pp. 313–327.

23. C. F. Stroebel, *QR: The Quieting Reflex: A Six-Second Technique for Coping with Stress Anytime, Anywhere* (New York: Putnam, 1982).

24. P. Reich et al., "Acute Psychological Disturbance Preceding Life-Threatening Arrhythmias," *Journal of the American Medical Association* Vol. 246 (1981): pp. 233–235.

25. N. Burks and B. Martin, "Everyday Problems and Life Change Events: Ongoing Versus Acute Sources of Stress," *Journal of Human Stress* Vol. 11 (1985): pp. 27–35.

26. A. D. Kanner et al., "Comparison of Two Modes of Stress Measurement: Daily Hassles and Uplifts Versus Major Life Events," *Journal of Behavioral Medicine* Vol. 4 (1981): pp. 1–39.

27. As quoted in D. Goleman, "Positive Denial: The Case for Not Facing Reality," *Psychology Today* Vol. 13 (1979): pp. 44–60.

28. R. Smoley, "My Mind Plays Tricks on Me," *Gnosis* Vol. 19 (1991): p. 12.

29. L. Dossey, "The Trickster," p. 14.

30. W. E. McClane and D. D. Singer, "The Effective Use of Humor in Organization Development," *Organization Development Journal* Vol. 9 (1991): pp. 67–72.

31. F. Safford, "Humor as an Aid in Gerontological Education," *Gerontology and Geriatrics Education* Vol. 11 (1991): pp. 27–37.

32. B. Schlesinger, "Lasting Marriages in the 1980s," *Conciliation Courts Review* Vol. 20 (1982): pp. 43–49.

33. J. Abrams, *The Shadow in America* (Novato, California: Nataraj Publishers, 1994), p. 214.

34. S. Prasinos and B. I. Tittler, "The Family Relationships of Humor-Oriented Adolescents," *Journal of Personality* Vol. 47 (1981): pp. 295–305.

35. A. A. Berger, "Humor: An Introduction," *American Behavioral Scientist* Vol. 30 (1987): pp. 6–15.

36. O. Nevo, "Does One Ever Really Laugh at One's Own Expense?" *Journal of Personality and Social Psychology* Vol. 49 (1985): pp. 799–807.

37. J. S. Mio and A. C. Graesser, "Humor, Language, and Metaphor," *Metaphor and Symbolic Activity* Vol. 6 (1991): pp. 87–102.

38. L. Deckers and R. T. Buttram, "Humor as a Response to Incongruities with or Between Schemata," *Humor: International Journal of Humor Research* Vol. 3 (1990), pp. 53–64.

39. J. L. Carroll, "The Relationship Between Humor Appreciation and Perceived Physical Health," *Psychology: A Journal of Human Behavior* Vol. 27 (1990): pp. 34–37.

40. T. Schill and M. S. O'Laughlin, "Humor Preference and Coping with Stress," *Psychological Reports* Vol. 55 (1984): pp. 309–310.

41. A. Ziv, "The Effect of Humor on Aggression Catharsis in the Classroom," *Journal of Psychology* Vol. 121 (1987): pp. 359–364.

42. K. M. Dillon, B. Minchoof, and K. H. Baker, "Positive Emotional States and Enhancement of the Immune System," *International Journal of Psychiatry in Medicine* Vol. 15 (1985–86): pp. 13–17.

43. M. S. George, "Brain Activity During Transient Sadness and Happiness in Healthy Women," *American Journal of Psychiatry* Vol. 152 (1995): pp. 341–351.

44. P. Wooten, *Compassionate Laughter: Jest for Your Health* (Salt Lake City, Utah: Commune-A-Key Publishing, 1996).

45. R. H. Blythe, quoted in R. Lewis in "Infant Joy," *Parabola* Vol. 12 (1987): p. 47.

46. J. Böhme, quoted in "Holy Laughter," *Parabola* Vol. 4 (1979): p. 51.

47. N. Cousins, *Head First* (New York: E. P. Dutton, 1989), p. 127.

Chapter 11: HEALING FROM THE HEART

1. D. Benor, "Survey of Spiritual Healing," *Complementary Medical Research* Vol. 4 (1990): pp. 9–33.

2. L. Dossey, "The Great Wait: In Praise of Doing Nothing," *Alternative Therapies* Vol. 2 (1996): pp. 8–14.

3. M. K. Klaus et al., "Maternal Assistance and Support in Labor: Father, Nurse, Midwife, or Doula?" *Journal of Clinical Consulting Obstetrical Gynecology* Vol. 4 (1992): pp. 211–217.

4. For a summary of the research on the healing brain, see D. Goleman and J. Gurin, *Mind/Body Medicine* (Yonkers, New York: Consumer Reports Books, 1993).

5. A. Storr, *Churchill's Black Dog, Kafka's Mice, and Other Phenomena of the Human Mind* (New York: Grove Press, 1988).

6. N. Cousins, *Anatomy of an Illness* (New York: Bantam Books, 1981).

7. B. Siegel, *Peace, Love and Healing* (New York: Harper and Row, 1989).

8. A. Storr, *Churchill's Black Dog*, p. 5.

9. A. L. Rowse, *The Early Churchills* (London: Macmillan, 1967): p. 120.

10. *Ibid.,* p. 252.

11. K. R. Jamison, "Manic-Depressive Illness and Creativity," *Scientific American* Vol. 23 (1995): pp. 62–67.

12. This is a partial quote from one of John Keats' many letters to friends that contained references to his concept of "negative capability" as a way of dealing with life and being able to realize the bitterness of life while at the same realizing its magnificent opportunities. As quoted in J. Jones and W. Wilson, *An Incomplete Education* (New York: Ballantine Books, 1987), pp. 244–245.

13. G. I. Engel, "Sudden and Rapid Death During Psychological Stress: Folk Lore or Folk Wisdom?" *Annals of Internal Medicine* Vol. 74 (1977): pp. 771–782.

14. Study by George L. Engel at the University of Rochester School of Medicine as quoted in L. Dossey, "In Praise of Unhappiness," *Alternative Therapies* Vol. 2 (1996): pp. 7–10.

15. G. Orwell, quoted in T. Miller, *How to Want What You Have* (New York: Henry Holt, 1994): p. 226.

16. *The American College Dictionary* (New York: Random House, 1960): p. 1102.

17. J. E. Blalock, "The Immune System as a Sensory Organ," *Journal of Immunology* Vol. 1132 (1984): pp. 1067–1070.

18. S. Metal'nikov and V. Chrine, "The Role of Conditioned Reflexes in Immunity," *Annals of the Pasteur Institute* Vol. 40 (1926): pp. 893–900.

19. S. Vincent and J. Thompson, "The Effects of Music on Human Blood Pressure," *Lancet* Vol. 1 (1929): pp. 534–537.

20. B. Bason and B. Celler, "Control of the Heart Rate by External Stimuli," *Nature* Vol. 4 (1972): pp. 279–280.

21. D. Aldridge, "The Music of the Body: Music Therapy in Medical Settings," *Advances* Vol. 9 (1993): pp. 17–35.

22. The concepts of disease as "bad systemic timing" and the attempt to impose clock time on personal physiology are discussed by C. Helman in "Heart Disease and the Cultural Construction of Time: The Type A Behavior Pattern as a

Western Culture-Bound Syndrome," *Social Science and Medicine* Vol. 25 (1987): pp. 969–979.

23. R. Gerber, *Vibrational Medicine* (Santa Fe, New Mexico: Bear and Company, 1988), p. 369.

24. *Ibid.,* p. 378.

25. C. B. Pert, "The Wisdom of the Receptors: Neuropeptides, the Emotions, and BodyMind," *Advances* Vol. 3 (1986): pp. 8–16.

26. Personal communication with C. B. Pert, May 7, 1997.

27. C. B. Pert, "The Wisdom of the Receptors," p. 9.

28. *Ibid.,* p. 12.

29. *Ibid.,* p. 16.

30. C. B. Pert et al., "Neuropeptides and Their Receptors: A Psychosomatic Network," *Journal of Immunology* Vol. 135 (1985): pp. 820S–826S.

31. As described in N. Cousins, *Head First* (New York: E. P. Dutton, 1989), p. 277.

32. D. C. McClelland, "Some Reflections on the Two Psychologies of Love," *Journal of Personality* Vol. 54 (1986): pp. 334–353.

33. H. Dreher, *The Immune Power Personality* (New York: Dutton Books, 1995), p. 216.

34. D. C. McClelland, "Inhibited Power Motivation and High Blood Pressure in Men," *Journal of Abnormal Psychology* Vol. 88 (1979): pp. 182–190.

35. D. C. McClelland and J. B. Jemmott, "Power Motivation, Stress, and Physical Illness," *Journal of Human Stress* Vol. 6 (1980): pp. 6–15.

36. D. C. McClelland and C. Kirshnit, "The Effect of Motivational Arousal Through Films on Salivary Immuno-globulin A," *Psychology and Health* Vol. 2 (1988): pp. 31–52.

37. Studies on affiliative trust are summarized in D. C. McClelland, "Motivational Factors in Health and Disease," *American Psychologist* Vol. 44 (1989): pp. 675–683.

38. C. B. Pert, "The Wisdom of the Receptors," p. 16.

Bibliography

"Thus, the task is not so much to see what no one yet has seen, but to think what nobody yet has thought about that which everybody sees."

— SCHOPENHAUER

Abell, G. O., and B. Singer. *Science and the Paranormal.* New York: Charles Scribner's Sons, 1981.

Abrams, J. *The Shadow in America.* Novato, California: Nataraj Publishers, 1994.

Achterberg, J. *Imagery in Healing.* Boston: Shambhala, 1985.

Ackerman, D. *The Natural History of the Senses.* New York: Random House, 1990.

Aldridge, D. "Is There Evidence of Spiritual Healing?" *Advances,* vol. 9. (1993): pp. 4–21.

———. "The Music of the Body: Music Therapy in Medical Settings." *Advances,* vol. 9. (1993): pp. 17–35.

Allan, R. "Introduction: The Emergence of Cardiac Psychology." In *Heart and Mind,* edited by R. Allen and S. Scheidt. Washington, D.C.: The American Psychological Association, 1996.

Allan, R. and S. Scheidt, eds. *Heart and Mind.* Washington, D.C.: American Psychological Association, 1996.

Allen, K. M., et al. "Presence of Human Friends and Pet Dogs as Moderators of Autonomic Response to Stress in Women." *Journal of Personality and Social Psychology,* vol. 61 (1991): pp. 582–589.

The American College Dictionary. New York: Random House, 1960.

The American Medical Association Encyclopedia. New York: Random House, 1989.

Andrykowski, M. A., M. Brady, and P. J. Henslee-Downey. "Psychosocial Factors Predictive of Survival After Allogeneic Bone Marrow Transplantation for Leukemia." *Psychosomatic Medicine,* vol. 56 (1994): pp. 432–439.

Antonovsky, A. *Unraveling the Mystery of Health: How People Manage Stress and Stay Well.* San Francisco: Jossey-Bass, 1987.

Armour, J., and J. Aradell, eds. *Neurocardiology.* New York: Oxford University Press, 1994.

Atkinson, R. C., and R. M. Shiffrin. "Human Memory: A Proposed System and Its Control Processes." In *The Psychology of Learning and Motivation: Advances in Research and Theory,* vol. 2, edited by K. W. Spence, pp. 89–195. New York: Academic Press, 1968.

Axel, R. "The Molecular Logic of Smell." *Scientific American,* vol. 273 (1995): pp. 154–159.

Bandura, A. *Social Foundations of Thought and Action: A Social-Cognitive Theory.* Englewood Cliffs, New Jersey: Prentice-Hall, 1986.

Bard, S. R. "Healing the Heart: An Interview with Dean Ornish, M. D." *Noetic Sciences Review,* vol. 20 (1991): pp. 5–13.

Baron, R. A. *Psychology* 2nd ed. Boston: Allyn and Bacon, 1992.

Barrie, J. M. *Peter Pan. Act I.* 1928.

Bartusiak, M. "Beeper Man." *Discover.* (November 1980): p. 57.

Bason, B., and B. Celler. "Control of the Heart Rate by External Stimuli." *Nature,* vol. 4 (1972): pp. 279–280.

Becker, R. O. *Cross Currents.* Los Angeles: Jeremy P. Tarcher, 1990.

Becker, R. O., and G. Selden. *The Body Electric.* New York: Morrow, 1985.

Beinfield, H., and E. Korngold *Between Heaven and Earth: A Guide to Chinese Medicine.* New York: Ballantine Books, 1991.

———. "Chinese Traditional Medicine: An Introductory Overview." *Alternative Therapies,* vol. 1 (1995): pp. 44–52.

Benor, D. *Healing Research: Holistic Energy Medicine and Spiritual Healing.* Munich, Germany: Helilz Verlag, 1993.

———. "Survey of Spiritual Healing." *Complementary Medical Research,* vol. 4 (1990): pp. 9–33.

Benson, H. *Beyond the Relaxation Response.* New York: Times Books, 1984.

Bentov, I. *Stalking the Wild Pendulum: On the Mechanics of Consciousness.* New York: Bantam Books: 1979.

Berger, A. A. "Humor: An Introduction." *American Behavioral Scientist,* vol. 30 (1987): pp. 6–15.

Berkowitz, L. "Frustration-Aggression Hypothesis: Examination and Reformation." *Psychological Bulletin,* vol. 106 (1989): pp. 59–73.

Bernard, C. *An Introduction to the Study of Experimental Medicine.* New York: Macmillan, 1927.

Bernard, J., and L. Sontag. "Fetal Reactions to Sound." *Journal of Genetic Psychology,* vol. 70 (1947): pp. 209–210.

Biggs, J., and F. Peat. "David Bohm's Looking-Glass Map." In *Looking-Glass Universe: The Emerging Science of Wholeness,* edited by J. Biggs and F. Peat. New York: Simon and Schuster, 1984.

Blalock, J. E. "The Immune System as a Sensory Organ." *Journal of Immunology,* vol. 1132 (1984): pp. 1067–1070.

Blythe, R. H. Quoted in R. Lewis. "Infant Joy." *Parabola,* vol. 12 (1987): p. 47.

Bohm, D. *Wholeness and the Implicate Order.* London: Routledge and Kegan Paul, 1980.

Böhme, J. Quoted in "Holy Laughter." *Parabola,* vol. 4 (1979): p. 51.

Bornstein, R. F. "Exposure and Affect: Overview and Meta-Analysis of Research." *Psychological Bulletin,* vol. 106 (1986): pp. 265–289.

Bosnak, R. *A Little Course in Dreams.* Boston: Shambhala, 1993.

Boyce, W. T. C., C. Schaefer, and C. Uitti. "Permanence and Change: Psychosocial Factors in the Outcome of Adolescent Pregnancy." *Social Science and Medicine,* vol. 21 (1985): p. 1281.

Braud, W. "Distant Mental Influence on Rate of Hemolysis on Human Red Blood Cells." *Journal of the American Society for Psychical Research,* vol. 84 (1990): pp. 1–24.

Braud, W., and W. Schlitz. "Methodology for the Objective Study of Transpersonal Imagery." *Journal of Scientific Exploration,* vol. 3 (1989): pp. 43–63.

Brodie, R. *Virus of the Mind.* Seattle: Integral Press, 1996.

Brown, R. A., and J. Kulik. "Flashbulb Memories." *Cognition,* vol. 5 (1977): pp. 73–99.

Bunzel, B., B. Schmidi-Mohl, A. Grundbock, and G. Wollenek. "Does Changing the Heart Mean Changing Personality? A Retrospective Inquiry of 47 Heart Transplant Patients." *Quality of Life Research,* vol. 1 (1992): pp. 251–256.

Burell, G., et al. "Modification of Type A Behavior Patterns in Post-Myocardial Infarction Patients: A Route to Cardiac Rehabilitation." *International Journal of Behavioral Medicine,* vol. 1 (1994): pp. 32–54.

Burks, N., and B. Martin. "Everyday Problems and Life Change Events: Ongoing Versus Acute Sources of Stress." *Journal of Human Stress,* vol. 11 (1985): pp. 27–36.

Byrd, R. C. "Positive Therapeutic Effects of Intercessory Prayer in a Coronary Care Unit Population." *Southern Medical Journal,* vol. 81 (1988): pp. 826–829.

Campbell, D., ed. *Music, Physician for Times to Come.* Wheaton, Illinois: Quest Publishers, 1991.

Cantin, M., and J. Genest. "The Heart as an Endocrine Gland." *Scientific American,* vol. 254 (1986): p. 76.

Carroll, J. L. "The Relationship Between Humor Appreciation and Perceived Physical Health." *Psychology: A Journal of Human Behavior,* vol. 27 (1990): pp. 34–37.

Cassidy, M. "Energy and Integrated Medicine." *Advances,* vol. 12 (1996): pp. 25–27.

Cassiere, E. *The Philosophy of the Enlightenment.* Princeton, New Jersey: Princeton University Press, 1951.

Castelnuovo-Tedesco, P. "Cardiac Surgeons Look at Transplantation: Interviews with Drs. Cleveland, Cooley, DeBakey, Hallman, and Rochelle." *Seminars in Psychiatry,* vol. 3 (1971): pp. 5–16.

———. "Ego Viscidities in Response to Replacement of Body Parts." *Psychoanalysis Quarterly,* vol. 47 (1978): pp. 381–397.

———. "Psychoanalytic Considerations in a Case of Cardiac Transplantation." In *The World Biennial of Psychiatry and Psychotherapy,* edited by S. Arieti. New York: Basic Books, 1971.

———. "Psychological Implications of Changes in Body Image." In *Psychonephrology 2,* edited by N. Levi. New York: Plenum, 1981.

Chalmers, D. J. "The Puzzle of Conscious Experience." *Scientific American,* vol. 273 (1995): pp. 80–86.

Chamoers, D. J. *The Conscious Mind: In Search of a Fundamental Theory.* New York: Oxford University Press, 1996.

Childre, D. L. *Freeze Frame.* Boulder Creek, California: Planetary Publications, 1994.

Chopra, D. *Ageless Body, Timeless Mind.* New York: Harmony Books, 1993.

Clarke, J. "SQUIDS." *Scientific American,* August 1994, pp. 46–53.

Colen, B. D. "Organ Concert." *Time,* Fall 1996, pp. 71–74.

Coles, M. G. H., G. Gratton, and M. Fabini. "Event-Related Brain Potentials." In *Principles of Psychophysiology: Physical, Social, and Inferential Elements,* edited by J. T. Cacioppo and L. G. Tassinary. New York: Cambridge University Press, 1990.

Condon, J. W., and W. D. Crano. "Inferred Evaluation and the Relation Between Attitude Similarity and Interpersonal Attraction." *Journal of Personality and Social Psychology,* vol. 54 (1988): pp. 789–797.

Cooke, R. "Cell Transplants Can Alter Behavior." *The Detroit News,* Monday, March 10, 1997, p. E1.

Cousins, N. *Anatomy of an Illness.* New York: Bantam Books, 1981.

———. *Head First.* New York: E. P. Dutton, 1989.

Csikszentmihalyi, M. *The Evolving Self.* New York: HarperCollins, 1993.

———. *Flow: The Psychology of Optimal Experience.* New York: Harper and Row, 1990.

Dawkins, R. *The Selfish Gene: New Edition.* New York: Oxford University Press, 1989.

DeBusk, R. F. "Sexual Activity Triggering Myocardial Infarction: One Less Thing to Worry About." *Journal of the American Medical Association,* vol. 275 (1996): pp. 1447–1448.

Deckers, L., and R. T. Buttram. "Humor as a Response to Incongruities with or Between Schemata." *Humor: International Journal of Humor Research,* vol. 3 (1990): pp. 53–64.

Deikman, A. "Deautomatization and the Mystic Experience." *Psychiatry,* vol. 29 (1966): pp. 329–343.

de la Pena, A. M. *The Psychobiology of Cancer.* South Hadley, Massachusetts: J. F. Berfin, Publishers, 1983.

Descartes, R. *The Philosophical Works of Descartes.* Translated by E. S. Haldane and G. R. T. Ross. New York: Cambridge University Press, 1970.

Dillon, K. M., B. Minchoof, and K. H. Baker. "Positive Emotional States and Enhancement of the Immune System." *International Journal of Psychiatry in Medicine,* vol. 15. (1985–86): pp. 13–17.

Dion, K. L., and K. K. Dion. "Belief in a Just World and Physical Attractiveness Stereotyping." *Journal of Personality and Social Psychology,* vol. 52 (1987): pp. 775–780.

Dixon, N. F. "Humor: A Cognitive Alternative to Stress?" In *Stress and Anxiety,* vol. 7, edited by I. G. Sarason and C. D. Spielberger, pp. 76–93. Washington, D.C.: Hemisphere, 1980.

Dossey, L. "The Forces of Healing: Reflections on Energy, Consciousness, and the Beef Stroganoff Principle." *Alternative Therapies,* vol. 3 (1997) pp. 8–16.

————. "The Great Wait: In Praise of Doing Nothing." *Alternative Therapies,* vol. 2 (1996): pp. 8–14.

————. *Healing Words: The Power of Prayer and the Practice of Medicine.* San Francisco: Harper San Francisco, 1993.

————. "In Praise of Unhappiness." *Alternative Therapies,* vol. 2 (1996): pp. 7–10.

————. "Lessons from Twins: Of Nature, Nurture, and Consciousness." *Alternative Therapies,* vol. 3 (1997): pp. 8–15.

————. "More on the Phenomenon of 'Loading.'" *Advances,* vol. 11 (1995): pp. 48–49.

————. *Prayer Is Good Medicine.* New York: HarperCollins, 1996.

————. "Running Scared: How We Hide from Who We Are." *Advances,* vol. 3 (1997): pp. 8–15.

————. "The Trickster: Medicine's Forgotten Character." *Alternative Therapies,* vol. 2 (1996): pp. 6–14.

————. "What's Love Got to Do With It?" *Advances,* vol. 2 (1996): pp. 8–15.

Dreher, H. *The Immune Power Personality.* New York: Dutton Books, 1995.

Dubos, R. *Mirage of Health.* New York: Harper, 1959.

Dunne, B. J. and R. G. Jahn. *Consciousness and Anomalous Physical Phenomenon Technical Notes.* Princeton, New Jersey: Princeton University Press, 1995.

Eccles, J. *The Brain and the Unity of Conscious Experience.* Oxford: Oxford University Press, 1961.

Eisenbud, J. *Parapsychology and the Unconscious.* Berkeley, California: North Atlantic Books, 1984.

Eisler, R. *The Chalice and the Blade.* San Francisco: Harper and Row, 1987.

Eliot, A. "The Hermit's Message." *Noetic Sciences Review,* vol. 42 (1997) pp. 29–33.

Eliot, R. S., and D. Breo. *Is It Worth Dying For?* Toronto and New York: Bantam, 1984.

Engel, G. I. "Sudden and Rapid Death During Psychological Stress: Folk Lore or Folk Wisdom?" *Annals of Internal Medicine,* vol. 74 (1987): pp. 771–782.

Faulkner, W. "Nobel Prize Acceptance Speech." Quoted in A. R. Damasio. *Descartes' Error: Emotion, Reason, and the Human Brain.* New York: Avon Books, 1994.

Ficino, M. *Commentary on Plato's Symposium on Love.* Translated by J. Sears. Dallas: Spring Publications, 1985.

Fisher, H. E. *Anatomy of Love: The Natural History of Monogamy, Adultery, and Divorce.* New York: W. W. Norton, 1992.

Fisher, J. "Is There a Need for Cardiac Psychology? The View of a Practicing Cardiologist." In *Heart and Mind: The Practice of Cardiac Psychology,* edited by R. Allan and S. Scheidt. Washington, D.C.: American Psychological Association, 1996.

Fox, M. *A Spirituality Named Compassion.* San Francisco: Harper and Row, 1979.

Fraser, J. T. *Time: The Familiar Stranger.* Redmond, Washington: Tempus Books of Microsoft Press, 1987.

Fredrickson, M. "Behavioral Aspects of Cardiovascular Reaction in Essential Hypertension." In *Biological and Psychological Factors in Cardiovascular Disease,* edited by T. H. Schmidt et al., pp. 418–446. Berlin: Springer-Verlag, 1985.

Freeman, A., D. Watts, and R. Karp. "Evaluation of Cardiac Transplant Candidates." *Psychosomatics,* vol. 25 (1984): pp. 197–207.

Freidman, H. S., et al. "Psychosocial and Behavioral Predictors of Longevity." *The American Psychologist,* vol. 50 (1995): pp. 69–78.

Friedman, M., N. Fleisschmann, and V. A. Price. "Diagnosis of Type A Behavior Pattern." In *Heart and Mind,* edited by R. Allan and S. Scheidt, pp. 179–195. Washington, D.C.: American Psychological Association, 1996.

Friedman, M., and R. H. Rosenman. "Association of Specific Overt Behavior Pattern with Blood and Cardiovascular Findings: Blood Cholesterol Level, Blood Clotting Time, Incidence of Arcus Senilis, and Clinical Coronary Artery Disease." *Journal of the American Medical Association,* vol. 169 (1959): pp. 1286–1296.

Frieson, R. I., and S. B. Lippman. "Heart Transplant Patients Rejected on Psychiatric Indications." *Psychosomatics,* vol. 28 (1987): pp. 347–355.

Fry, W. Jr., and W. Allen. *Make 'Em Laugh: Life Studies of Comedy Writers.* Palo Alto, California: Science and Behavior Books, 1975.

Fry, W. Jr., and M. Langsath. *Crying: The Mystery of Tears.* New York: Harper and Row, 1985.

Gardner, H. *Frames of Intelligence: The Theory of Multiple Intelligences,* 2nd ed. New York: Basic Books, 1993.

George, M. S. "Brain Activity During Transient Sadness and Happiness in Healthy Women." *American Journal of Psychiatry,* vol. 152 (1995): pp. 341–351.

Gerber, R. *Vibrational Medicine.* Santa Fe, New Mexico: Bear and Company, 1988.

Gerzon, R. *Finding Serenity in the Age of Anxiety.* New York: Macmillan, 1997.

Gilligan, C. *In a Different Voice: Psychological Theory and Women's Development.* Cambridge, Massachusetts: Harvard University Press, 1988.

Gilligan, C., and J. Attanucci. "Two Moral Orientations." In *Mapping the Moral Domain: A Contribution of Women's Thinking to Psychological Theory and Education,* edited by C. Gilligan, J. V. Ward, and J. M. Taylor. Cambridge, Massachusetts: Harvard University Press, 1986.

Gleick, J. *Chaos: Making a New Science.* New York: Penguin Books, 1988.

Goethals, G. R. "Fabrication and Ignoring Social Reality: Self-Serving Estimates of Consensus." In *Relative Deprivation and Social Comparison: The Ontario Symposium on Social Cognition IV,* edited by J. Olson et al. Hillsdale, New Jersey: Lawrence Erlbaum Associates, 1986.

Goldberger, A. L., V. Bhargava, and B. J. West. "Nonlinear Dynamics of the Heartbeat." *Physica,* vol. 17D (1985): pp. 207–214.

Goleman, D. *Emotional Intelligence.* New York: Bantam Books, 1995.

———. "Positive Denial: The Case for Not Facing Reality." *Psychology Today,* vol. 13 (1979): pp. 44–60.

Goleman, D., and J. Gurin. *Mind/Body Medicine.* Yonkers, New York: Consumer Reports Books, 1993.

Goswawi, A. "The Idealistic Interpretation of Quantum Mechanics." *Physics Essays,* vol. 2 (1989): pp. 385–400.

Gottman, J. *What Predicts Divorce: The Relationship Between Marital Processes and Marital Outcomes.* Hillsdale, New Jersey: Lawrence Erlbaum Associates, 1993.

———. *Why Marriages Succeed or Fail.* New York: Simon and Schuster, 1994.

Grad, B. "Some Biological Effects of Laying On of Hands and Their Implications." In *Dimensions in Holistic Healing: New Frontiers in the Treatment of the Whole Person,* edited by B. Otton and R. Knight, pp. 199–212. Chicago: Nelson Hall, 1979.

Green, E. E., et al. "Anomalous Electrostatic Phenomena in Exceptional Subjects." *Subtle Energies,* vol. 12 (1996): pp. 69–94.

Groff-Halifax, J. "Hex Death." In *Parapsychology and Anthropology: Proceedings of an International Conference Held in London, England, August 29–31, 1973,* edited by A. Angoff and D. Barth, pp. 59–79. New York: Parapsychology Foundation, 1973.

Grotjahn, M. *Beyond Laughter: Humor and the Subconscious.* New York: McGraw-Hill, 1957.

Haan, N. *Coping and Defending: Processes of Self-Environment Organization.* New York: Academic Press, 1977.

Haber, S. "The Professions and Higher Education in American: A Historical View." In *Higher Education and the Labor Market,* edited by M. Gordon, pp. 131–142. New York: McGraw Hill, 1974.

Hackett, T. P. and N. Cassem. "Development of a Qualitative Rating Scale to Assess Denial." *Journal of Psychosomatic Research,* vol. 18 (1974), pp. 93–100.

Hackett, T. P., N. H. Cassem, and H. A. Wishnie. "The Coronary Care Unit: An Appraisal of Its Psychological Hazards." *New England Journal of Medicine,* vol. 279 (1968): p. 1365.

Hameroff, S. R., and R. Penrose. "Orchestrated Reduction of Quantum Coherence in Brain Microtubules: A Model for Consciousness." In *Toward a Science of Consciousness: The First Tucson Discussions and Debates,* edited by S. R. Hameroff, A. Kaszniak, and A. C. Scott, pp. 131–142. Cambridge, Massachusetts: MIT Press, 1996.

Hartmann, F. *Paraclesus: Life and Prophecies.* Blauvelt, New York: Teiner Books, 1973.

Harvey, W. *Anatomical Studies on the Motion of the Heart and Blood.* Translated by C. D. Leake. Springfield, Illinois: Charles C. Thomas, 1928. (Originally published in 1628.)

Hearne, K. M. "A Nationwide Mass Dream-Telepathy Experiment." *Journal of the Society for Psychical Research,* vol. 55 (1989): pp. 271–274.

Heinberg, R. *Memories and Visions of Paradise.* Los Angeles: Jeremy P. Tarcher, 1989.

Helman, C. "Heart Disease and the Cultural Construction of Time: The Type A Behavior Pattern as a Western Culture-Bound Syndrome." *Social Science and Medicine,* vol. 25 (1987): pp. 969–979.

Herbert, N. *Quantum Reality.* New York: Anchor Books, 1987.

Hess, E. H. *The Tell-Tale Eye.* New York: Van Nostrand Reinhold, 1975.

Heuer, F., and D. Reisberg. "Vivid Memories of Emotional Events: The Accuracy of Remembered Minutiae." *Memory and Cognition,* vol. 18 (1990): pp. 496–506.

Hilgard, E. R. *Divided Consciousness: Multiple Controls in Human Thought and Action.* New York: Wiley, 1977.

Hillman, J. *The Soul's Code.* New York: Random House, 1996.

Hockenbury, D. H., and S. E. Hockenbury. *Psychology.* New York: Worth Publishers, 1997.

Hocrine, C. *Nutrition Plan for High Blood Pressure.* San Francisco: Jove Publications, 1977.

Holden, C. "Identical Twins Reared Apart." *Science,* vol. 207 (1980): pp. 1323–1328.

Holst, S. *Prose for Dancing.* Barrytown, New York: Station Hill Press, 1983.

Horrigan, B. "Stuart Hameroff: Consciousness and Microtubules in a Quantum World." *Alternative Therapies,* vol. 3 (1997): pp. 70–75.

Hotson, J., and T. Pedely. "The Neurological Complications of Cardiac Transplantation. *Brain,* vol. 99 (1976): pp. 673–694.

Huang, M., et al. "Identification of Novel Catecholamine-Containing Cells Not Associated with Sympathetic Neurons in Cardiac Muscle." *Circulation,* vol. 92 (1995): pp. 1–59.

Jackson, D. D. "Reunion of Identical Twins, Raised Apart, Reveals Some Astonishing Similarities." *Smithsonian,* October 1980, pp. 48–56.

Jahn, R. G. "Information, Consciousness, and Health." *Alternative Therapies,* vol. 2 (1996): pp. 32–38.

Jahn, R. G., and B. J. Dunne. *Margins of Reality: The Role of Consciousness in the Physical World.* New York: Harcourt Brace Jovanovich, 1987.

James, W. *Psychology: Briefer Course.* New York: Holt, 1890.

Jameson, D., and L. Hurvic. "Essay Concerning Color Constancy." *Annual Review of Psychology,* vol. 40 (1989): pp. 55–73.

Jamison, K. R. "Manic-Depressive Illness and Creativity." *Scientific American,* vol. 23 (1995): pp. 62–67.

Jasnoski, M. L., and J. Kugler. "Relaxation, Imagery, and Neuroimmunomodulation." *Annals of the New York Academy of Science,* vol. 496 (1987): pp. 723–730.

Jeffreys, D. "Have These Transplant Patients Inherited the Donor's Character?" *London Daily Mail,* June 4, 1996, p. 51.

Jensen, E. W. "The Families' Routine Inventory." *Social Science and Medicine,* vol. 7 (1983): pp. 210–211.

Jones, J., and W. Wilson. *An Incomplete Education.* New York: Ballantine Books, 1987.

Josephon, B. D., and F. Pallikari-Virus. "Biological Utilization of Quantum Nonlocality." *Foundations of Physics,* vol. 21 (1991): pp. 197–207.

Joy, W. Brugh. *Joy's Way.* Los Angeles: Jeremy P. Tarcher, 1978.

Jung, C. *Memories, Dreams, and Refections.* Translated by R. Winston and C. Sinston. New York: Vintage Books, 1963.

———. "Synchronicity: An Acausal Connecting Principle." In *Collected Works,* vol. 8. Princeton, New Jersey: Princeton University Press, 1973.

Kabat-Zinn, J. *Full Catastrophe Living.* New York: Delta, 1990.

Kafka, F. *The Trial.* New York: Schocken Books, 1974.

Kagan, J. *Galen's Prophecy.* New York: HarperCollins, 1994.

Kaminer, W. *I'm Dysfunctional—You're Dysfunctional.* New York: Addison-Wesley, 1992.

Kanner, A. D., et al. "Comparison of Two Modes of Stress Measurement: Daily Hassles and Uplifts Versus Major Life Events." *Journal of Behavioral Medicine,* vol. 4 (1981): pp. 1–39.

Karagulla, S. *Breakthrough to Creativity.* Marina Del Ray, California: De Vorss, 1967.

Kaznacheev, V. P., S. P. Shurin, et al. "Distant Intercellular Interaction in a System of Two Tissue Cultures." *Psychoenergetic Systems,* vol. 1 (1976): pp. 141–142.

Klaus, M. K., et al. "Maternal Assistance and Support in Labor: Father, Nurse, Midwife, or Doula?" *Journal of Clinical Consulting Obstetrical Gynecology,* vol. 4 (1992): pp. 211–217.

Klein, A. *The Healing Power of Humor.* Los Angeles: Jeremy P. Tarcher, 1988.

Kornfield, J. *A Path with Heart.* New York: Bantam Books, 1993.

Kraft, L. A. "Clinical Psychiatric Aspects of a Cardiac Transplantation Program." Lecture, *Annual Southern Psychiatry Association Meeting,* October 1969.

———. "Psychiatric Complications of Cardiac Transplantation." *Seminars in Psychiatry,* vol. 3 (1971): pp. 89–97.

Kuhn, W. F., B. Myers, A. F. Brennan, et al. "Psychopathology in Heart

Transplant Candidates." *Journal of Heart Transplant,* vol. 7 (1988): pp. 223–226.

Lacey, J., and B. Lacey. "Conversations Between Heart and Brain." *Bulletin of the National Institute of Mental Health.* Rockville, Maryland: March 1987.

Laskow, L. *Healing with Love: The Art of Holoenergetic Healing.* New York: HarperCollins, 1992.

Laszlo, E. *The Interconnected Universe: Conceptual Foundations of Transdisciplinary Unified Theory.* Singapore: World Scientific Publishing, 1995.

Laver, A. B. "Precursors of Psychology in Ancient Egypt." *Journal of the History of the Behavioral Sciences,* vol. 8 (1989): pp. 181–195.

Lazarus, R. S., and S. Delongis. "Psychological Stress and Coping in Aging." *American Psychologist,* vol. 38 (1983): pp. 245–253.

Leonard, G. "The End of Sex." In *The Fireside Treasury of Light,* edited by M. O. Kelly. New York: Simon and Schuster, 1990.

LeShan, L., and H. Maragenau. *Einstein's Space and Van Gogh's Sky.* New York: Collier Books, 1982.

Lettiere, A. L. "Toward a Philosophy of Science in Women's Health Research." *Journal of Scientific Exploration,* vol. 10 (1996): pp. 535–545.

Levine, B. H. *Your Body Believes Every Word You Say.* Boulder Creek, California: Aslan Publishing, 1991.

Liden, R. C., and T. R. Mitchel. "Ingratiatory Behaviors in Organizational Settings." *Academy of Management Review,* vol. 13 (1988): pp. 572–587.

Lin, H., R. Cohen, M. Cohen, and B. Campton, eds. *Secrets and Benefits of Internal Qigong Cultivation.* Malvern, Pennsylvania: Amber Leaf Press, 1997.

Locke, J. *An Essay Concerning Human Understanding.* New York: Oxford University Press, 1956. (Originally published in 1690.)

Lough, M. E., A. M. Lindsay, J. A. Shinn, and N. A. Stolts. "Life Satisfaction Following Heart Transplantation." *Journal of Heart Transplant,* vol. 4 (1985): pp. 381–385.

Lunde, D. T. "Psychiatric Complications of Heart Transplants." *American Journal of Psychiatry,* vol. 124 (1968): pp. 1190–1195.

Lynch, J. J. *The Broken Heart: The Medical Consequences of a Broken Heart.* New York: Basic Books, 1979.

Lynn, S. J., and J. W. Rhue. "The Fantasy-Prone Person: Hypnosis, Imagination and Creativity." *Journal of Personality and Social Psychology,* vol. 51 (1986), pp. 404–408.

Mackay, M. C., and L. Glass. "Oscillation and Chaos in Physiological Control Systems." *Science,* vol. 197 (1977): p. 287.

MacLean, P. "On the Evolution of Three Mentalities." In *New Dimensions in Psychiatry: A World View,* vol. II, edited by S. Arieti and G. Chrznowki. New York: Wiley, 1977.

Mai, F. M. "Graft and Donor Denial in Heart Transplant Recipients." *American Journal of Psychiatry,* vol. 143 (1986): pp. 1159–1161.

———. "Psychiatric Aspects of Cardiac Transplantation: Preoperative Evaluation and Postoperative Sequelae." *British Medical Journal,* vol. 292 (1986): pp. 311–313.

Mai, F. M., and J. Burley. "The Psychosocial Aspects of Heart Transplantation." *Transplantation Today,* vol. 2 (1985): pp. 16–21.

Mai, F. M., N. McKenzie, and W. Kostuk. "Laison Psychiatry in a Heart Transplant Unit (Abstract)." *Psychosomatic Medicine,* vol. 41 (1884): pp. 910–916.

Malmivuo, J., and R. Plosney. *Bioelectromagnetics.* New York: Oxford University Press, 1995.

Marek, G. R. *Toscanini.* London: Vision Press, 1975.

Martin, J., and M. T. Jessell. "The Sensory System." In *Essentials of Neural Science and Behavior,* edited by E. R. Kandel, J. H. Schwartz, and T. M. Jessell. Norwalk, Connecticut: Appleton and Lange, 1995.

Maslow, A. *The Farther Reaches of Human Nature.* New York: Penguin, 1971.

Maslow, B. G. *Abraham Maslow: A Memorial Volume.* Monterey, California: Brooks-Cole, 1972.

Matthews, K. A., et al. "Are Cardiovascular Responses to Behavioral Stressors a Stable Individual Difference Variable in Childhood?" *Psychophysiology,* vol. 24 (1987): pp. 464–473.

McClane, W. E., and D. D. Singer. "The Effective Use of Humor in Organizational Development." *Organizational Development Journal,* vol. 9 (1991): pp. 67–72.

McClelland, D. C. "Inhibited Power Motivation and High Blood Pressure in Men." *Journal of Abnormal Psychology,* vol. 88 (1979): pp. 182–190.

———. "Motivational Factors in Health and Disease." *American Psychologist,* vol. 44 (1989): pp. 675–683.

————. "Some Reflections on the Two Psychologies of Love." *Journal of Personality,* vol. 54 (1986): pp. 334–353.

McClelland, D. C., and J. B. Jemmott. "Power Motivation, Stress, and Physical Illness." *Journal of Human Stress,* vol. 6 (1980): pp. 6–15.

McClelland, D. C., and C. Kirshnit. "The Effect of Motivational Arousal Through Films on Salivary Immuno-Globulin A." *Psychology and Health,* vol. 2 (1988): pp. 31–52.

McCormick, A., and D. McCormick. *Horse Sense and the Human Heart: Discovering Wisdom, Healing, and Spiritual Growth.* Deerfield Park, Florida: Health Communications, 1997.

McCrae, R. R. "Situational Determinants of Coping Responses: Loss, Threat, and Challenge." *Journal of Personality and Social Psychology,* vol. 46 (1984): pp. 919–928.

McCraty, R. *Stress Medicine.* 1997, in press.

McCraty, R., and A. Watkins. *Autonomic Assessment Report Interpretation Guide.* Boulder Creek, California: Institute of HeartMath, 1996.

McCraty, R., et al. "The Effects of Emotions on Short-Term Heart Rate Variability: Using Power Spectrum Analysis." *American Journal of Cardiology,* vol. 76 (1995): pp. 1089–1093.

McCraty, R., M. Atkinson, and W. A. Tiller. "New Electrophysiological Correlates Associated with Intentional Heart Focus." *Subtle Energies,* vol. 4 (1995): pp. 251–268.

Mead, S. *The Lively Experiment: The Shaping of Christianity in America.* New York: Harper and Row, 1963.

Mendelssohn, W., M. Maczaj, and J. Holt. "Bupirone Administration to Sleep Apnea Patients." *Journal of Clinical Psychopharmacology,* vol. 23 (1991): pp. 71–72.

Merton, R. K. *The Sociology of Science.* Chicago: University of Chicago Press, 1973.

Meserve, H. C. "The Matter of the Heart." *Journal of Religion and Health,* vol. 23 (1984): pp. 263–267.

Metal'nikov, S. and V. Chrine. "The Role of Conditioned Reflexes in Immunity." *Annals of the Pasteur Institute,* vol. 40 (1926): pp. 893–900.

Miller, G. "The Magical Number Seven, Plus or Minus Two. Some Limits on Our Capacity for Processing Information." *Psychological Review,* vol. 101 (1986): pp. 343–352.

Miller, J. B. "The Development of Women's Sense of Self." *Work in Progress.* Wellsley, Massachusetts: The Stone Center, 1984.

Miller, J. G. *Living Systems.* New York: McGraw-Hill, 1978.

Miller, T. *How to Want What You Have.* New York: Henry Holt, 1994.

Mio, J. S., and A. C. Graesser. "Humor, Language, and Metaphor." *Metaphor and Symbolic Activity,* vol. 6 (1991): pp. 87–102.

Moore, T. *Care of the Soul.* New York: HarperPerennial, 1992.

———. *The Re-Enchantment of Everyday Life.* New York: HarperCollins, 1996.

Moss, T. *The Body Electric.* Los Angeles: Jeremy P. Tarcher, 1979.

———. "Puzzles and Promises." *Osteopathic Physician,* vol. 4 (1976): pp. 30–37.

Motoyama, H. *Theories of the Chakras.* Wheaton, Illinois: Theosophical Publishing House, 1981.

Motz, J. "Everyone an Energy Healer: The TREAT V Conference in Santa Fe." *Advance,* vol. 9 (1993): pp. 95–98.

———. "What Energy 'Knows' " *Advances,* vol. 12 (1996): pp. 33–35.

Mulcahy, R., L. Daley, I. Graham, and N. Hickey. "Level of Education, Coronary Risk Factors, and Cardiovascular Disease." *Irish Medical Journal,* vol. 7 (1984): pp. 316–318.

Muller, J. E., et al. "Triggering Myocardial Infarction by Sexual Activity: Low Absolute Risk and Prevention by Regular Physical Exertion?" *Journal of the American Medical Association,* vol. 275 (1996): pp. 1405–1409.

Murphy, M., and S. Donovan, eds. *The Physical and Psychological Effects of Meditation.* Sausalito, California: Institute of Noetic Sciences, 1997.

Neisser, V., and N. Harsch. "Phantom Flashbulbs: False Recollections of Hearing the News About the Challenger." In *Affect and Accuracy in Recall: Studies of Flashbulb Memories,* edited by E. Windgrad and V. Neisser. New York: Cambridge University Press, 1992.

Nesse, R. M., and G. C. Williams. *Why We Get Sick: The New Science of Darwinian Medicine.* New York: Random House, 1994.

Neuser, J. "Personality and Survival Time After Bone Marrow Transplantation." *Journal of Psychosomatic Research,* vol. 32 (1988): pp. 451–455.

Nevo, O. "Does One Ever Really Laugh at One's Own Expense?" *Journal of Personality and Social Psychology,* vol. 49 (1985): pp. 799–807.

Niebuhr, R. *Discerning the Signs of the Times.* Quoted in L. Dossey. "Now You Are Fit to Live: Humor and Health." *Alternative Therapies,* vol. 2 (1996): p. 11.

Norris, P. A. "Clinical Psychoneuroimmunology," In *Biofeedback: Principles and Practice for Clinicians,* edited by K. J. V. Basmahjian. Baltimore: Williams and Wilkins, 1988.

Nuland, S. B. *The Wisdom of the Body.* New York: Alfred A. Knopf, 1997.

Ohno, S., and M. Jabara. "Repeats of Base Oligomers ($N = 3n + - 1$ or 2) as Immortal Coding Sequences of the Primeval World: Construction of Coding Sequences Is Based upon the Principle of Musical Composition." *Chemical Scripta,* 26B. (1986): pp. 43–49.

Ohno, S., and M. Ohno. "The All-Pervasive Principle of Repetitious Recurrence Governs Not Only During Sequence Sontrionic but Also Human Endeavor in Musical Composition." *Immunogenetics,* vol. 24 (1986): pp. 71–78.

Ornish, D. M. "Can Lifestyle Change Reverse Coronary Heart Disease? The Lifestyle Heart Trial." *Lancet,* vol. 336 (1990): pp. 129–133.

Ornstein, R. *The Roots of Self.* San Francisco: Harper San Francisco, 1993.

Ornstein, R., and P. Erlich. *New World, New Mind.* New York: Doubleday, 1989.

Ornstein, R., and D. Sobel. *Healthy Pleasures.* Reading, Massachusetts: Addison-Wesley, 1993.

Orwell, G. Quoted in T. Miller. *How to Want What You Have,* p. 226. New York: Henry Holt, 1994.

Osler, W. *Lectures on Angina Pectoris and Allied States.* New York: Appleton-Century-Crofts, 1897.

———. "The Lumelian Lectures in Angina Pectoris." *Lancet* (1910).

Ozer, E. M., and A. Bandura. "Mechanisms Governing Empowerment Effects: A Self-Efficacy Analysis." *Journal of Personality and Social Psychology,* vol. 58 (1990): pp. 472–486.

Paddison, S. *The Hidden Power of the Heart.* Boulder Creek, California: Planetary Publications, 1992.

Pearce, J. C. *Evolution's End: Claiming the Potential of Our Intelligence.* San Francisco: Harper San Francisco, 1992.

Pearsall, P. *A Healing Intimacy: The Power of Loving Connections* New York: Crown, 1994.

———. *Making Miracles.* New York: Avon Books, 1991.

———. *The Pleasure Prescription: To Love, To Work, To Play—Life in the Balance.* Alameda, California: Hunter House Publishers, 1996.

———. *Super Marital Sex: Loving for Life.* New York: Doubleday, 1987.

———. *Ten Laws of Lasting Love.* New York: Simon and Schuster, 1993.

Penfield, W. *The Mystery of the Mind.* Princeton, New Jersey: Princeton University Press, 1975.

Peoch, R. "Psychokinetic Action of Young Chicks on the Path of an Illuminated Source." *Journal of Scientific Exploration,* vol. 9 (1995): pp. 223–229.

Pert, C. B., et al. "Neuropeptides and Their Receptors. A Psychosomatic Network." *Journal of Immunology,* vol. 135 (1985): pp. 820S–826S.

———. "The Wisdom of the Receptors: Neuropeptides, the Emotions, and BodyMind." *Advances,* vol. 3 (1986): pp. 8–16.

Piaget, J. *The Origins of Intelligence in Children.* New York: International Universities Press, 1952.

Plato. *The Collected Deluges.* E. Hamilton and H. Cairns, eds. New York: Pantheon Books, 1961.

Plotkin, H. *Darwin, Machines, and the Nature of Knowledge.* Cambridge, Massachusetts: Harvard University Press, 1993.

Polkinghorne, J. "Can a Scientist Pray?" In *Explorations in Science and Theology.* London: The Royal Society for the Encouragement of Arts, Manufactures, and Commerce, 1993, pp. 17–22.

Popp, F. A., U. Warnke, H. L. Koenig, and W. Peshka. *Electro-Magnetic Bioinformation.* Baltimore, Maryland: Urban and Schwarzenberg, 1989.

Poppel, E. "Oscillations as Possible Basis for Time Perception." In *The Study of Time: Proceedings of the First Conference of the International Society for the Study of Time,* edited by J. T. Fraser et al. Oberwolfach, West Germany. New York: Springer-Verlag, 1969.

Powell, L. H. "The Hook: A Metaphor for Gaining Control of Emotional Reactivity." In *Heart and Mind: The Practice of Cardiac Psychology,* edited by R. Allan and S. Scheidt. Washington, D.C.: American Psychological Association (1996): pp. 313–327.

Prasinos, S., and B. I. Tittler. "The Family Relationships of Humor-Oriented Adolescents." *Journal of Personality,* vol. 47 (1981): pp. 295–305.

Pribram, K. H. *Languages of the Brain.* Monterey, California: Wadsworth Publishing, 1977.

Pribram, K. H., and J. S. King, eds. *Brain and Values: Behavioral Neurodynamics,* vol. 5. Hillsdale, New Jersey: Lawrence Erlbaum Associates, 1996.

Price, G. R. "Science and the Supernatural." *Science,* vol. 122 (1955): pp. 359–367.

Puthoff, H. E. "Technological Problems, Bold Possibilities." *Advances,* vol. 12 (1996): pp. 35–36.

Ragan, P. A., W. Wang, and S. R. Eisenberg, "Magnetically Induced Currents in the Canine Heart: A Finite Element Study." *IEEE Transactions on Biomedical Engineering,* vol. 42 (1995): pp. 110–115.

Rauch, J. B., and K. K. Kneen. "Accepting the Gift of Life: Heart Transplant Recipients' Post-Operative Adaptive Tasks." *Social Work Health Care,* vol. 14 (1989): pp. 47–59.

Rechtschaffen, S., "Shifting Time: How to Pace Your Life to Natural Rhythms." *Noetic Sciences Review,* vol. 42 (1997): pp. 19–21.

———. *Timeshifting.* New York: Doubleday, 1996.

Reich, P., et al. "Acute Psychological Disturbance Preceding Life-Threatening Arrhythmias." *Journal of the American Medical Association,* vol. 246 (1981): pp. 233–235.

Rein, G., and R. McCraty. "Long-Term Effects of Compassion on Salivary IgA." *Psychosomatic Medicine,* vol. 56 (1994): pp. 171–172.

Rein, G., R. M. McCraty, and M. Atkinson. "Effects of Positive and Negative Emotions on Salivary IgA." *Journal of Advanced Medicine,* vol. 8 (1995): pp. 87–105.

Rhine, G. "A Psychokinetic Effect on Neurotransmitter Metabolism: Alterations in the Degradative Enzyme Monoamine Oxidase." In *Research in Parapsychology,* edited by D. H. Weiner and D. Radin, pp. 77–80. Metuchen, New Jersey: Scarecrow Press, 1985.

Rhine, J. B., and S. R. Feather. "The Study of Cases of 'Psi-Training' in Animals." *Journal of Parapsychology,* vol. 1 (1962): pp. 1–21.

Rhine, L. E. "Psychological Processing in ESP Experiments Part I: Waking Experiences." *Journal of Parapsychology,* vol. 29 (1962): pp. 88–111.

Rifkin, J. *Time Wars.* New York: Henry Holt, 1987.

Robbins, J. *Reclaiming Our Health.* Tiburon, California: H. J. Kramer, 1996.

Roediger, H. L., and K. B. McDermott. "Creating False Memories: Remembering Words Not Presented in Lists." *Journal of Experimental Psychology: Learning, Memory, and Cognition,* vol. 21 (1995): pp. 803–814.

Roszak, T., M. E. Gomes, and A. D. Kanner. *Ecopsychology.* San Francisco: Sierra Club Books, 1995.

Rowse, A. L. *The Early Churchills*. London: Macmillan, 1967.

Rubik, B. "Energy Medicine and the Unifying Concept of Information in Energy Medicine." *Alternative Therapies,* vol. 1 (1995): pp. 34–39.

————, ed. *The Interrelationship Between Mind and Matter.* Philadelphia: Center for Frontier Sciences at Temple University, 1992.

Russek, Linda G., and G. E. Schwartz. "Energy Cardiology: A Dynamical Energy Systems Approach for Integrating Conventional and Alternative Medicine." *Advances,* vol. 12 (1996): pp. 4–24.

————. "Energy, Information, and the Essence of Integrated Medicine." *Advances,* vol. 13 (1997): pp. 74–77.

————. "Interpersonal Heart-Brain Registration and the Perception of Parental Love: A 42-Year Follow-Up of the Harvard Mastery of Stress Study." *Subtle Energies,* vol. 5 (1996): pp. 36–45.

————. "Narrative Descriptions of Parental Love and Caring Predict Health Status in Midlife: A 35-Year Follow-Up of the Harvard Mastery of Stress Study." *Alternative Therapies,* vol. 2 (1996): pp. 55–62.

————. "Perceptions of Parental Caring Predict Health Status in Midlife: A 35-Year Follow-Up Study of the Harvard Stress Study." *Psychosomatic Medicine,* vol. 59 (1997): pp. 144–149.

Safford, F. "Humor as an Aid in Gerontological Education." *Gerontology and Geriatrics Education,* vol. 11 (1991): pp. 27–37.

Safire, W., and L. Safire. *Words of Wisdom.* New York: Simon and Schuster, 1989.

Sanderson, I. "Editorial: A Fifth Force." *Pursuit,* vol. 5 (1972): p. 4.

Sapolsky, R. M. *Why Zebras Don't Get Ulcers.* New York: W. H. Freeman, 1994.

Schacter, D. L. *Searching for Memory.* New York: BasicBooks, 1996.

Schill, T., and M. S. O'Laughlin. "Humor Preference and Coping with Stress." *Psychological Reports,* vol. 55 (1984): pp. 309–310.

Schlesinger, B. "Lasting Marriages in the 1980s." *Conciliation Courts Review,* vol. 20 (1982): pp. 43–49.

Schlitz, M. J. "Intentionality and Intuition and Their Clinical Implications: A Challenge for Science and Medicine." *Advances,* vol. 2 (1996): pp. 58–66.

Schlitz, M., and N. Lewis. "Meditation East and West." *Noetic Sciences Review,* vol. 42 (1997): pp. 34–38.

Schwartz, B. E. "Possible Telesomatic Reactions." *Journal of the Medical Society of New Jersey,* vol. 64 (1973): pp. 600–603.

Schwartz, G. "Information and Energy: The Soul and Spirit of Mind-Body Medicine." *Advances,* vol. 13 (1997): pp. 75–77.

———. "Soul Is to Spirit as Information Is to Energy: A Theoretical Note and Poem." *Bridges,* vol. 5 (1994).

Schwartz, G., and L. G. Russek. "Do All Dynamical Systems Have Memory? Implications of the Systemic Memory Hypothesis for Science and Society." In *Brain and Values: Behavioral Neurodynamics,* vol. 5, edited by K. H. Pribam and J. S. King. Hillsdale, New Jersey, Lawrence Erlbaum Associates, 1996.

———. "Dynamical Energy Systems and Modern Physics: Fostering the Science and Spirit of Complementary and Alternative Medicine." *Alternative Therapies in Health and Medicine.* In Press.

———. "Energy Cardiology: A Dynamical Energy Systems Approach for Integrating Conventional and Alternative Medicine." *Advances,* vol. 12 (1996): pp. 4–24.

———. "Neurotherapy and the Heart: The Challenge of Energy Cardiology." *Journal of Neurotherapy,* vol. 1 (1996): pp. 1–11.

Sheldrake, R. *A New Science of Life.* Los Angeles: Jeremy P. Tarcher, 1981.

———. *The Presence of the Past.* New York: Random House, 1981.

Shelly, M. W. *Frankenstein; or, the Modern Prometheus.* New York: Oxford University Press, 1969. (Originally published in 1818.)

Siebert, C. "Carol Palumbo Waits for Her Heart." *New York Times Magazine,* April 13, 1997.

Siegel, B. "Emotions, Energy, and Healing." *Advances,* vol. 13 (1997): pp. 4–5.

———. *Peace, Love and Healing.* New York: Harper and Row, 1989.

Sivin, N. *Traditional Medicine in Contemporary China.* Ann Arbor: University of Michigan Press, 1987.

Skinner, B. F. *Beyond Freedom and Dignity.* New York: Bantam Books, 1971.

Smoley, R. "My Mind Plays Tricks on Me." *Gnosis,* vol. 19 (1991): p. 12.

Sobel, D., and R. Ornstein. "Sexual Activity and Heart Attack: Not to Worry." *Mind/Body Health Newsletter,* vol. 5 (1996): pp. 2–3.

Solomon, R. L. "The Opponent Process in Acquired Motivation." In *The Physiological Mechanisms of Motivation,* edited by D. W. Pfaff. New York: Springer-Verlag, 1982.

Sperry, R. W. *Science and Moral Priority.* New York: Columbia University Press, 1982.

Stent, G. "Prematurity and Uniqueness in Scientific Discovery." *Scientific American,* December 1972, pp. 84–93.

Sternberg, R. J., and M. Barnes, eds. *The Psychology of Love.* New Haven, Connecticut: Yale University Press, 1988.

Stone, L. *The Family, Sex, and Marriage in England, 1500–1800.* New York: Harper and Row, 1977.

Storr, A. *Churchill's Black Dog, Kafka's Mice, and Other Phenomena of the Human Mind.* New York: Grove Press, 1988.

Straus, M. B. *Familiar Medical Quotations.* Boston: Little, Brown, 1968.

Streltzer, J., M. Moe, E. Yanagida, et al. "Coping with Transplant Failure: Grief and Denial." *International Journal of Psychiatry and Medicine,* vol. 13 (1983): pp. 97–106.

Stroebel, C. F. *QR: The Quieting Reflex: A Six-Second Technique for Coping with Stress Anytime, Anywhere.* New York: Putnam, 1982.

Stroink, G. "Principles of Cardiomagneticism." In *Advances in Biomedical Engineering,* edited by S. J. Williamson et al., pp. 47–57. New York: Plenum Press, 1989.

Sylvia, C., and B. Novak. *A Change of Heart.* Boston: Little, Brown, 1997.

Syme, S. L. "Social Support and Risk Reduction." *Mobius,* vol. 4 (1984): pp. 44–54.

Swerdlow, J. L. "Quiet Miracles of the Mind." *National Geographic,* vol. 187 (1995): pp. 2–41.

Tabler, J. B., and R. I. Frieson. "Sexual Concerns After Heart Transplantation." *Journal of Heart and Lung Transplant,* vol. 9 (1990): pp. 397–493.

Targ, R., and H. I. Puthoff. *Mind-Reach.* New York: Dell, 1977.

———. "Scanning the Issue." *Proceedings of the IEEE,* vol. 14 (1976): p. 291.

Tart, C. T. *Living the Mindful Life: A Handbook for Living in the Present Moment.* Boston: Shambhala, 1994.

Teich, H. "Sun and Moon." *Parabola,* vol. 19 (1994): pp. 55–58.

Tennant, C. "Parental Loss in Childhood: Its Effect in Adult Life." *Archives of General Psychiatry,* vol. 45 (1988): pp. 1045–1050.

Tennen, H., and G. Affleck. "Blaming Others for Threatening Events." *Psychological Bulletin,* vol. 108 (1990): pp. 209–232.

Terman, L. M., and M. H. Ogsden. *Genetic Studies of Genius: The Gifted Children Grow Up,* vol. 4. Stanford, California: Stanford University Press, 1947.

Thomas, A., S. Chess, and H. G. Birch. "The Origins of Personality." *Scientific American,* vol. 223 (1970): pp. 102–104.

Tiller, W. A., R. McCraty, and M. Atkinson. "Cardiac Coherence: A New, Noninvasive Measure of Autonomic Nervous System Disorder." *Alternative Therapies,* vol. 2 (1996): pp. 52–65.

Tipler, F. *The Physics of Immortality.* New York: Macmillan, 1994.

Toms, M. *At the Leading Edge.* Burdett, New York: Larson Publications, 1991.

Treffil, J. *Sharks Have No Bones.* New York: Simon and Schuster, 1992.

Tulvin, E., and D. M. Thompson. "Encoding Specificity and Retrieval Processes in Episodic Memory." *Psychological Review,* vol. 80 (1973): pp. 352–373.

Turner, J. R. "Individual Difference in Heart-Rate Response During Behavioral Challenge." *Psychophysiology,* vol. 26 (1989): pp. 497–505.

Tylor, E. B. *Primitive Culture,* vol. 1. London: 1871.

Ullman, M., and L. Krasner. *Dream Telepathy.* New York: Macmillan, 1973.

Villaire, M. "Second Annual Alternative Therapies Symposium Explores the Forces of Healing." *Alternative Therapies,* vol. 3 (1997): pp. 27–29.

Vincent, S., and J. Thompson. "The Effects of Music on the Human Blood Pressure." *Lancet,* vol. 1 (1929): pp. 534–537.

Voelker, R. "Puppy Love Can Be Therapeutic, Too." *Journal of the American Medical Association,* vol. 274 (1995): pp. 1897–1899.

von Bertalanffy, L. *General Systems Theory.* New York: Braziller, 1968.

von Helmholtz, H. Quoted in M. Murphy, *The Future of the Body,* p. 345. Los Angeles: Jeremy P. Tarcher, 1992.

Wakai, R. T., M. Wang, and C. B. Martin. "Spatio-Temporal Properties of the Fetal Magnetocardiogram." *American Journal of Obstetrics and Gynecology,* vol. _ (1994): pp. 770–776.

Watkins, A. D. "Intention and Electromagnetic Activity of the Heart." *Advances,* vol. 12 (1996): pp. 35–36.

———. "Medicine and the Heart's Energy." *Advances,* vol. 13 (1997): pp. 70–74.

———. "Letter to the Editor." *Advances,* vol. 13 (1997): p. 3.

Watson, L. *Lifetide: The Biology of Consciousness.* New York: Simon and Schuster, 1980.

Watts, A. "Odyssey of Aldous Huxley." *Original Live Recordings on Com-*

parative Philosophy. San Anselmo, California: The Electronic University, 1995.

Webster's Third New International Dictionary. Springfield, Massachusetts: Merriam Webster, 1993.

Wentzel, M. "Voices of Their Ancestors." *Sheraton's Hawai'i.* Summer 1997.

West, M. A. "Traditional and Psychological Perspectives on Meditation." In *The Psychology of Meditation,* edited by M. A. West. New York: Oxford University Press, 1987.

White, J. *The Meeting of Science and Spirit.* New York: Paragon House, 1990.

Wilentz, J. S. *The Senses of Man.* New York: Thomas Crowell, 1968.

Williams, R. *The Trusting Heart: Great News About Type A Behavior.* New York: Times Books, 1989.

Williams, R., and V. Williams. *Anger Kills.* New York: HarperPerennial, 1993.

Woodmansee, J. J. "The Pupil Response as a Measure of Social Attitudes." In *Attitude Measurement,* edited by G. F. Summer. Chicago: Rand-McNally, 1970.

Woodward, K. "Talking to God." *Newsweek,* January 6, 1992, pp. 38–44.

Wooten, P. *Compassionate Laughter: Jest for Your Health.* Salt Lake City, Utah: Commune-A-Key Publishing, 1996.

Zilbergeld, B., and A. A. Lazarus. *Mind Power.* Boston: Little, Brown, 1987.

Zilborg, G. *A History of Medical Psychology.* New York: W. W. Norton, 1941.

Ziv, A. "The Effect of Humor on Aggression Catharsis in the Classroom." *Journal of Psychology,* vol. 121 (1987): pp. 359–364.

Zohar, D. *The Quantum Self: Human Nature and Consciousness Defined by the New Physics.* New York: William Morrow, 1990.

Index